Handbook of Clinical Pathology

Contributors

Paul M. Allison, MD
Assistant Professor of Pathology
University of Texas Southwestern
Medical School, Dallas
Hemostasis

L. Maximilian Buja, MD
Professor and Chairman of Pathology
University of Texas Medical School,
Houston
Myocardial Injury: Laboratory Tests,
Plasma Lipoproteins

Edwin H. Eigenbrodt, MD
Professor of Pathology
University of Texas Medical School,
Houston
Intestinal Malabsorption Function Tests,
Gastric Secretion Tests, Liver Function
Tests, Renal Function Tests

Jose A. Hernandez, MD
Associate Professor of Pathology
University of Texas Southwestern
Medical School, Dallas
Erythrocyte Disorders,
Leukocyte Disorders

J. H. Keffer, MD, Editor
Professor of Pathology
University of Texas Southwestern
Medical School, Dallas
Pregnancy Tests, Myocardial Injury:
Laboratory Tests, Exocrine Pancreas Tests,
Diabetes Mellitus and Hypoglycemia:
Laboratory Tests, Acid-Base Balance:
Laboratory Tests, Calcium and
Phosphorus Metabolism, Thyroid Function
Tests, Adrenocortical Function Tests,
Pituitary Function Tests

Mary F. Lipscomb, MD
Professor of Pathology
University of Texas Southwestern
Medical School, Dallas
Infectious Disease: Immunologic Tests,
Syphilis: Serologic Tests, Synovial Fluid,
Connective Tissue Disease Tests

Robert W. McKenna, MD, Editor
Professor and Vice Chairman
of Pathology
University of Texas Southwestern
Medical School, Dallas
Erythrocyte Disorders, Leukocyte
Disorders, Hemostasis

Paul J. Orsulak, PhD
Professor of Psychiatry and Pathology
University of Texas Southwestern
Medical School, Dallas
Therapeutic Drug Monitoring, Toxicology
and Substance Abuse Testing

Julie S. Sandstad, MD, Senior Editor
Assistant Professor of Pathology
University of Texas Southwestern
Medical School, Dallas
The Physician and the Laboratory,
Tumor Biomarkers

Nancy R. Schneider, MD, PhD
Assistant Professor of Pathology
University of Texas Southwestern
Medical School, Dallas
Clinical Cytogenetics

Paul M. Southern, MD
Professor of Pathology and
Internal Medicine
University of Texas Southwestern
Medical School, Dallas
Infectious Disease: General Laboratory
Tests, Cerebrospinal Fluid

Laurie J. Sutor, MD
Assistant Professor of Pathology
University of Texas Southwestern
Medical School, Dallas
Infectious Disease: Immunologic Tests,
Blood Bank Tests and Blood
Component Usage

Arthur G. Weinberg, MD
Professor of Pathology
University of Texas Southwestern
Medical School, Dallas
Urinalysis

Handbook of Clinical Pathology

Edited by

Julie S. Sandstad, MD
Assistant Professor of Pathology

Robert W. McKenna, MD
Professor and Vice Chairman of Pathology

J. H. Keffer, MD
Professor of Pathology

University of Texas Southwestern Medical School
Dallas

American Society of Clinical Pathologists
Chicago

Acquisitions & Development: Joshua Weikersheimer
Editor: Philip Rogers
Production Manager: Lisa Pollak
Designer: Jennifer Sabella
Cover: illustration courtesy of The Bettmann Archive

 Printed on recycled paper.

Notice

Trade Names and equipment and supplies described herein are included as suggestions only. In no way does their inclusion constitute an endorsement by the American Society of Clinical Pathologists. The ASCP did not test the equipment, supplies, or procedures and, therefore, urges all readers to read and follow all manufacturers' instructions and package insert warnings concerning the proper and safe use of products.

Library of Congress Cataloging-in-Publication Data

Handbook of clinical pathology / editors, Julie Sandstad, Robert McKenna,
    Joseph Keffer.
    p. 288
Includes bibliographical references and index.
    ISBN 0-89189-314-8
    1. Diagnosis, Laboratory—Handbooks, manuals, etc. I. Sandstad, Julie, 1945- .
II. McKenna, Robert, 1940- . III. Keffer, Joseph H, 1936- .
    [DNLM: 1. Pathology, Clinical—methods—handbooks. QY 39 H236]
RB38.2.H36 1992
616.07'5—dc20
DNLM/DLC   91-26137
for Library of Congress   CIP

Printed in the United States of America.

96 95   5

Contents

Preface

This handbook is meant to be a handy, succinct reference covering most issues related to the clinical laboratory.

We presume a basic science knowledge of some disciplines. We cannot exhaustively cover any topic. Hence, we hope to bridge the gap between basic science knowledge and advanced understanding of clinical disease.

This handbook is meant for medical students, to supplement their pathology course and aid during their clinical years, and for residents as they gain confidence with their skills. If others find it useful, we are pleased.

We acknowledge the work of those who wrote before us, specifically Merill Shore, MD, who compiled the first Southwestern Medical School Handbook in the 1970s under the leadership of Vernie Stembridge, MD. We thank those who contributed greatly to chapters: Rita Gander, PhD (Infectious Disease: General Laboratory Tests, Cerebrospinal Fluid); Paul Van Dreal, PhD (Pregnancy: Related Tests, Exocrine Pancreas Tests, Diabetes Mellitus and Hypoglycemia: Laboratory Tests, Calcium and Phosphorous Metabolism, Adrenocortical Function Tests). We applaud the excellent work of Beverly Shackelford, layout editor, and Debbie Watts, word processor typist.

We take responsibility for errors, and welcome feedback.

J. S. Sandstad, MD
Senior Editor

Abbreviations

ACTH: adrenocorticotropic hormone
ADH: antidiuretic hormone
AFP: alpha-fetoprotein
AIDS: acquired immunodeficiency syndrome
ALL: acute lymphocytic leukemia
ALP: alkaline phosphatase
ALT: alanine aminotransferase
AMP: adenosine monophosphate
ANA: antinuclear antibody
ANLL: acute nonlymphocytic leukemia
anti-HAV: antibody to hepatitis A virus
anti-HBC: antibody to hepatitis B core antigen
anti-HBe: antibody to hepatitis B e antigen
anti-HBs: antibody to hepatitis B surface antigen
anti-HCV: antibody to hepatitis C virus
ASO: antistreptolysin O
AST: aspartate aminotransferase
BAO: basal acid output
ßHCG: ß–human chorionic gonadotropin
BPH: benign prostatic hyperplasia
BUN: blood urea nitrogen
C1inh: C1 esterase inhibitor
CBC: complete blood count
CCK-PZ: cholecystokinin and pancreozymin
CDC: Centers for Disease Control
CEA: carcinoembryonic antigen
CGD: chronic granulomatous disease
CK: creatine kinase
CML: chronic myeloid leukemia

CMV: cytomegalovirus
CSF: cerebrospinal fluid
CT: computed tomography
DDAVP: desmopressin
DIC: disseminated intravascular coagulation
DM: diabetes mellitus
DNA: deoxyribonucleic acid
DNase B: deoxyribonuclease B
dsDNA: double-stranded DNA
EA: early antigen
EBNA: EBV-associated nuclear antigen
EBV: Epstein-Barr virus
EDTA: ethylenediaminetetraacetic acid
ELISA: enzyme-linked immunosorbent assay
ENA: extractable nuclear antigen
FEP: free erythrocyte protoporphyrin
FSH: follicle-stimulating hormone
FT_4: free thyroxine
FTA-Abs: fluorescent treponemal antibody absorption test
G6PD: glucose-6-phosphate dehydrogenase
GFR: glomerular filtration rate
GGT: γ-glutamyltransferase
GI: gastrointestinal
GSH: group, screen, and hold
HBeAg: hepatitis B e antigen
HBsAg: hepatitis B surface antigen
HCAg: hepatitis C antigen
HCG: human chorionic gonadotropin
HCT: hematocrit
HDL: high-density lipoprotein
HGB: hemoglobin
5-HIAA: 5-hydroxyindoleacetic acid
HIV: human immunodeficiency virus
HLA: human leukocyte antigen
HMWK: high-molecular-weight kininogen
HPF: high-power field
HVA: homovanillic acid
KOH: potassium chloride
LD: lactate dehydrogenase
LDL: low-density lipoprotein
LH: luteinizing hormone
MAO: maximal acid output
MCH: mean cell hemoglobin
MCHC: mean cell hemoglobin concentration
MCV: mean cell volume
MHA-TP: microhemagglutination assay for *Treponema pallidum* antibodies
MoAb: monoclonal antibody
MRI: magnetic resonance imaging

MSAFP: maternal serum alpha-fetoprotein
NCCLS: National Committee for Clinical Laboratory Standards
NCEP: National Cholesterol Education Program
NIH: National Institutes of Health
17-OHCS: 17-hydroxycorticosteroids
PABA: *p*-aminobenzoic acid
PAP: prostatic-fraction acid phosphatase
PCP: phencyclidine
PL: plasma lipid
PNH: paroxysmal nocturnal hemoglobinuria
PSA: prostate-specific antigen
PT: prothrombin time
PTH: parathyroid hormone
PTT: partial thromboplastin time
RBC: red blood cell
RDW: red cell distribution width
RMSF: Rocky Mountain spotted fever
RNA: ribonucleic acid
RPR: rapid plasma reagin
RSV: respiratory syncytial virus
SGOT: serum glutamic-oxaloacetic transaminase
SGPT: serum glutamate pyruvate transaminase
SLE: systemic lupus erythematosus
STD: sexually transmitted disease
T_3: triiodothyronine
T_4: thyroxine
TBG: thyroxine-binding globulin
TDM: therapeutic drug monitoring
TIBC: total iron-binding capacity
tPA: tissue plasminogen activator
TRH: thyrotropin-releasing hormone
TSH: thryoid-stimulating hormone
TSI: total serum iron
TU: Todd units
VCA: viral capsid antibody
VDRL: Venereal Disease Research Laboratory
VLDL: very-low-density lipoprotein
VMA: vanillylmandelic acid
vWD: von Willebrand disease
vWF: von Willebrand factor
WBC: white blood cell

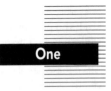

One

The Physician and the Laboratory

Key Points

1. Effectively using the clinical laboratory is a learned skill. One cannot be both a superb diagnostician and a mediocre laboratory user.
2. Laboratory normal values and patient laboratory results are not "truth."
3. The sensitivity of a particular test tells you the probability that a person with the disease in question will have an abnormal laboratory result.
4. The specificity of a particular test tells you the probability that a person without the disease in question will have a normal laboratory result.
5. Sensitivity and specificity can be greatly affected by the prevalence of a disease. Using sensitivity and specificity in conjunction with prevalence, the predictive value of a test can be established.

Background

Using the clinical laboratory is a learned skill, just as is using a stethoscope or reflex hammer. Through wise clinical judgment you decide on your patient's appropriate bodily specimen, collect it, and present it for assay or examination by laboratory experts, after which you have data to move forward the diagnostic or therapeutic process. Laboratory data are so valuable because, along with a patient's history and physical examination, evidence is building, usually in a cost-effective manner, to confirm or refute the differential diagnosis.

The hospital laboratory is directed by a physician (usually a pathologist) with special training in the areas of chemistry, hematology, microbiology, virology, computer science, immunology, blood bank, coagulation, or cytogenetics. The pathologist must also be versed in management and personnel strategies, hospital finance, and governmental regulations to operate an efficient laboratory. Larger laboratories have divisions, each directed by a different physician specializing in one area, eg, immunology. Many laboratories have personnel at the doctorate level who play an integral role in bringing the basic science of their discipline to a clinical level. The technologists performing laboratory tests are under extraordinary pressure to perform their tasks perfectly to produce accurate and precise data. All of these people can be valuable resources to help you use the laboratory as efficiently as possible. In addition, clerical personnel, messengers, and others are necessary to provide the 24-hour operation essential in our health care system.

This group of highly trained personnel using complex analytical services must function as a team in a somewhat rigid system to meet every clinician's need every minute of the day. Murphy's Law can, and often will, intercede at every level—the order must be written, the clerk must transfer it to the appropriate laboratory slips, the sample must be drawn from the correct patient, at the correct time, under known pretest conditions, and the sample must be transported to the laboratory. Like the birth of a healthy baby after 9 months of developing under exact conditions, it is sometimes amazing that the proper test results ever reach the physician but, happily, they usually do. By understanding both the tests you order and how their results come about, you will be in a better position to judge their validity and utilize the data clinically.

Clinical laboratories, like most other areas in medicine, are going through a transition period, attempting to respond to governmental and private forces limiting the expansion of health care costs in this country. To this end, it becomes imperative that laboratorians, pathologists in particular, provide ongoing education for their clinician colleagues so that the laboratory can be used most effectively for diagnosis and follow-up. Medical school is the logical starting point for helping future clinicians begin to learn what the laboratory can and cannot, or should not, do.

The concepts of normal values, sensitivity, specificity, predictive value, the test setting, and test purposes all need to be mastered before laboratory data are interpreted. A presentation of these concepts follows.

Normal Values, Accuracy, and Precision

For each test that a laboratory performs, normal values have been established. These usually consist of a range of values with a given quantitation, eg, mg/dL, that sets the minimum and the maximum values that a patient can have and still be considered healthy, within the normal limits for that test. It is important to understand that normal value ranges can change depending on the patient population used as subjects from which the normal values are derived. In other words, a range of normal values for a given test is not "truth." Not all patients outside a normal range will have disease and, conversely, even some patients that show a laboratory value within a normal range will have the disease being considered. If you run a number of independent laboratory tests on a phlebotomized, healthy person, there is an increasing probability of getting an abnormal test result the more tests you order. For example, if 20 independent laboratory tests are performed on the serum of a healthy person (not an unlikely number of tests if a general chemistry battery is ordered), there is a greater than 60% probability that at least one of the laboratory values will be outside the range of normal for that given test (a false positive). Obviously, your job as the clinician will be to determine whether that abnormal test result is relevant to your patient.

Often, normal values have been obtained by performing clinical laboratory tests on a statistically appropriate number of healthy volunteers. These people are often hospital personnel or volunteer blood donors. The values obtained for these people are not always applicable as "normal" for comparison with sick people of all ages. Furthermore, statistical methods used to establish "normal ranges" have usually assumed a normal, gaussian (bell-shaped) distribution curve, when in fact a skewed distribution may better reflect reality. Don't forget: reference ranges differ among laboratories depending on the analytical method and units used to report results. Your laboratory has a list of the values.

What is meant by "normal" should be considered as well. At least four types have been suggested: (1) the individual normal, or values obtained from a patient in his or her usual or standard state; (2) the ideal normal, or values obtained from a population in optimum health; (3) the cohort normal, or values from a population similar to, or representative of, the patient; and (4) the general population normal, or values derived from samples of the overall population from which the patient comes. Most physicians use a general population normal in their everyday interpretation of laboratory data, even though the other types of "normal" might be more accurate standards. What no one really knows are the test value ranges for specific individuals, in both health and disease. It would be ideal to be able to compare a test result in a patient with his or her own values while well and with values in similar patients with the same disease. You must develop, through clinical experience, your own range of "normal" values as well as "action" values (the values at which in a given clinical situation you intervene clinically on the patient's behalf).

Interpretation of laboratory data is more than a comparison with "normal" values; the laboratory test setting also needs attention. For instance, a physician should be cognizant of patient conditions (diet, exercise habits, prescribed and self-obtained drug intake, emotional background, circadian rhythms, and occupation) and of sample collection, factors that can affect the final laboratory result. For instance, postphlebotomy red blood cell hemolysis causes a higher serum potassium level than is accurate for the patient.

Use the following list to assess possible causes of test result error, misinterpretation, or misuse:

1. Although rare, inadvertent human error can occur at any point from ordering, obtaining, and labeling the specimen to accessioning, analyzing, and reporting in the laboratory.
2. Physiological states, normal or abnormal, in your patient may affect test results, eg, pregnancy and a child's normal growth increase serum alkaline phosphatase levels.
3. The patient sample, if improperly handled, can affect test results, eg, all fluids that contain cells need to be refrigerated or preserved to prevent cytolysis.
4. Small fluctuations in serial test results may simply reflect expected laboratory analytical variability, and so can be ignored; other test result fluctuations are clinically important.
5. Laboratory test results are just numbers unless they are interpreted based on your patient's clinical findings plus an understanding of normal values and disease prevalence.

A physician must critically interpret a laboratory test result and not accept it as fact. Laboratory results are not truth.

Accuracy is a measure of the true value of the item being determined. Agreement of test results with patient conditions is the best measure of accuracy, because accuracy is difficult to assess in the clinical laboratory. Precision, on the other hand, is well monitored by the laboratory. Precision, or reproducibility, is a measure of the deviation of test results when performed over and over again under the same conditions. Various quality control materials are used by laboratories to monitor precision. Physicians should visit the clinical laboratory and inspect posted quality control charts to become aware of expected day-to-day fluctuations in results for tests they use often and rely on heavily for their particular patient population.

Sensitivity, Specificity, and Predictive Value

The sensitivity of a test is an expression of the probability that a result will be positive in the presence of disease. Sensitivity (SEN), therefore, is the percentage of true-positive (TP) results, where FN indicates the number of false negatives:

$$SEN=TP/(TP+FN)$$

The specificity of a test is an expression of the probability that a result will be negative in the absence of disease. Specificity (SPEC), then, is the percentage of true-negative (TN) results, where FP indicates the number of false positives:

$$SPEC=TN/(TN+FP)$$

Perfect specificity and sensitivity are virtually impossible to obtain for any laboratory test, and that's when diagnostic acumen comes into play.

A powerful tool to evaluate laboratory tests relating to your patient's clinical situation is the predictive value of a test result. Simply stated, the predictive value (PV) of a positive (or negative) test is the ratio of the true-positive (TP) (or true-negative [TN]) results to all positive (TP+FP) (or negative [TN+FN]) results:

$$PV(+) = TP/(TP+FP)$$
$$PV(-) = TN/(TN+FN)$$

The power of this statistical tool comes from the fact that predictive value takes into account the prevalence of a disease in your patient's particular setting. The following example should clarify these terms (see also Table 1.1) :

A laboratory test is both 95% sensitive (95% of all people with the disease have a positive or abnormal test result; 5% of the people with this disease have a negative test result) and 95% specific (95% of all people without the disease have a negative or normal test result; 5% of the people without the disease have a positive test result). This test is used to screen for disease A, which is relatively rare (1% prevalence). Therefore, a group of 100,000 people would contain 1000 people with disease A and 99,000 people without disease A. If all of these 100,000 people are tested, 950 people with disease A (95% of 1,000) and 4950 people without disease A (5% of 99,000) will have positive test results. There will be a total of 5900 positive test results. Hence, the predictive value of a positive result

Table 1.1 Predictive Value of a Test Result.

Total people in sample	100,000
Prevalence of disease A	1%
People with disease A	1000
People without disease A	99,000
Sensitivity	95%
Specificity	95%

Test	People With Disease A	People Without Disease A	Total
Positive (Abnormal result)	950 (95% of 1000) True positives	4950 (5% of 99,000) False positives	5900
Negative (Normal result)	50 (5% of 1000) False negatives	94,050 (95% of 99,000) True negatives	94,100
Total	1000	99,000	100,000

PV(+) = 950/(950 + 4950) = 16%

with this laboratory test for disease A in this population will be 950/5900, or 16%. In other words, only 16% of all positive test results will indicate disease A. If, however, the prevalence of disease A among the tested persons had been 50%, the predictive value of the test's positive results would have been 95%.

The prevalence of a disease greatly affects predictive values. Since exact prevalence figures are unavailable for many diseases, it is possible only to estimate the predictive value for tests used to screen most diseases. By carefully selecting the patients to be tested (principally by using good clinical judgment), physicians can greatly increase the predictive values of the laboratory tests they use.

Optimum Laboratory Utilization

Much has been written about the apparent overutilization of the laboratory and the attendant increased health care costs. Overutilization can mean mindless use of "routine" laboratory orders, useless repetition of orders on the same patient so that daily blood drawing actually causes a drop in hemoglobin concentration in a patient, little attention to how one diagnostic procedure can affect others, increased length of hospital stay—the list goes on.

At the inception of learning about laboratory use, in medical school, we need to appreciate each test ordered as an individual cost to the patient. When medical students are polled about laboratory costs, only a small percent can closely estimate what the laboratory charges the patient to perform the assay. No laboratory or diagnostic test should be ordered without the physician's awareness of what that test will cost the patient monetarily, physically, and emotionally. Get a list of laboratory test charges from the laboratories you use.

Although the clinical laboratory test could be considered another form of physical diagnosis, laboratory tests have limitations, and the laboratory is not an infinite resource. Furthermore, physicians should become aware of tests that are particularly suited for their patient's problem and use only those tests. Random screening bears little fruit compared with the thoughtful ordering of a few indicated laboratory tests. A complete history and properly performed physical examination should be made before a laboratory test is ordered except in an emergency. Skilled and experienced physicians use the clinical laboratory to confirm or exclude a possible diagnosis. The naive physician relies on the laboratory to screen patients for disease. Before ordering any laboratory test a physician should ask these questions:

1. Will the results of this test change my diagnosis, prognosis, or therapy?
2. Will the results of this test provide a better understanding of the disease process in my patient?
3. What do I expect this test result to tell me, and will it benefit my patient to learn it?

Physicians in clinical practice should open lines of communication with the laboratory. They should use the clinical pathologist as a consultant in test ordering and also provide clinical feedback to the pathologist. When problems about availability or interpretation of laboratory tests develop, the physician should immediately consult with the clinical laboratory. A test value too often is considered a "lab error" when that value could be calling attention to an important clinical fact. Clinical laboratories, however, are not infallible, and test results that diverge from the clinical picture should be reported to the laboratory.

Reference

Burke MD. Cost-effective laboratory testing. *Post Grad Med.* 1981;69:191-202.

```
═══════════
─────────────
═══════════
─────────────
███████ Two ███████
─────────────
═══════════
─────────────
═══════════
```

Clinical Cytogenetics

Key Points

1. Cytogenetic analysis requires living cells. Therefore, follow instructions for specimen collection and transport scrupulously.
2. Six of every 1000 neonates have a constitutional chromosome abnormality. Constitutional chromosome abnormalities are important causes of birth defects, mental retardation, and infertility.
3. Cytogenetic analysis of bone marrow has become routine in chronic myeloid leukemia, acute leukemias, and myelodysplasias because of the diagnostic and prognostic value of specific acquired chromosome abnormalities.
4. Prenatal cytogenetic diagnosis should be offered to every pregnant woman 35 years or older because the risk of a baby with trisomy increases significantly with advanced maternal age.

Background

There are only two normal cytogenetic test results:

> 46,XX: normal female karyotype
> 46,XY: normal male karyotype

Small structural chromosomal variations occur in some normal individuals; these variant chromosomes may be included in the notation of a normal karyotype. Examples:

> 46,XX,21s+: normal female karyotype with large satellites on chromosome 21 (normal variant)
> 46,XY,9qh+: normal male karyotype with large heterochromatic region of chromosome 9 (normal variant)

Table 2.1 Standard Cytogenetic Notation.

ace	Acentric fragment (also see f)
del	Deletion
der	Derivative chromosome
dic	Dicentric
dup	Duplication
f	Fragment (also see ace)
fra	Fragile site
h	Secondary constriction (heterochromatin)
i	Isochromosome
ins	Insertion
inv	Inversion
mar	Marker chromosome
minus (-)	Loss of
p	Short arm of chromosome
parentheses ( )	Used to surround structurally altered chromosome(s) or breakpoint(s)
Ph¹ or Ph	Philadelphia chromosome
plus (+)	Gain of
q	Long arm of chromosome
question mark (?)	Indicates questionable identification of chromosome or chromosome structure
r	Ring chromosome
s	Satellite
semicolon (;)	Separates chromosomes and chromosome regions in structural rearrangements involving more than one chromosome
slant line or solidus (/)	Separates cell lines in describing mosaics or chimeras
t	Translocation
ter	Terminal (end of chromosome)

Staining techniques produce a unique pattern of transverse light and dark bands on each chromosome and each band, by convention, is numbered. Locations of structural chromosome abnormalities are designated according to the chromosome (number), arm (letter), and band (number) involved.

Standard cytogenetic notation used in reporting results and examples of cytogenetic nomenclature and notation are provided in Tables 2.1 and 2.2.

Disease States

Chromosome abnormalities are either (1) constitutional (congenital) and may be detected pre/postnatally or (2) acquired and associated with tumors.

Constitutional Chromosome Abnormalities

Patients with constitutional chromosome abnormalities (Table 2.3) are not only seen by pediatricians and obstetricians, but are also seen (and, it is hoped, recognized) by physicians in virtually every medical specialty. Chromosome abnormalities are of two basic types: (1) **numerical** (too many or too few chromosomes) and (2) **structural** (the result of chromatin breakage with loss, gain, or rearrange-

Table 2.2 Examples of Cytogenetic Nomenclature and Notation.

Normal: 46,XX
         46,XY

Aneuploidy: 45,X (Monosomy X)
              47,XY,+18 (Trisomy 18)
              50,XY,+6,+14,+20,+21 (Hyperdiploidy)

Deletion: 46,XY,5p-
  Terminal: 46,XY,del(5)(p14)
  Interstitial: 46,XY,del(5)(q21q31)

Inversion:
  Paracentric: 46,XX,inv(3)(q21q26)
  Pericentric: 46,XX,inv(16)(p13q22)
Isochromosome: 46,X,i(Xq)

Translocation: 46,XY,t(9;22)(q34;q11)
  Interpretation: 46,XY,-9,-22,+der(9),+der(22)t(9;22)(q34;q11)

Mosaic (more than one cell line):
     45,X/46,X,Xp-
     46,XY/46,XY,t(9;22)(q34;q11)/46,XY,t(9;22),-17,+i(17q)

Marker: 47,XY,+mar
      46,XX,-7,-12,+mar1,+mar2

---

ment of chromosomal material). Although the vast majority of cytogenetically abnormal conceptions result in embryonic or fetal death (50% of spontaneous abortions have a chromosome abnormality), constitutional chromosome abnormalities are present in 6 of every 1000 newborns. Two of these 6 are unbalanced autosomal abnormalities (eg, Down syndrome), 2 are sex chromosome abnormalities (eg, Klinefelter syndrome), and 2 are balanced autosomal abnormalities (phenotypically normal carriers who have increased risk of cytogenetically abnormal progeny and pregnancy loss). Diagnosis of a constitutional chromosome abnormality not only suggests appropriate management and accurate prognosis, but is essential for genetic counseling.

The clinical syndromes associated with the more common constitutional chromosome abnormalities are familiar to most physicians; their phenotypes, epidemiology, and natural history are well described (see references and Table 2.3). The phenotypes of constitutional autosomal cytogenetic abnormalities range from multiple, severe malformations (eg, trisomy 18) to mild or no dysmorphisms (eg, a small deletion); however, virtually all include some degree of mental retardation. Therefore, any unexplained developmental delay is an indication for cytogenetic evaluation.

Examples of other liveborn autosomal trisomies include trisomy 8 mosaicism, trisomy 9 mosaicism, trisomy 4p, trisomy 9p, partial trisomy 10q, trisomy 20p, and partial trisomy (or tetrasomy) 22 (cat-eye syndrome).

Other sex chromosome aneuploidies include 47,XXX; 48,XXXX; 48,XXYY or 48,XXXY; and 47,XYY.

Chromosome deletions associated with recognizable syndromes include 4p- (Wolf syndrome); 5p- (cri du chat syndrome); 9p-; 11p- (aniridia/Wilms' tumor); 13q- (with or without retinoblastoma); 18p-; and 18q-. Syndromes in which a

Table 2.3 Some Common Constitutional Chromosome Abnormalities.

Common Name	Examples of Common Karyotype(s)	Incidence	Common Phenotypic Features
Down syndrome (trisomy 21)	47,XX,+21 46,XY,-14,+t(14q21q)	1/700 births	Hypotonia, upward slanted eyes, epicanthal folds, flat face, simian creases, congenital heart defect, mental retardation
Trisomy 18	47,XY,+18 46,XX/47,XX,+18	1/4000-5000 births	Severe growth retardation, micrognathia, congenital heart defect, overlapping fingers, rocker-bottom feet, limited survival
Trisomy 13	47,XY,+13 46,XX-14,+t(13q14q)	1/5000 births	Cleft lip/palate, polydactyly, microphthalmia, congenital heart defect, holoprosencephaly, limited survival
Turner syndrome	45,X 46,X, abnormal X 45,X/46,X, abnormal X	1/3000-5000 females	Newborn edema of hands and feet, webbed neck, short stature, cubitus valgus, absent puberty
Klinefelter syndrome	47,XXY	1/500 males	Hypogonadism, possible gynecomastia, long legs
Fragile X syndrome	46,fra(X),Y	1/2500 births	Mental retardation, large chin, ears, testes, possible autistic behavior

tiny chromosomal deletion is sometimes but not always found include Prader-Willi syndrome (15q-), Miller-Dieker (lissencephaly) syndrome (17p-), Langer-Giedion syndrome (8q-), and DiGeorge anomaly (22q-).

Indications for Prenatal Constitutional Chromosome Analysis. Prenatal diagnosis of constitutional chromosome abnormalities is possible in most cases and should be offered to all patients who are at increased risk of cytogenetically abnormal progeny.

Specimen: Amniotic fluid, chorionic villus sample, or percutaneous umbilical cord blood sample.
1. Advanced maternal age
   Women older than 34 years have three times greater risk than younger women of having a baby with trisomy. For example, the risk of a liveborn trisomy 21 child is about 1 in 1500 below age 30, 1 in 370 at age 35, and 1 in 100 at age 40.

2. Low maternal serum alpha-fetoprotein (MSAFP)
   Although most women with low MSAFP have normal fetuses, about one third of women carrying a fetus with trisomy have low MSAFP.
3. Parental carrier of a balanced chromosome abnormality
   For example, balanced reciprocal translocation, Robertsonian translocation, inversion
4. Previous child with chromosome abnormality
5. Carrier of X-linked genetic disorder (to determine fetal sex)
   Other indications for prenatal diagnosis include a previous child with neural tube defect, high MSAFP, and parental carriers of a recessive mutant gene (eg, sickle hemoglobin, Tay-Sachs disease).

Indications for Postnatal Constitutional Chromosome Analysis.

Specimen: Blood or solid tissue.
1. Multiple congenital anomalies
2. Unexplained mental retardation and/or developmental delay
3. Suspected aneuploidy
   For example, trisomy 21 (Down syndrome), trisomy 18, trisomy 13
4. Suspected unbalanced autosome
   For example, cri du chat syndrome, Prader-Willi syndrome
5. Suspected sex chromosome abnormality
   For example, Turner syndrome, Klinefelter syndrome
6. Suspected fragile X syndrome
7. Suspected chromosome-breakage syndrome
   For example, ataxia-telangiectasia, Bloom syndrome, Fanconi anemia, xeroderma pigmentosum. Note: Many laboratories do not have the special induction systems required to diagnose the chromosome-breakage syndromes. Consult with the laboratory director before sending a specimen.
8. Infertility
   Rule out sex chromosome abnormality, carrier of balanced abnormality.
9. Multiple spontaneous abortions
   Rule out carrier of balanced abnormality; both partners should be evaluated.
10. Relative of a child with chromosome translocation or other structural chromosome abnormality

Acquired Chromosome Abnormalities

Cytogenetic abnormalities, often multiple, are acquired by most tumor cells; the abnormalities are present only in the neoplastic cells and not in the non-neoplastic tissues of the patient's body. Many of these cytogenetic changes are nonrandom and are specific for a particular type or subtype of neoplasm. In hematologic disorders, their identification in neoplastic cells provides important independent prognostic information about the patient's disease, and in some instances may be the single most important factor in predicting outcome. In many kinds of leukemias and some other hematologic disorders, cytogenetic analysis of a specimen of bone marrow is a routine part of the diagnostic workup. Establishment of

Table 2.4 Prognostic Associations of ALL Chromosomes.

Good prognosis
  Hyperdiploidy, 51-60 chromosomes

Intermediate prognosis
  Hyperdiploidy, 47-50 chromosomes
  del(6q)
  Normal chromosomes

Poor prognosis
  Any translocation; most frequent: t(8;14),t(4;11),t(9;22),t(1;19)
  Near-haploidy; hypodiploidy

Undetermined
  del(12p); others

such clinically meaningful associations has begun for cytogenetic changes in chronic lymphoproliferative disorders, lymphomas, and solid tumors.

The following are indications for cytogenetic analysis of bone marrow:

1. Any acute leukemia, lymphocytic (ALL) (Table 2.4) or nonlymphocytic (ANLL) (Tables 2.5 and 2.6), at diagnosis
2. Chronic myeloid leukemia (CML) at diagnosis (presence or absence of Philadelphia chromosome)
3. Myelodysplastic states at diagnosis (Table 2.7)
4. Remission of acute leukemia (to evaluate ablation of cytogenetically abnormal clone[s])
5. Relapse of acute leukemia (to evaluate clonal evolution)
6. More aggressive or unstable phase of CML or myelodysplastic state (to evaluate conversion to "blast crisis" or acute leukemia)
7. Aplastic anemia vs "aleukemic leukemia" in a child
8. To assess engraftment of other-sex donor bone marrow after transplant
9. To diagnosis rapidly a critically ill newborn with suspected aneuploidy

Table 2.5 Common Chromosome Abnormalities in ANLL.

Chromosome Abnormality	FAB Subgroup(s)
t(9;22)	M1
t(8;21)	M2
t(15;17)	M3
inv(16),t(16;V),del(16q)	M4
del(11q),t(11q;V)	M4, M5
ins(3q),inv(3q),t(3q)	Thrombocytosis, abnormal megakaryocytes
+8	M1, M2, M4, M5, M6
-7	Secondary ANLL
-5/5q-	Secondary ANLL

V = variable chromosomes

Table 2.6 Prognostic Associations of ANLL Chromosomes.

Good prognosis
  inv(16), abnormal 16q
  t(8;21)

Intermediate prognosis
  Normal chromosomes*
  Trisomy 8
  Translocations t(6;9), t(11q;V), t(9;22),t(15;17),45,X,-Y

Poor Prognosis
  Monosomy 7 or del(7q); monosomy 5 or del(5q)
  Multiple chromosome defects
  Hyperdiploidy

Undetermined
  inv(3); others

* Conflicting data concerning prognostic implications of apparently normal chromosomes almost certainly reflect an admixture of undetected chromosome abnormalities with karyotypes that are truly normal.

Specimen Information

All specimens for chromosome analysis must be collected and handled to preserve living cells capable of cell division. Aseptic technique must be used because cells will be grown in culture medium for days or even weeks. A working diagnosis or pertinent history indicating the reason for cytogenetic evaluation must be provided with the specimen; this information determines which culture systems, staining techniques, and methods of analysis will be used.

Blood

Routine cytogenetic studies are performed on blood specimens, specifically the lymphocytes. Special studies that require special culture and staining techniques, such as fragile X screening and high-resolution banding to detect small deletions, are done on blood specimens.

Table 2.7 Prognostic Associations of Myelodysplastic State Chromosomes.

Good prognosis
  Normal chromosomes
  del(5q) alone

Intermediate prognosis
  Trisomy 8

Poor prognosis
  Monosomy 7 or del(7q)
  Multiple chromosome abnormalities

Undetermined
  Monosomy 5 (in secondary myelodysplastic state); others

Blood (venous, arterial, or capillary) must be collected in preservative-free sodium heparin (green-top vacutainer tube or heparinized syringe or capillary tube); all other anticoagulants inhibit cell division. About 2 mL of blood is the minimum necessary for routine evaluation; more (5-10 mL) is necessary for special studies. The specimen should remain at room temperature until delivered to the cytogenetics laboratory. Heart blood (autopsy) or umbilical cord blood (stillborns, perinatal deaths, fetal blood sampling) may be submitted.

Spontaneously dividing cells are not present in normal blood; therefore, blood must be cultured with a mitogen that stimulates lymphocytes to divide. Dividing cells are most abundant 66 to 72 hours after stimulation. Therefore, stat cytogenetic results are not possible from any specimen except bone marrow. Results from blood specimens are routinely available in 5 to 10 days. In certain cases, preliminary results can be provided in $2^{1}/2$ days if a rapid result is mandatory and if arranged in advance with the laboratory. Results of special studies may not be available for 2 or more weeks.

Solid Tissue

If chromosomal analysis of blood does not yield an unequivocal result, examination of other tissues (cell types) is necessary (eg, to exclude mosaicism). Culturing of solid tissue (which usually produces fibroblast cultures) is also useful for examination of fetal and autopsy material when blood is not available or useable.

A small piece (eg, 0.3x0.3x0.3 cm) of tissue should be obtained aseptically. A 2- to 3-mm punch biopsy of skin is most commonly submitted for chromosome analysis. Postmortem organ specimens such as lung or kidney may be used within 24 hours of death. All specimens should be transported to the cytogenetics laboratory as soon as possible in sterile tissue culture medium. Sterile saline can be used when medium is unavailable if the specimen will reach the cytogenetics laboratory within a few hours. Solid tissue specimens should be refrigerated (not frozen!) in tissue culture medium overnight if immediate transport to the cytogenetics laboratory is not possible.

Results from solid tissue specimens are available in 3 to 5 weeks, dependent on tissue growth in culture flasks.

Bone Marrow

At least 1 to 2 mL of aspirated marrow drawn into a syringe wetted with preservative-free sodium heparin is required. The specimen should be transported immediately, at room temperature, to the cytogenetics laboratory. If the specimen must be sent a long distance or overnight, the heparinized bone marrow should be mixed with sterile tissue culture medium as soon as it is collected.

In samples from patients with hematologic disorders, dividing cells may be examined directly from the specimen without culture, and/or after overnight and/or 48-hour culture. A direct examination, particularly useful in ALL, is usually possible only if the specimen is received in the cytogenetics laboratory before 1 PM. Preliminary results are telephoned to the physician in 2 to 4 days; a final report takes about 2 weeks.

Because spontaneously dividing cells are present in normal bone marrow, a bone marrow chromosome analysis can be used for rapid diagnosis of chromosome aneuploidy in cases of critically ill newborns with multiple congenital anomalies when a conventionally performed 48- or 72-hour blood culture with mitogen could delay a critical decision regarding surgery or resuscitation of the infant. Results from such an analysis, when successful, are available in 6 hours; however, analyzable dividing cells are not found in one third of such specimens. Therefore, a specimen of blood for conventional culture with mitogen should be submitted with this type of bone marrow specimen.

Note that only numerical chromosome abnormalities (aneuploidy) can be reliably detected in neonatal bone marrow specimens. Bone marrow should not be sent for cytogenetic diagnosis if an abnormality of chromosome structure such as translocation, deletion, or duplication is suspected. Blood should be used.

Amniotic Fluid
Cells from amniotic fluid obtained by transabdominal amniocentesis at 14 to 20 weeks of gestation are grown in culture and used for prenatal diagnosis. About 20 mL of amniotic fluid should be submitted at room temperature in a sterile syringe, sterile centrifuge tube, or other sterile container. Results are available in 10 to 21 days.

Chorionic Villus Sample
A small biopsy of chorionic villi, obtained transcervically in the first trimester of pregnancy or transabdominally in the first or second trimester, can be cultured and used for prenatal diagnosis. At least 10 mg of villi (excluding decidua) is required; 25 mg is optimal. The specimen should be transported to the cytogenetics laboratory immediately in sterile tissue culture medium at room temperature. Results are available in 8 to 14 days. Results from a direct (uncultured) preparation may be available in 1 to 2 days, but recent data show that direct results are less reliable than those from cultured chorionic villus sample cells.

Other Specimens
Cytogenetic analysis of specimens such as solid tumors and effusions is also possible in some laboratories. Contact the laboratory director for instructions concerning specimen collection and transport.

Charges
Cytogenetic procedures and analysis are still very labor-intensive and are therefore expensive tests. Charges range from approximately $300 to $900.

References

Cotran RS, Kumar V, Robbins SL. *Pathologic Basis of Disease*. 4th ed. Philadelphia, Pa: WB Saunders Co; 1989.

Gelehrter TD, Collins FS. *Principles of Medical Genetics*. Baltimore, Md: Williams & Wilkins; 1990.

Harnden DG, Klinger HP, eds. *ISCN 1985: An International System for Human Cytogenetic Nomenclature*. Basel, Switzerland: S Karger; 1985.

Heim S, Mitelman F. *Cancer Cytogenetics*. New York, NY: Alan R Liss Co Inc; 1987.

Jones KL. *Smith's Recognizable Patterns of Human Malformation.* 4th ed. Philadelphia, Pa: WB Saunders Co; 1988.

Milunsky A, ed. *Genetic Disorders and the Fetus.* 2nd ed. New York, NY: Plenum Press; 1986.

Nussbaum RL, Ledbetter DH. The fragile X syndrome. In: Scriver CR, Beaudet AL, Sly WS, Valle D, eds. *The Metabolic Basis of Inherited Disease.* 6th ed. New York, NY: McGraw-Hill Inc; 1989:327-341.

Schinzel A. *Catalogue of Unbalanced Chromosome Aberrations in Man.* New York, NY: Walter de Gruyter; 1984.

Thompson MW, McInnes RR, Willard HF. *Thompson and Thompson Genetics in Medicine.* 5th ed. Philadelphia, Pa: WB Saunders Co; 1991.

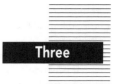

Three

Infectious Disease:
General Laboratory Tests

Key Points

1. Collection of specimens for microbiological diagnosis of infectious diseases requires thoughtful planning, extreme caution in the acquisition process, and rapid transport to the laboratory for it to be meaningful.
2. Often, diagnostic information can be rapidly obtained by staining smears of directly acquired specimens (pus, sputum, body fluids) with various stains (Gram's, Giemsa, etc) and examining them microscopically.
3. Anyone suspected of having bacteremia or fungemia should have three properly collected blood culture specimens cultured during the first 24 hours of diagnostic evaluation.

Background

The process of diagnosis in infectious diseases begins with a complete medical history and a thorough physical examination. Based on findings from these procedures, the physician then turns to the clinical microbiology, virology, and immunology laboratories for assistance in identifying responsible pathogenic microorganisms.

Proper Specimen

A proper specimen for identification of pathogenic microorganisms is one appropriate to the clinical stage of infection. For instance, cultures of lesions from acute infections usually yield more organisms than cultures from chronic lesions. Many specimens are useless because they are contaminated with indigenous or transient microbial flora. An adequate amount of specimen (ideally several milliliters) must be submitted for all of the diagnostic procedures to be performed. If only a small amount of material can be obtained, a list of priorities for microbiological testing should be submitted.

Specimens from deep, closed, normally sterile body areas are often the best ones for microbiological examination. These include deep tissues, joints, and pleural, peritoneal, and other body spaces. They are satisfactory for both anaerobic and aerobic bacteriological and most virological studies. Specimens are collected either by surgical excision or by closed needle aspiration. Portions of several lesions, if present, as well as several portions of large lesions (eg, wall and center of an abscess cavity) should be sampled. If closed needle aspiration is performed, the site of percutaneous needle aspiration must be thoroughly disinfected with 70% alcohol and iodine or an iodophor.

Some specimens are obtained from deep body areas via a communicating pathway, such as the oropharynx, urethra, cervix uteri, and sinus tracts. Such specimens may be appropriate for aerobic, but not anaerobic, bacteriology since they contain a normal anaerobic flora. Sometimes the communicating pathway can be bypassed to obtain a specimen, as with suprapubic aspiration of the urinary bladder or transtracheal aspiration of the upper airways. Results from specimens contaminated by the microflora of the communicating pathway are difficult to interpret.

Some body areas are heavily contaminated with indigenous microflora. Specimens from the mouth, throat, gastrointestinal stomata, fissures, fistulas, and superficial wounds are unlikely to yield meaningful microbiological data unless a specific bacterial pathogen is being sought or the base of the wound can be sampled via an uncontaminated approach. In superficial wounds, the base of the lesion should be aspirated and/or biopsy should be performed after appropriate disinfection. The margins or adjacent undermined areas should be sampled also. Swabs should be avoided. Although handy, they give less satisfactory results than aspirates or biopsy specimens because the sample size is smaller, the specimen is often dried by the air, and some substances in swabs may inhibit bacterial growth (eg, fatty acids on cotton swabs inhibit *Neisseria gonorrhoeae*).

Transportation of Specimens

Proper transportation of specimens is crucial for accurate outcome. Before leaving the bedside, all specimens and requisitions must be completely labeled with patient and specimen data, the date and time collected, the name of the responsible physician, pertinent clinical data (including antimicrobial therapy and working diagnosis), and the type of procedure desired from the laboratory. All specimens should then be transported to the laboratory as rapidly as possible, using appropriate containers for specimen transport. Do not use cotton-plugged or loosely stoppered containers that may leak. Urine should be refrigerated if there is a delay in transportation. Anaerobic specimens must be transported in either gassed-out tubes or evacuated and capped syringes or transport media kept at room temperature. All swabs, except those for routine throat culture that are self-contained, should be transported in sterile tubes containing transport media. Specimens for viral culture should be transported in appropriate transport media and at the temperature appropriate to the specimen type and the agent(s) suspected (cytomegalovirus [CMV] and respiratory syncytial virus [RSV] will not survive freezing).

Specific Specimens and Associated Infectious Diseases

Blood

Blood cultures are collected to document bacteremia or fungemia, which may be transient, intermittent, or continuous. Transient bacteremia is associated with manipulation of infected or contaminated tissues (eg, tonsillectomy, dental procedures) and those occurring during the early phases of some bacterial infections (eg, pneumococcal pneumonia). Continuous bacteremia is uncommon but may be a feature of early typhoid fever or brucellosis, and is the rule in intravascular infections such as infective endocarditis or in patients who are severely immunocompromised (eg, *Mycobacterium avium-intracellulare* bacteremia in patients with acquired immunodeficiency syndrome [AIDS]).

Blood cultures are indicated in patients who experience a sudden change in clinical parameters, such as pulse rate, temperature, prostration, or hypotension, and in all febrile patients with chills, serious illness, suspected infective endocarditis, immunosuppression, or in whom bacteremia is a possibility but no cause is apparent. Two or three sets of blood cultures within a 24-hour period are usually satisfactory to document bacteremia. The collection of a single set is unacceptable because intermittent bacteremia may be missed and possible culture contamination will be less well documented. Collection of four or more sets is rarely helpful and "overphlebotomizes" the patient. A relatively large volume of blood (20-30 mL in adults) is ideal because of the low number of bacteria per milliliter present in the blood of most patients with bacteremia.

The ideal time for blood culture collection is just prior to the anticipated onset of a chill. Because chills are difficult to predict, a more practical optimum time is either just as the patient's temperature begins to rise or at the onset of a chill.

Blood cultures should be collected by percutaneous venipuncture after meticulous disinfection of the skin surrounding the puncture site. Both aerobic and anaerobic bottles must be inoculated so that the resultant dilution ratio of blood to broth is approximately 1:10. Some laboratories also incorporate an Isolator™ (Wampole Laboratories, Division of Carter-Wallace Inc, Cranbury, NJ) tube (lysis centrifugation, followed by inoculation of solid media) as a part of a blood culture "set." Most clinical laboratories notify physicians of positive blood cultures as soon as results are confirmed. Patients suspected of having endocarditis or brucellosis should be reported to laboratory personnel so that the patient's cultures can be kept an extended time. Also, cultures from patients with AIDS are held longer because of the frequency with which they are infected with such pathogens as *Mycobacterium* species, yeasts, and systemic fungi. Approximately 10% of all bacteremias are polymicrobial. Several microorganisms—notably *Bacillus*, *Corynebacterium*, and *Propionibacterium* species, and *Staphylococcus epidermidis*—are commonly found in blood cultures as the result of skin contamination. These microorganisms at times may be implicated in severe infections. Positive blood cultures involving these microorganisms, therefore, must be carefully evaluated.

Cerebrospinal Fluid

Acute bacterial meningitis is a medical emergency that must be diagnosed and treated as soon as possible. Cerebrospinal fluid (CSF) should be collected as soon as this diagnosis is considered. Strict aseptic technique is imperative during the lumbar puncture procedure. As much CSF as is reasonable should be collected. Concurrent blood cultures should always be collected, because 50% to 90% of patients with acute bacterial meningitis also have bacteremia. CSF must be transported immediately and without refrigeration to the clinical laboratory. Many microorganisms that cause meningitis (eg, *Neisseria meningitidis*) are fastidious and will not survive at temperatures below 37°C. CSF is itself a good culture medium. It can be incubated either before or after subcultures have been performed on solid media.

In addition to cytological and chemical tests on CSF (discussed in Chapter 12), certain microbiological tests are required in suspected cases of meningitis. Concentrated CSF is examined microscopically with Gram's stain, acridine orange (if a fluorescence microscope is available), and methylene blue. Sometimes, stainable but nonviable microorganisms are identified. In partially treated meningitis gram-positive microorganisms may stain gram-negative. All CSF specimens are cultured aerobically. Anaerobic meningitis is uncommon. If unusual microorganisms (eg, fungi, *Leptospira*) are suspected, the clinical laboratory should be notified before the specimens are collected.

Other techniques may be used in the rapid diagnosis of meningitis. Detection of microbial antigens in CSF by latex particle agglutination can be extremely valuable. In cases of suspected fungal meningitis, an india ink preparation or a latex particle agglutination test may establish the diagnosis of cryptococcal meningitis. Parasitic organisms that cause primary amebic meningoencephalitis (eg, *Naegleria*) can be identified by characteristic ameboid movements during examination of wet-mount preparations of CSF or by Giemsa-stained smears of CSF.

Urine

Urine and sputum are examples of specimens obtained after passage through a communicating pathway. In each case, the communicating pathway (the urethra for urine and the oropharynx for sputum) contains indigenous microbial flora that contaminate the specimen. Because of the relative ease in reducing the contamination, cultures of voided urine are more reliable than cultures of expectorated sputum.

Normally a clean-voided midstream specimen is collected, which requires cleansing and disinfecting the external urethral meatus and genitalia. The urine specimen is caught in a sterile container during voiding and in midstream and promptly transported to the laboratory. Because clean-voided midstream urine specimens are reliable specimens for detection of bacteriuria, physicians should make every effort to collect and transport these specimens properly.

Under certain circumstances a urine specimen may be obtained by suprapubic aspiration of the urinary bladder. This specimen is indicated in some infants and small children, adults in whom cultures of clean-voided midstream specimens have yielded equivocal results, and patients with suspected anaerobic bacteriuria. As in any case of closed needle aspiration of a deep body cavity, strict aseptic technique is essential.

A third type of urine specimen is that obtained after instrumentation, usually catheterization or cystoscopic examination. Catheterization for the sole purpose of obtaining a urine specimen is discouraged, because of the risk of resultant bacteriuria. Urine may be collected from indwelling catheters by aseptically aspirating urine through the disinfected wall of the catheter, but not from the drainage bag or tube. Foley catheter tips should not be submitted for culture.

Reports of urine culture should state not only the name of the microorganism(s) isolated but also the approximate colony count. Nonquantitative urine cultures are never indicated. Colony counts are essential for establishing the presence of significant bacteriuria. Colony counts of 100,000 per milliliter or greater are indicative of infection, while counts exceeding 50,000 per milliliter are indicative of probable infection. Some experts require at least two colony counts equal to or greater than 100,000 to establish a diagnosis of urinary tract infection in women. Additionally, the "acute urethral syndrome" (symptomatic pyuria) in young women may be associated with fewer than 10,000 organisms per milliliter.

The presence of a microorganism in any quantity in urine obtained by suprapubic aspiration is significant. Up to one third of urinary tract infections are associated with colony counts between 10,000 and 100,000. Low colony counts of clinical significance occur in patients receiving antibiotic therapy, and rarely in patients with either an obstructed ureter or an infection due to a fastidious organism. Most urinary tract infections are caused by a single species. True polymicrobial urinary tract infections occur only in patients with either chronic indwelling urethral catheters or chronic, high-grade urinary tract obstruction (eg, calculi).

Respiratory Tract Specimens

Ear. Microorganisms associated with acute otitis media are usually limited to a few species, predominantly *Streptococcus pneumoniae*, *Haemophilus influenzae*, and *Moraxella catarrhalis*. Routine tympanocentesis to obtain middle ear fluid for bacterial culture is not indicated in uncomplicated cases. Patients with severe or atypical symptoms, immunosuppressed patients, and patients who fail to respond to therapy may benefit from culture of their middle ear fluid.

Nasopharynx. Because of its heavy indigenous microbial flora, culture of the nasopharynx is useful only when a specific bacterial pathogen is being sought. Nasopharyngeal specimens are used to identify carriers of certain bacteria (eg, *Staphylococcus aureus*, *N meningitidis*). Specimens for the diagnosis of pertussis are best obtained from the nasopharynx by swab, loop, or aspiration. These specimens must be cultured by inoculation onto special media immediately after collection. Rapid diagnosis of pertussis by fluorescent antibody identification of the bacteria ("pertussis prep") in material from the nasopharynx is also available.

Throat. Throat specimens should be cultured only when a particular organism is being sought. The most common microorganisms sought are *Bordetella pertussis*, *N gonorrhoeae*, *N meningitidis*, *Corynebacterium diphtheriae*, and *Streptococcus pyogenes* (group A). The diagnosis of pertussis is best made from nasopharyngeal specimens. Gonococcal pharyngitis can be diagnosed by throat culture, but the clinical microbiology laboratory must be notified if this diagnosis is suspected because it is inoculated on different media. Suspicion of diphtheria also requires that the laboratory be notified, and specimens from such patients should include a swab of any membrane present.

The most commonly requested throat culture is for identification of *S pyogenes*. Throat cultures are useful because a diagnosis of streptococcal pharyngitis cannot be made reliably on clinical grounds alone. Thorough sampling of the throat is needed to ensure a proper specimen. The posterior pharynx, tonsils or tonsillar pillars, the area behind the uvula, and any areas of purulence, inflammation, or ulceration must be swabbed. Most patients with streptococcal pharyngitis have a positive throat culture, thus, a negative culture is helpful in excluding this diagnosis. Some patients with a light growth of *S pyogenes* fail to demonstrate an antibody response to the microorganism, and these individuals may represent carriers rather than patients with true streptococcal infection. Direct tests to detect antigens of group A streptococci are also available, and are especially useful in pediatric outpatient practices. These are less sensitive than culture, thus optimal procedure requires that cultures be done when the direct antigen test is negative.

Attempts to isolate viral agents from the nasopharynx or throat should be directed towards specific agents, such as enterovirus, influenza and parainfluenza viruses, RSV, adenovirus, and herpes simplex virus. Nasopharyngeal swabs, throat washes, throat swabs, or swabs or scrapings of unroofed vesicular lesions or ulcers should be placed into appropriate viral transport media and sent to the laboratory promptly at the appropriate temperature (consult the laboratory in advance).

Sputum. Bacterial cultures of sputum are frequently ordered, but their value is questionable. Many patients with pneumococcal pneumonia do not have these bacteria in their sputum, and up to 20% of healthy individuals may be pharyngeal carriers of pneumococci at any given time. Expectorated sputum is frequently contaminated by oropharyngeal microbial flora; thus, interpretation of sputum cultures is difficult. In addition to (and some experts insist, instead of) a sputum culture, microscopic examination of a Gram's-stained smear helps to identify certain important microorganisms, such as the pneumococcus. Sputum should be obtained early in the morning under the supervision of a nurse, respiratory therapist, or physician. Sputum obtained should be inspected for pus and/or blood, and this material should be examined microscopically. The presence of many leukocytes and few epithelial cells indicates that the original sputum specimen probably does contain material from the lower respiratory tract. Large numbers of squamous epithelial cells indicate that the material is contaminated by oropharyngeal secretions and is unsuitable for culture.

There are several alternatives to expectorated sputum. All must be obtained by invasive procedures that involve risks. Direct endotracheal or endobronchial aspiration, bronchial brushings, bronchoalveolar lavage or biopsy materials, and needle aspiration of a pulmonary infiltrate under fluoroscopic control produce reasonably good specimens. Transtracheal aspiration is also of potential value. Because of significant risks involved with the procedure, transtracheal aspiration should be performed only when strongly indicated, and then only by an experienced individual.

All patients with suspected lower respiratory tract infection should have concurrent blood cultures. If a pleural effusion is present, the effusion should be aspirated and cultured.

Lower respiratory tract infections are sometimes caused by viruses, rickettsiae, chlamydiae, *Mycoplasma pneumoniae*, parasites, and *Legionella* species. These agents cannot be isolated routinely and identified from sputum specimens. They require special media and techniques for isolation and/or identification.

Gastrointestinal Tract Specimens

Mouth. Bacterial cultures of the mouth, periodontal lesions, or saliva are rarely useful. If actinomycosis is suspected, the clinical microbiology laboratory should be contacted for instructions about specimen collection. Thrush (oral candidiasis) and Vincent's angina can be diagnosed by examination of stained smears from scrapings of suspected lesions.

Feces. Fecal (stool) cultures are helpful in the diagnosis of certain types of diarrhea. Clinical microbiology laboratories should be able to isolate and identify *Salmonella*, *Shigella*, and *Campylobacter* species. Most laboratories will search for *Vibrio* and *Yersinia* if requested by the physician. At present there are no easy means of identifying enterohemorrhagic, enterotoxigenic, enteroinvasive, enteroadherent, or "enteropathogenic" serotypes of *Escherichia coli* in the clinical microbiology laboratory. Enterohemmorrhagic *E coli* can be sought by a variety of screening procedures, but these are not "routine" tests. Tests to detect antigens of rotavirus are available in most hospitals. Recently, *Cryptosporidium* has been implicated as a cause of diarrhea, particularly in immunocompromised hosts. This organism can be detected by various noncultural methods, particularly acid-fast– and immunofluorescence-stained smears of feces.

Genital Tract Specimens

Urethra. In men, Gram's-stained smears of urethral exudate or discharge are both sensitive and specific for the diagnosis of gonorrhea. The finding of five or more leukocytes per high-power field indicates urethritis. The diagnosis of gonorrhea is confirmed by finding typical gram-negative diplococci within neutrophils. If gonorrhea is suspected but the smears are negative, a culture of the urethral discharge for *N gonorrhoeae* should be made. Cultures of the throat and/or anal crypts for this microorganism may be indicated. In women, Gram's-stained smears of vaginal or cervical discharge are not reliable for the diagnosis of gonorrhea. Cultures of the cervical os (obtained during speculum examination) and the anal crypts for *N gonorrhoeae* are indicated in all women suspected of having gonorrhea. Since members of the *Neisseria* species are fastidious organisms, culture material ideally should be plated at the bedside onto Thayer-Martin (or similar) agar that has been warmed previously to body temperature. These plates must then either be transported immediately to the clinical microbiology laboratory or be placed in a CO_2 incubator (or candle extinction jar) in a peripheral laboratory.

Genitalia. The diagnosis of syphilis is suspected when there are painless, ulcerative genital lesions. Because most genital ulcerations cannot be diagnosed on clinical grounds alone, it is imperative to exclude syphilis by serologic tests in all cases of genital ulcerations. A discussion of the serologic tests for syphilis is included elsewhere (Chapter 5). A useful method for the rapid diagnosis of syphilis is darkfield microscopy of genital ulcers. The yield depends on the stage of disease as well as on whether antimicrobial agents have been administered.

Chancroid is caused by *Haemophilus ducreyi*. Cultural isolation requires special media, and identification of this microorganism is difficult (but not impossible); Gram's-stained smears of fresh exudate from the genital lesions will often show the typical pairs and short chains of gram-negative coccobacilli. Culture of *Chlamydia trachomatis* can be accomplished in some laboratories by inoculation of urethral, cervical, or rectal (occasionally throat) and conjunctival specimens onto certain tissue culture cell lines. This procedure is not widely available. Detection of antigens of *C trachomatis* from these specimens can also be accomplished by immunofluorescence or by enzyme immunoassay procedures. Lymphogranuloma venereum, a specific syndrome caused by some serovars of *C trachomatis*, is usually diagnosed by serologic means. The best test for diagnosis of granuloma inguinale is direct examination of a Wright's- or Giemsa-stained smear of tissue from the margin of a genital ulcer. The finding of small, straight or curved, pleomorphic bacilli with rounded ends and characteristic polar granules ("safety pin" appearance) within mononuclear cells is typical of this infection. It has been thought that *Calymmatobacterium granulomatis* is the etiologic agent of granuloma inguinale, but this causal relationship remains to be established firmly, as the organism has never been isolated regularly from patients with this syndrome. All of these diseases must be differentiated from syphilis by the appropriate serologic tests for syphilis.

Genital infections with *Trichomonas vaginalis* are often symptomatic in women but asymptomatic in men. Vaginal discharge or urethral or prostatic secretions can be examined directly by microscopy after mixing the body fluid in normal saline. Culture techniques are also available.

Infection with the genital herpes simplex virus characteristically produces painful genital ulcerations. The virus can be demonstrated by culture of fluid from the ulcers and can be demonstrated by direct immunoassays. As with all genital ulcerations, appropriate serologic tests for syphilis must be performed.

Besides *Neisseria* and *Trichomonas*, four other microorganisms may be associated with sexually transmitted diseases (STDs) and cause urethritis, vaginitis, or cervicitis. *Candida albicans* can be identified either by culture or by microscopic examination of the discharge fluid. *Gardnerella vaginalis* may be associated with bacterial vaginosis, although no causal link has been established. Its presence can be inferred by cytologic preparations showing the presence of "clue cells." *C trachomatis* is a common cause of nongonococcal urethritis and cervicitis. *Chlamydia* can be detected in cervical or male urethral smears containing epithelial cells with appropriate paranuclear cytoplasmic inclusions. A fluorescent monoclonal antibody preparation is available that will detect the presence of *C trachomatis* antigen. *Mycoplasma hominis* and *Ureaplasma urealyticum* may also be associated with these STDs. They require special culture procedures for recovery. Several species of small, curved, gram-negative anaerobic organisms (*Mobiluncus* species) have also been found in association with bacterial vaginosis. No etiologic role for those anaerobes has been established. The absence of normal vaginal flora (particularly *Lactobacillus* species) on stained smears of vaginal specimens is also an indicator of bacterial vaginosis.

Exudates, Tissues, and Wounds

Pus from undrained abscesses and from pericardial, pleural, peritoneal, and synovial fluids is best obtained by closed needle aspiration through disinfected skin. Direct smears and cultures should be made. If anaerobic infection is suspected, the aspirated material must be submitted in either a stoppered syringe or a gassed-out sterile tube. Swabs should not be used to obtain pus or fluid for microbiological study. These same rules apply to pus obtained after surgical incision and drainage of an abscess. Proper material from deep communicating suppurations is difficult to obtain, because the communicating pathway usually contains a microbial flora of its own. Attempts to disinfect the communication may be successful, but cultures of curettings or biopsy specimens of the suppurative lesions that bypass these sinus tracks are superior.

Submission of tissue either from surgery or from a postmortem examination requires forethought by the person collecting the tissue. Adequate material that represents the suspected infectious process should be obtained. Swabs are rarely indicated. If fluid is obtained, the entire collection (not just a few milliliters) should be submitted.

Exudates, drainage fluid, and other material from skin, soft tissue, and superficial wounds are usually heavily contaminated with an indigenous microbial flora. This material is best submitted only if a particular pathogen is suspected. Direct examination of Gram's-stained smears is useful. The typical material submitted includes swabs of pus, closed needle aspirations from cellulitis or bullae, punch biopsy specimens of skin and subcutaneous infections, and semiquantitative cultures of burn eschars. In addition, intravenous and intra-arterial catheter tips are often submitted in cases of suspected catheter-induced bacteremia. Semiquantitative cultures of these catheter tips should be made by laboratory personnel.

Skin

Tuberculin skin tests are useful in identifying patients with tuberculous infections, both active and dormant. Tuberculin (or purified protein derivative) is a protein fraction of *Mycobacterium tuberculosis*. When administered intradermally, it triggers the release of several lymphokines, which in turn cause progressive edema and accumulation of sensitized lymphocytes, leading to a localized thickening of the skin noted after 24 to 72 hours. Intermediate-strength tuberculin, containing 5 tuberculin units of purified protein derivative, produces a positive reaction in the majority of persons infected with *M tuberculosis*. False-negative results occur in 15% to 20% of persons tested. These individuals usually have nonfunctional sensitized T lymphocytes due to chronic illness, a large effusion, or immunosuppression caused by underlying disease/therapeutic agents. Positive tuberculin skin tests indicate the presence of tuberculous infection, but they do not distinguish between active and dormant infections. This distinction must be made by clinical, roentgenographic, and other means. When applying tuberculin skin tests it is always appropriate to apply other skin test antigens as "controls." These include antigens made from mumps virus, *Candida* species, *Trichophyton* species, or others. Most adults have had exposures to these antigens and will react to them unless they have skin-test anergy due to one or more of the conditions mentioned previously.

The best laboratory evidence for active tuberculosis is positive culture of clinical material such as sputum, gastric aspirates, urine, CSF, serous effusion, tissue biopsy specimens, and pus from abscess or sinuses. Most clinical material is examined first by acid-fast stains, which are not as sensitive as cultural isolation and identification of the microorganism. Multiple cultures are often necessary to recover the microorganism, especially in patients with early tuberculous infections, tuberculous pleural effusions, small and/or noncavitary pulmonary lesions, and old or chronic tuberculous lesions. Because of the presence of acid-fast indigenous nonpathogens, gastric aspirates, urine, and urethral specimens are not satisfactory for routine acid-fast stains.

Interpretation

Direct microscopic examination of body fluids, exudates, and tissues can be very useful. Characteristic microorganisms may be identified by examining wet mounts or using stains of dried smears.

Wet Mounts

Darkfield Microscopy. Darkfield microscopy is a technique for identification of *Treponema pallidum* in superficial lesions of primary or secondary (rarely latent) syphilis. Lesions must first have any superficial crusts removed. The surface of the lesion is abraded until bleeding occurs. Excess blood is removed until serous exudate appears. Additional exudate is expressed by pressure on the base of the lesion. A coverslip is touched to the exudate and placed on a microscope slide. The slide must be kept moist en route to the laboratory, which is done by putting it into a petri dish along with a moist gauze sponge. The slide is examined with a darkfield microscope at medium (eg, 450x) magnification for the characteristic "corkscrew" motility of pathogenic treponemes. Avoid use of detergents or surface antiseptics, because they may inactivate spirochetes.

Potassium Hydroxide Preparation. Potassium hydroxide (KOH) preparation is used to diagnose superficial mycoses. Specimens are placed on a slide in a drop of 10% KOH. A coverslip is applied and the preparation is cleared by gentle heating. The preparation is examined under low (40x to 100x) magnification for the presence of hyphae and spores.

India Ink Preparation. India ink preparation is used to identify microorganisms with large, prominent capsules (eg, *Cryptococcus*) in CSF.

Stool or Duodenal Drainage. Wet mounts of stool or duodenal drainage using saline or iodine-stained mounts are useful in the diagnosis of intestinal protozoal and helminthic infections.

Motility. Wet mounts for motility are useful in identifying characteristically motile microorganisms. Wet mounts of blood may be examined for the presence of microfilaria or trypanosomes, and wet mounts of vaginal exudate may reveal the presence of *Trichomonas vaginalis*. Similar preparations of liquid stool samples may assist in diagnosis of enterocolitis due to *Campylobacter* or *Vibrio* species.

Stained Smears

Gram's. Gram's stain is the best stain for the rapid diagnosis of bacterial infections. It may be used with exudates, normally sterile body fluids, tissue and biopsy specimens, purulent eye drainage, transtracheal aspirates, urethral discharge from males, and uncentrifuged urine samples. Gram's-stained smears of older surgical and traumatic wounds are useful for presumptively anaerobic infections if characteristic organisms are present. Sputum smears are probably better than cultures in the diagnosis of pneumococcal pneumonia. Examples of the use of Gram's-stained smears include Vincent's angina, diphtheria, gas gangrene, staphylococcal abscesses, gonococcal urethritis, bacterial meningitis, urinary tract infection, chancroid, and inflammatory or necrotizing enterocolitis.

Methylene Blue. Methylene blue stain is a useful adjunct to Gram's stain in examining specimens for bacterial infection. It preserves bacterial morphology better than Gram's stain. It is not, however, a substitute for Gram's stain.

Giemsa, Wright's, and Iodine. Giemsa, Wright's, and iodine stains may be useful for chlamydial infections of the eye, urethra, and cervix. Iodine stains are used to identify intestinal parasites. Giemsa and Wright's stains are used for granuloma inguinale, cytomegalovirus in urine, poxviruses and herpes viruses from vesicular fluid, parasites of the blood and respiratory tract, amebic meningoencephalitis, and *Borrelia* species that cause relapsing fever. Giemsa stain is useful in recognizing *Pneumocystis carinii* in bronchial washings or bronchoalveolar lavage specimens.

Acid-Fast. Acid-fast stains are useful in identifying mycobacteria and related organisms. These include Kinyoun, Ziehl-Neelsen, and fluorochrome stains (eg, auramine and auramine-rhodamine). Approximately 10,000 mycobacteria per milliliter are necessary to be identified in acid-fast–stained smears. Smears are likely to be positive, therefore, only in patients who are expelling large numbers of mycobacteria.

Sputum is the most common specimen used for acid-fast–stained smears. It may be spontaneously produced, or induced. For some patients (eg, children, debilitated persons) sputum production may be impossible. Gastric aspirates, therefore, are obtained just after these patients awaken in the morning. Unlike sputum, gastric aspirates may contain saprophytic mycobacteria that may be confused with *M tuberculosis* in an acid-fast–stained smear. Hence, culture is the preferred usage of gastric aspirates for tuberculosis. The same is true of urine, which may contain nonpathogenic mycobacteria.

The intestinal coccidian parasites, *Cryptosporidium* species and *Isospora belli*, which cause gastrointestinal symptoms (particularly severe in immunocompromised persons), can also be stained by acid-fast methods.

A modified acid-fast stain occasionally may be used to identify *Nocardia* in smears of clinical material. This modified stain uses mineral acid instead of acid-alcohol as the decolorizing agent.

Acridine Orange. Acridine orange stain is used to identify bacteria in specimens with low numbers of organisms (10,000 colony-forming units per milliliter is the lower limit of detection for this stain, while approximately 100,000 colony-forming units per milliliter is the lower limit of detection by Gram's stain). Fluorescence microscopy is necessary. Such specimens as blood cultures, urine, or CSF may be examined. Bacteria fluoresce a bright orange color, while leukocytes appear pale green. A positive acridine orange–stained smear can be confirmed by staining the same slide with Gram's stain and reexamining it.

Modified Methylene Blue. Modified methylene blue stain utilizes methylene blue and basic fuchsin. It is of value in identifying pathogens in tissues of immunocompromised individuals. The stain will reveal the presence of bacteria, yeasts, fungal hyphae, *Pneumocystis carinii*, viral inclusions, and other pathogens. An example of its use would be to make a "touch-prep" of fresh lung tissue at the time of open biopsy. Hasten the air drying of the slide by waving it around several times. It is also useful for detecting *Cryptosporidium* in fecal specimens.

Other Methods

Immune Microscopy. Immune microscopy uses specific antibody preparations labeled with fluorescent dyes and examined by fluorescence microscopy. Rapid diagnosis can be made for rabies, herpetic encephalitis, Legionnaires' disease, chlamydial infections, pertussis, and viral respiratory tract infections.

Electron Microscopy. Electron microscopy has limited but valuable usefulness in clinical microbiology. It is usually reserved for diagnosis of viral infections such as rotavirus gastroenteritis, smallpox, and viral hepatitis.

Detection of Microbial Antigens. Detection of microbial antigens by latex particle agglutination is useful to identify bacterial antigens in body fluids such as *Cryptococcus neoformans* antigen in CSF, serum, and urine, and causative microorganisms of meningitis in CSF, ie, *S pneumoniae*, *N meningitidis*, group B streptococci, and *H influenzae*. Enzyme-linked immunosorbent assay (ELISA) and coagglutination methods can also be used for antigen detection and identification.

Immunologic techniques may be used to identify viral and fungal antigens because they allow rapid diagnosis of serious diseases whose causative agents are not easily or rapidly cultured.

Antimicrobial Susceptibility Testing

An important function of the clinical microbiology laboratory is to determine in vitro if a patient's pathogenic microorganisms are susceptible to antimicrobial agents and to establish adequate dosage of these agents. Microorganisms tested in this way generally include rapidly growing bacteria, which contribute to an infectious process but whose susceptibility cannot be predicted solely on the basis of their identity. These bacteria include species of *Staphylococcus*, facultative gram-negative fermentative and nonfermentative bacilli, certain anaerobic bacteria, and, occasionally, unusual pathogens. The latter group would commonly be involved in infections in immunocompromised hosts. Other species (eg, *Haemophilus* species, *S pneumoniae*, *N gonorrhoeae*, *Enterococcus* species, *M catarrhalis*) should be tested in a more limited fashion, such as by screening for ß-lactamase production, other forms of penicillin resistance, or high-level aminoglycoside resistance.

Routine susceptibility tests are not indicated for pathogens whose history of response to various agents has been predictable (eg, *S pyogenes*, *N meningitidis*). The testing of *M tuberculosis* is indicated to "first line" antituberculous agents, and in the case of resistance to any of those, to "second line" drugs. The latter is generally performed in a reference laboratory. Routine testing of yeasts and other fungi is not currently recommended; there are no well-standardized tests available, and test-to-test variability is such that results cannot always be trusted. If testing of fungi seems clinically warranted, the tests should be done in a laboratory that specializes in antifungal susceptibility tests. Very few laboratories are prepared to do susceptibility tests on such organisms as *Chlamydia* species, *Mycoplasma* species, or viruses. At present, such testing should be done only in highly selected, problematic cases.

Factors involved in the selection of antimicrobial agents for therapeutic purposes include considerations of the in vitro susceptibility of the infecting organism(s), pharmacological properties of the antimicrobial agents, the nature of the underlying pathological process, the immunologic status of the host, and prior clinical experiences in the treatment of infections by the same species. Only the susceptibility in vitro is subject to direct testing. However, one must recognize that this is only one factor to be considered, and that the actual tests are done in a setting outside the host.

In recent years most laboratories in the United States and Canada, and increasingly in other parts of the developed world, have come to rely on the recommendations of the National Committee for Clinical Laboratory Standards (NCCLS) for performance of antimicrobial susceptibility tests. This organization has a variety of committees composed of experts in the field, who supervise such testing, and who propose methods for performing, controlling, reporting, and interpreting these tests. These recommendations are published and revised regularly. It is currently the practice for most clinical laboratory inspecting and accrediting agencies to expect that antimicrobial susceptibility testing be done in accordance with NCCLS recommendations.

The testing of rapidly growing bacteria for susceptibility to antimicrobial agents can be done by a variety of documented, standardized methods. These include agar (disk) diffusion (also known as the Bauer-Kirby test), agar dilution (the incorporation of concentrations of antimicrobials in agar), broth microdilution (the incorporation of various concentrations of antimicrobials in broth in plates usually containing 96 wells), broth macrodilution (the incorporation of various concentrations of antimicrobials in small test tubes), or by several commercially available automated or mechanized systems. Some of the latter are versions of broth microdilution tests, while others are unique and based on different formats. Whichever test method is used in a laboratory, it must be done in a standardized fashion, controlled by testing specific strains of bacteria with known susceptibility patterns, and reported in a standardized format accompanied by interpretive guidelines. All of these features are prescribed in various documents published by the NCCLS.

References

Bartlett RC. Cost and usefulness of clinical microbiology services. *Eur J Clin Microbiol.* 1985;4:375-378.

Detection of microbial pathogens in the blood stream. Proceedings of a symposium held in Phoenix, Arizona, November 19-20, 1987. *Lab Med.* September 1988;(suppl):1-38.

Illstrup DM, Washington JA II. The importance of volume of blood cultured in the detection of bacteremia and fungemia. *Diagn Microbiol Infect Dis.* 1983;1:107-110.

Neu HC. Cost effective blood cultures—is it possible or impossible to modify behavior? *Infect Control.* 1986;7:32-33.

Roberts FJ, Geere IW, Coldman A. A three-year study of positive blood cultures, with emphasis on prognosis. *Rev Infect Dis.* 1991;13:34-46.

Weinstein MP, Reller LB, Murphy JR, Lichtenstein KA. The clinical significance of positive blood cultures: a comprehensive analysis of 500 episodes of bacteremia and fungemia in adults. I. Laboratory and epidemiologic observations. *Rev Infect Dis.* 1983;5:35-53.

Young DW. Improving laboratory usage: a review. *Postgrad Med J.* 1988;64:283-289.

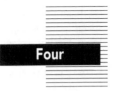
Four

Infectious Disease: Immunologic Tests

Key Points

1. In suspected poststreptococcal disease, the antistreptolysin O (ASO) antibody test most sensitively detects prior pharyngeal disease, while the deoxyribonuclease B (DNase B) test is most sensitive for prior skin infections.
2. Diagnosis of Lyme disease in nonendemic areas or in endemic areas when erythema chronicum migrans is not present usually requires detecting an antibody to *Borrelia burgdorferi*. However, this test has limited sensitivity and specificity.
3. In suspected whooping cough, a direct fluorescence test on nasopharyngeal smears is sensitive and specific for detecting *Bordetella pertussis*.
4. In suspected cryptococcal meningitis, an antigen detection test on cerebrospinal fluid (CSF) is a sensitive, rapid test for diagnosis.
5. In amebic liver abscesses, serum antibodies to *Entamoeba histolytica* can be detected in 85% to 90% of cases.
6. The best laboratory test to help confirm toxoplasmosis is a serum antibody test; nearly all patients with toxoplasmosis, including acquired immunodeficiency syndrome (AIDS) patients with toxoplasma encephalitis, will have significant titers.
7. In infectious mononucleosis, specific heterophile antibodies are detected in 90% of typical cases; specific antibody tests for Epstein-Barr virus should be ordered to confirm possible heterophile-negative cases, but other agents should also be considered.
8. In suspected human immunodeficiency virus (HIV) infection, a screening enzyme-linked immunosorbent assay (ELISA) test must be followed by a confirmatory Western blot. Remember, a "window period" exists when an HIV-infected (and infectious) patient tests negative for HIV antibodies.

Background

Antibody detection tests for the diagnosis of infectious disease usually require a pair of serum specimens (conventionally labeled "acute" and "convalescent") to establish a diagnosis. A fourfold increase in antibody titer rather than a single specific titer is diagnostic. A single specimen may be useful in cases of chronic or long-standing infection or when a certain antibody titer is known to represent the average in a population with no recent exposure to the infectious agent. Cross-reactions occur and can cause confusion in test result interpretation. Culture is usually the best way to identify an etiologic infectious agent. Sometimes, however, the diagnosis of an infection cannot be made except by detecting the antibody as, for example, when microorganisms are present in an inaccessible body site (amebic liver abscess) or when there is great difficulty culturing the microorganism (rickettsia).

The use of antibodies of known specificity to identify intact infectious agents and/or their antigens is extremely useful for rapid diagnosis. Examples include the detection of hepatitis B antigen in serum (see Chapter 17) and identification of polysaccharide microorganism antigens in CSF of patients with meningitis.

Nonviral Diseases and Tests Used to Diagnose Them

Postinfectious Complications of Streptococcal Infections

Extracellular enzymes produced by *Streptococcus pyogenes* (group A) are used as antigens in serologic tests because antibodies to these enzymes appear in the circulation following group A streptococcal infections. These antibodies provide no protection against recurrent streptococcal infection, however. The antibodies most commonly tested for are ASO and anti–DNase B. Streptozyme, a commercial antigen preparation, is sometimes used to measure antibodies against five different streptococcal enzymes.

Detection of serum antibodies to streptococcal extracellular products is confirmation of recent streptococcal infection in patients suspected of having either acute rheumatic fever or acute glomerulonephritis. These tests are of no value, however, in the diagnosis of acute streptococcal infections, which should be diagnosed by directly identifying the streptococcus in clinical material either by culture or using a rapid antigen detection test.

Antistreptolysin O. Instead of the usual twofold serial tube dilution method of units (1:2, 1:4, etc), a more closely spaced dilutional scheme in Todd units (TU) is traditionally used to report ASO results. Normal values for ASO titers vary with the age group tested. Children less than 1 year old usually have titers of 50 TU or less. Preschool children from 1 to 4 years old and normal adults almost always have titers less than 125 TU. In contrast, in school-age children the upper limit of normal is 166 TU.

Ideally, the titers from acute and convalescent serum specimens, obtained 14 to 21 days apart, should be compared. A rise in titer of at least two dilution tubes (eg, 125-333 TU) is evidence of recent streptococcal infection, regardless of the absolute titer levels or the age of the patient. Less information is obtained if a single ASO titer is compared with normal control values. A single low ASO titer (≤50 TU) is more reliable in ruling out a recent streptococcal infection than a single elevated titer is in implicating one. Most patients with uncomplicated streptococcal pharyngitis have ASO titers above 125 TU. If rheumatic fever or glomerulonephritis is present, the ASO titer is generally over 250 TU. Approximately 65% of patients with streptococcal pyoderma (with or without glomerulonephritis) fail to develop streptolysin O antibodies. Thus, to diagnose poststreptococcal glomerulonephritis following a streptococcal pyoderma, anti-DNase B is the test of choice.

Anti-DNase B. A dilutional scheme similar to that used for the ASO is the usual reporting method. Normal individuals may have up to 250 units. Elevated titers are found in 91% of patients with streptococcal pyoderma and in 54% of patients with streptococcal pharyngitis.

Streptozyme. This is a commercial preparation of sheep erythrocytes sensitized with multiple streptococcal products. The test has greater sensitivity than any single antibody determination (91%). However, its specificity is much less (there is a 25% false-positive rate), which limits its utility.

Lyme Disease

In areas of the country where Lyme disease is endemic, the diagnosis is readily made in a patient who has the classic lesions of erythema chronicum migrans. When the presentation is not classic or in any case outside an endemic area, laboratory confirmation is required, usually the identification of a serum antibody to the causative agent, *B burgdorferi*. Unfortunately, the antibody detection tests that are currently available have relatively low sensitivity and specificity. Early in the disease IgM antibodies develop, but they may be undetectable in up to 50% of patients. Later in the disease, IgG antibodies can be consistently detected.

Unfortunately, the detection of antibodies does not necessarily indicate Lyme disease because (1) false positives are frequent in patients with antibodies to other agents, including the agents of syphilis and relapsing fever, and (2) 10% of asymptomatic individuals in endemic Lyme disease areas have *B burgdorferi* antibodies indicating that patients with joint, cardiac, or central nervous system symptoms suggestive of Lyme disease may simply have preexisting coincidental *B burgdorferi* antibodies. Other methods to diagnose Lyme disease, such as culture or direct detection of antigen in tissue including the use of the polymerase chain reaction, are either insensitive or not currently widely available.

Brucellosis and Tularemia

Brucellosis and tularemia are uncommon in the United States. Serologic tests are important in the diagnosis of these organisms because they are difficult to culture. Less than 50% of patients with brucellosis have positive blood cultures, and *Francisella tularensis* can only rarely be isolated from clinical material. Furthermore, because these infections are often confused with other febrile illnesses, prompt diagnosis and therapy may be delayed. *Brucella* antibody responses occur after infections with *Brucella abortus*, *Brucella suis*, or *Brucella melitensis*. *Brucella canis* infections require a different specific agglutination test antigen. Most uninfected individuals have titers of less than 1:160, and titers 1:160 or greater occur in about 95% of patients with brucellosis. Normal individuals usually have *F tularensis* antibody titers of less than 1:40. Even after successful therapy, elevated antibody titers may persist for life following infection with either brucellosis or tularemia. Antibodies to these two infectious agents cross-react, so both tests should be ordered if the clinical presentation suggests either infection is possible.

Bordetella pertussis

A rapid diagnosis (within 4 hours) of whooping cough can be made using direct immunofluorescence technique after obtaining exudate via nasopharyngeal swab. The exudate is spread on a slide and submitted to the laboratory, where it is stained using a fluorescein-conjugated antibody specific for the organism. In the first week of illness, this test is 60% to 90% sensitive and 90% specific. False positives may occur in a small number of cases. Cultures are even more sensitive, but growth and identification of the organism will take at least 3 days. The direct fluorescence test does not become negative until several days after the cultures become negative because the antibody detects nonviable as well as viable organisms.

Antigen Detection in Bacterial Meningitis

These tests utilize specific antibodies to capsular polysaccharide antigens of the infecting organisms. The tests should not be used in place of direct Gram's stain of spinal fluid and culture. However, they can identify the causative organism more rapidly than culture. Antigen detection tests may be particularly helpful when patients have received partial treatment before the diagnosis of meningitis has been entertained, because CSF cultures may be negative at this time. Antigen detection tests commonly available to test CSF include *Haemophilus influenzae*, type b; *Neisseria meningitidis*, groups A, B, C, Y, and W135; *Escherichia coli* K-1 antigen; and *Streptococcus pneumoniae* and *Streptococcus*, group B. Sensitivity for detection of these organisms in spinal fluid varies from 50% to 95%. Thus, negative tests should never be used to rule out the presence of bacterial meningitis.

In group B streptococcal septicemia, the capsular polysaccharide is concentrated in the urine. Therefore, in this systemic infection urine is the preferred specimen. Diagnosis of *H influenzae* pneumonia or cellulitis may also be facilitated by the identification of the relevant antigens in blood or urine, or both.

Fungal Infections

Fungi often grow slowly in culture (about 3 weeks). Therefore, rapid diagnosis routinely depends on direct detection of the organisms in tissue and body fluids, utilizing special stains and microscopy. In addition, antibody detection is used as an ancillary technique in the diagnosis of histoplasmosis, blastomycosis, coccidioidomycosis, and aspergillosis. Antibodies may be detected by immunodiffusion, complement fixation, or enzyme immunoassay. High titers usually indicate active disease, while low titers may indicate either active disease or old, quiescent disease. For *Coccidioides* infections a latex agglutination test to detect antibody is helpful for early active disease. In nonendemic areas, these tests are often sent to reference laboratories and interpretations are provided with reports. In patients with a previous remote exposure to histoplasmosis, skin testing increases already present antibody titers; therefore skin testing should not be performed on patients with suspected acute histoplasmosis.

The direct latex agglutination test for the detection of cryptococcal antigens in spinal fluid is extremely valuable because it is more sensitive than the india ink test designed to directly visualize the organisms in CSF and should be ordered in all cases of cryptococcal meningitis. The cryptococcal antigen test is both sensitive and specific, ie, nearly all culture-proven cases are positive, and nearly all true-negative patients are negative. In patients who are being adequately treated, the cultures will become negative before the antigen detection tests become negative. Falling titers indicate a response to treatment.

Parasitic Infections

Toxoplasma gondii. The etiologic agent of toxoplasmosis is neither readily cultured nor easily identified in tissue. Detection of antibody is the best way to confirm a clinical suspicion of the disease. The common method is an indirect immunofluorescence test that detects either IgM or IgG antibodies. Low titers may indicate either very early infection or past infection. However, high titers do not always indicate acute infection. Detection of IgM antibodies, because they form earlier in disease, is a more specific way to diagnose acute toxoplasmosis and is best performed using an ELISA. The IgM test should be ordered if the initial antibody titer is high in suspected cases of primary toxoplasmosis. *Toxoplasma* encephalitis is a relatively common entity in patients with AIDS and indicates reactivation infection; IgM antibodies are generally not elevated. Indeed, IgG antibodies may fail to increase although a titer of at least 1:64 nearly always exists in AIDS patients with *Toxoplasma* encephalitis.

Entamoeba histolytica. This is a common infecting agent in the Mexican-American population in the Southwestern United States. Most patients (>85%) with invasive amebiasis, including both dysentery and amebic liver abscess, have elevated antibody titers to the organism. Trophozoite and cyst detection in stools is the preferred way to diagnose dysentery. However, antibody detection is very helpful in confirming the clinical impression of amebic liver abscess because these patients frequently do not have amebae in their stools. Fever, a tender liver with an abscess by sonography, and a positive *E histolytica* antibody test (a titer of ≥1:128) in an individual from an endemic area are virtually diagnostic of an amebic liver abscess.

Other parasitic diseases that might be suspected in the United States for which antibody detection tests are generally available in reference laboratories are amebic meningoencephalitis, leishmaniasis, trichinellosis, Chagas disease, paragonimiasis, trypanosomiasis, cysticercosis, schistosomiasis, echinococcosis, and toxocariasis.

Rickettsial Infections

The most common rickettsial disease in the United States is Rocky Mountain spotted fever (RMSF), but murine (or endemic) typhus, Q fever, and rickettsial pox also occur. The organisms are not readily cultured. Latex agglutination tests for RMSF and endemic typhus are available. Antibodies are detectable 4 to 9 days after the onset of illness. A titer of ≥1:128 is diagnostic. A lower titer is suspicious and should be followed by repeated testing 7 to 10 days later. There may be some low level cross-reactivity of antibodies to other rickettsial diseases in these tests, but if Q fever or rickettsial pox are suspected, antibody tests for these diseases should be specifically requested.

Viral Diseases and Tests Used to Diagnose Them

Serologic tests for viral diseases should be performed in conjunction with attempts at virus isolation, and then the results should be evaluated using clinical and epidemiological information. Acute and convalescent sera showing a fourfold rise in antibody titer is diagnostic. In some cases a single elevated titer is helpful. For several viral diseases, eg, arbovirus infections, rubella, infectious mononucleosis, and hepatitis, culture is difficult or impossible and antibody detection is essential. Direct identification of the viral antigen in tissues or body fluids by immunologic techniques is available for hepatitis B, cytomegalovirus (CMV), herpes simplex, influenza A, and respiratory syncytial virus.

When ordering serologic tests, the suspected viral agent should be noted. For example, if an adult has a respiratory syndrome, antibodies to influenza A and B, adenovirus, and mycoplasma should be ordered. For congenital infections, the most common viral agents are herpes simplex, CMV, and rubella (other congenital infections include *Toxoplasma* and syphilis). Depending on the clinical syndrome and evidence of disease and/or positive antibody tests in the mother, the appropriate serologic tests should be ordered. A single serum sample is sufficient to order antibodies to all five of these common congenital infectious agents. If herpes or CMV is suspected, material for culture should be obtained as well.

Infectious Mononucleosis

In patients with the appropriate clinical syndrome and atypical lymphocytosis, the diagnosis of infectious mononucleosis can be confirmed with serum tests for either infectious mononucleosis–specific heterophile antibodies or with tests for Epstein-Barr virus (EBV) antibodies. A heterophile antibody is one that reacts with antigens common to tissues from different species. Heterophile antibodies specific for infectious mononucleosis are usually measured by rapid screening tests (such as the Monospot) that incorporate appropriate absorptions to help assure specificity. Nevertheless, false-positive screening tests occur in a small percentage of patients. If a patient has a positive heterophile antibody test but the clinical presentation fails to support the diagnosis of infectious mononucleosis, an EBV antibody detection test should be ordered to rule out the specific infection.

Infectious mononucleosis–specific heterophile antibodies develop in about 90% of young adults with symptoms and signs associated with the disease. The antibody appears after the first week or two of illness. Thus, a negative test should be repeated in 7 to 10 days if the clinical suspicion of infectious mononucleosis is high. The antibody usually disappears by 6 months. Fewer than 30% of children less than 2 years of age who develop EBV infection have specific heterophile antibodies. The percentage of children with EBV infections who develop positive screening tests increases with age; positive screening tests are more likely to occur in young children with more typical manifestations of infectious mononucleosis.

In heterophile-negative infectious mononucleosis, antibodies specific for EBV should be determined. There are at least eight antigen systems for detecting EBV antibody. Detection of antibody to viral capsid antigen (anti-VCA) is particularly useful. Anti-VCA appears at the end of the first week of the disease and eventually appears in 100% of infected patients. IgG anti-VCA persists for life, and low titers may indicate a prior rather than a current infection. IgM anti-VCA appears shortly before IgG anti-VCA and falls rapidly in early convalescence. Additional diagnostically useful antibodies are to early antigens (EA) and to EBV-associated nuclear antigens (EBNA). The presence in serum of anti-EA roughly parallels IgM anti-VCA; anti-EBNA rises during early convalescence and persists. An antibody pattern of positive IgG and IgM anti-VCA and anti-EA with negative anti-EBNA indicates early infection. Negative IgM anti-VCA and anti-EA, and positive IgG anti-VCA and anti-EBNA indicate past infection.

HIV Infections

The diagnosis of HIV infection should be made only by correlating clinical information with serologic findings. Nearly all patients with this infection to date have a history of high-risk exposure to HIV-infected persons, either through sexual or parenteral routes. Sole reliance on laboratory results may result in overdiagnosis or underdiagnosis of infection.

Two variants of HIV have been identified to date. HIV-1 is the virus prevalent in the United States, and most available tests identify exposure to this virus. HIV-2 is a related but distinct virus confined largely to infected persons in parts of sub-Saharan Africa and surrounding islands and parts of Europe. Both viruses are thought to be transmitted via similar routes and both can cause AIDS.

Many of the available tests for HIV rely on detection of antibody to the virus—a marker of infection produced by the body's immune system. After the acute episode of infection, a period of time elapses before antibody to the virus is made in sufficient quantity to be detected by a laboratory test. This "window period" lasts from 1 to 4 months in most infected people, but may be as brief as 2 weeks or as long as 3 years in rare cases. During this period, antibody cannot be detected but HIV viral antigen is present. Generally, as antibody levels increase, antigen levels decrease. The antibody will then persist throughout the course of the infection. It may disappear late in the disease, in the terminal stages of AIDS, as the patient's immune system no longer can generate adequate levels of immunoglobulin. HIV antigen may at this time be detected in increasing amounts in the serum. All persons with confirmed HIV antibody should be considered infectious because antibody to HIV does not signify the patient is noninfectious.

A diagnosis of AIDS or AIDS-related complex must be based on clinical findings. A diagnosis of AIDS may be rendered only when selected "indicator" diseases such as certain opportunistic infections or AIDS-related neoplasms occur in persons at risk for or with documentation of HIV infection.

Antibody to HIV-1. This test, available commercially in the United States since 1985, is the most commonly used screening test for patients at risk for HIV infection. The results are reported as "nonreactive" or "reactive." The test is performed by ELISA and takes 2 to 4 hours to complete. Most laboratories use a commercially prepared test kit that has viral antigen bound to a solid surface (plate well or bead) to which antibodies in the patient's serum bind. After a wash step, enzyme-linked antibody to human immunoglobulin (usually IgG) is added. A chromogenic substrate is added, on which the enzyme acts to produce a color change. The more HIV antibody bound to the antigen, the stronger the color change produced. The results are determined spectrophotometrically and compared with known controls. A cutoff value for each batch of tests is calculated depending on the readings of the controls. All specimens with optical density readings greater than the cutoff for that batch are called "reactive." The test is run once, and if a particular specimen is reactive the test should be repeated. To be reported as a reactive result, the sample should have been reactive at least two times (repeatably reactive).

Overall, the specificity and sensitivity of currently available tests are very high (>99%). However, false-positive results do occasionally occur, especially in young women in low-risk populations. Generally, an antibody in the serum of these patients will cross-react with one of the HIV antigens or one of the non–HIV-specific antigens in the in vitro culture system used to produce the viral antigen. False-positive results may also occur because of nonspecific immunoglobulin adherence in the test system.

Many of the current tests utilize a "whole virus lysate" as the source of antigen. This means that the HIV virus is grown in cell culture and a preparation of the whole virus is used when coating the beads or plates; thus, all viral antigens are available for detection of antibody. On the other hand, some manufacturers utilize recombinant HIV antigens. They have chosen one or a few individual HIV antigens and used recombinant viral material to coat their plates or beads. These tests may theoretically not detect all antibodies to HIV-associated antigens, but should be more specific and result in fewer false positives.

False-negative results may occur if the patient is tested too early in the course of infection, eg, before the patient has developed a sufficient quantity of antibody to the virus to be recognized by testing. False-negative results may also occur very late in disease, when production of all immunoglobulins is poor. Patients who have been massively transfused or have undergone plasma exchange may also have antibodies to HIV below detectable limits because of dilutional effects.

Because of the importance, both psychological and medical, often placed on the results of this test, a repeated test on a second sample of blood might be considered for all reactive results and any suspicious negative results. Samples occasionally get mislabeled, and technical errors in the laboratory do occur, although rarely.

All reactive results should be confirmed by a second, more specific method to eliminate any false-positive results. Most commonly, a Western immunoblot preparation (Western blot) is used for such confirmation, but other methods such as indirect immunofluorescence and radioimmunoprecipitation assay are also available in reference laboratories. Many laboratories will not report an HIV antibody test result until the confirmation study is completed.

The screening HIV-1 antibody tests currently available will also detect the presence of antibodies to HIV-2 in 30% to 90% of HIV-2–infected persons. However, if HIV-2 infection is suspected, a specific test for HIV-2 antibodies should be utilized.

Most HIV-1 antibody tests were designed for use with serum or plasma samples. Care should be taken in the interpretation of results if other body fluids (eg, CSF or urine) are tested with these assays. Appropriate positive and negative controls must be available. Some reference laboratories may offer testing of non-blood specimens. Postmortem blood may be tested by some ELISA tests, but the presence of significant hemolysis may interfere with the interpretation of the results.

Rapid HIV Antibody Tests. Recently, rapid methods of HIV antibody diagnosis have become available. These methods utilize latex agglutination or "dot immunobinding" techniques, requiring only minutes for completion. These tests are often used in nonlaboratory settings. Because nontechnical personnel may be performing these tests in emergent settings, without the benefit of quality control or quality assurance guidelines, and because these tests provide preliminary results not yet confirmed by a second method, the information gathered should be used with caution; no major therapeutic decisions should be based on their outcome. In addition, sensitivity and specificity may be lower with these methods.

Western Immunoblot. This test confirms the presence of HIV antibody in samples previously found reactive by screening tests. Western blots for both HIV-1 and HIV-2 are available. The Western blot is expensive and time-consuming and should not be used as a screening tool. HIV viral antigens are separated in an electrophoretic field on a polyacrylamide gel by size, then transferred from the electrophoretic gel to nitrocellulose paper strips. These strips are then incubated with patient's serum, and an enzyme-linked antibody to viral antigens is added, followed by a chromogenic substrate. The presence of antibody to specific viral antigens is demonstrated by the presence of stained bands at characteristic molecular weights.

The classic pattern of reactivity seen in full-blown HIV-1 infection shows nine bands of staining. Three bands represent antibody to the core protein molecules (*gag*): p17, p24, and p55. Three bands reflect antibodies to the envelope glycoproteins (*env*): gp41, gp120, and gp160. The final three bands are antibodies to the polymerase proteins (*pol*): p31, p51, and p66. The numbers refer to the molecular weight of the viral antigens in kilodaltons. Most infected persons have antibody to all of these viral antigens, and will demonstrate all the classic bands of staining on Western blotting. However, early and late in infection, certain persons may demonstrate only some of the expected bands. For example, late in disease, patients may lose antibody to the p24 antigen.

Different laboratories use slightly different interpretive criteria for evaluating HIV-1 Western blots. In many cases the variation in criteria is not significant. All laboratories will call a specimen nonreactive if no bands are present. The specimen will be called "indeterminate" if bands are present but the distribution does not meet their criteria for "reactive." Most infected persons will be reactive on Western blot by any criteria. Only those patients with incomplete patterns may be called indeterminate at one laboratory and reactive at another laboratory. The three most common sets of criteria to declare a specimen reactive for HIV antibodies are as follows: (1) criteria from the Centers for Disease Control and the Association of State, Territorial, and Public Health Laboratory Directors will call a blot reactive if two of the following bands are present—p24, gp41, or gp120/gp160; (2) the American Red Cross criteria considers a sample positive if one band from each of the three groups is available—one *env*, one *pol*, and one *gag* band; and (3) the Food and Drug Administration criteria allow a specimen to be called reactive if p24, p31, and either gp41 or gp120/gp160 are present. Combining the screening test result and the confirmatory test result allows a final determination of "positive," "negative," or "indeterminate."

Controversy exists as to the sensitivity and specificity of the Western blot. Most laboratories have no better method to use as a comparison. The Western blot may in rare cases detect HIV antibody in persons found negative by ELISA screening test.

A patient with a repeatably reactive ELISA and an indeterminate Western blot for HIV antibodies should have HIV testing repeated within 3 to 6 months. Progression of the Western blot pattern to include more HIV-associated bands suggests true infection. Persistence of one or two bands with no change over time suggests nonspecific reactivity.

HIV-1 Antigen. This test is performed by ELISA. However, this assay detects a specific viral antigen (p24) rather than HIV antibody. A neutralization step may be desirable to rule out nonspecific reactivity. Since p24 antigen appears within days to weeks of infection, its detection may be useful in early diagnosis, before significant levels of antibody are present. HIV antigen may disappear as antibody levels rise, or may persist along with HIV antibody. Late in disease, antigen levels often rise. Generally, this test is reported as "reactive" or "nonreactive." However, recently available commercial assays can report quantitative levels of antigen, which may be helpful in prognosis. Patients with persistent or rising levels of p24 antigen may be at risk for earlier disease progression.

HIV Infection in Infants. The serologic diagnosis of HIV infection in neonates born to HIV-seropositive mothers is difficult. Maternal HIV antibody of IgG class is passively transferred across the placenta to the fetus in such pregnancies, although only about one third of neonates are actually infected. Passively transferred anti-HIV can persist for up to 15 months; therefore, the HIV antibody tests are of little use in determining whether an infant is actually infected. The p24 antigen test may be of some diagnostic help, as may viral culture. However, negative results by these methods do not assure the absence of infection. More specialized tests such as the polymerase chain reaction and tests for IgA or IgM HIV antibody may be most rewarding, but are often not readily available.

Antibody to HIV-2. This test, similar to the test for HIV-1 antibodies, is now commercially available in the United States. It should be used for diagnosis of HIV-2 infection in persons at risk for exposure to the type 2 virus. It may be helpful in patients who demonstrate clinical evidence of AIDS with an atypical or negative serologic picture for HIV-1 and who may have had contact with persons in HIV-2 endemic areas. A combined ELISA assay that detects antibodies to both HIV-1 and HIV-2 is being developed and will be useful to screen blood donors.

Polymerase Chain Reaction. This expensive, sophisticated test using deoxyribonucleic acid (DNA) amplification techniques is available mainly in reference and research laboratories. Use of this test should be reserved for patients posing difficult diagnostic problems, such as a person suspected of HIV-1 infection, but with negative serological findings. Because of its expense and limited availability, the polymerase chain reaction assay is not well suited for mass screening. This test is very sensitive and can identify extremely small amounts of proviral DNA incorporated into host cells. It can be performed on blood or tissue, and looks for direct evidence of the virus, rather than antibody. False-positive results have been a problem in some laboratories because of the high risk of contamination of the test system.

HIV Viral Culture. This technique looks for direct evidence of HIV infection by infecting in vitro mononuclear cell lines and propagating the virus in the laboratory. Specimens of blood or tissue can be collected aseptically and grown in cell culture over a period of days to weeks. The presence of viable HIV is assessed in the culture cells and/or in the supernatant by detection of either reverse transcriptase activity or p24 antigen. This technique is not routinely available in all hospitals.

Patient Consent. Patient consent and counseling for HIV testing are important issues. Because of the unusually prominent social, psychological, financial, and legal issues surrounding HIV testing in this country, most hospitals have adopted policies defining procurement of patient consent prior to HIV testing. Some states have passed legislation regarding this issue. In addition, both pre-testing and post-testing counseling of patients are advocated by most organizations.

CD4 Cell Counts and CD4 to CD8 Ratio. Quantitating the number of cells in specific T lymphocyte subsets provides useful prognostic and therapeutic information for management of the HIV-infected patient. In addition, T-cell subset counts may help in the diagnosis of HIV infection in a patient with confusing serologic findings. Such subsets are defined by the kind of surface antigen expressed on the lymphocytes. Lymphocyte surface markers are detected by immunofluorescence staining of blood mononuclear cells and flow cytometry. The surface markers of most use in HIV infection are those for CD4 and CD8 found on T-helper (T4) and T-suppressor (T8) cells, respectively. Early in infection, the total numbers of T lymphocytes within both subsets are in the normal range. However, as the disease progresses, the total number of CD4 positive cells declines, and the ratio of CD4 cells to CD8 cells decreases. The normal range for the CD4 to CD8 ratio is about 0.9 to 3.0. Patients with advanced HIV disease usually have ratios less than 1.0. However, low ratios and even low CD4 counts are nonspecific and may be found in conditions other than HIV infection.

References

Dodd RY, Fang CT. The Western immunoblot procedure for HIV antibodies and its interpretation. *Arch Pathol Lab Med.* 1990;114:240-245.

Husson RN, Comeau AM, Hoff R. Diagnosis of human immunodeficiency virus infection in infants and children. *Pediatrics.* 1990;86:1-10.

Revision of the CDC surveillance case definition for acquired immunodeficiency syndrome. *MMWR*. 1987;36:3S-15S.

Rose NR, Friedman H, Fahey JL, eds. *Manual of Clinical Laboratory Immunology*. 3rd ed. Washington, DC: American Society for Microbiology. 1986.

Sninsky JJ, Kwok S. Detection of human immunodeficiency virus by the polymerase chain reaction. *Arch Pathol Lab Med*. 1990;114:259-262.

Update: serologic testing for antibody to human immunodeficiency virus. *MMWR*. 1988;36:833-840,845.

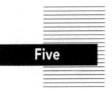
Syphilis: Serologic Tests

Key Points

1. In primary syphilis, both the commonly used nontreponemal (rapid plasma reagin [RPR] and Venereal Disease Research Laboratory [VDRL]) and treponemal (microhemagglutination assay for *Treponema pallidum* antibodies [MHA-TP]) tests may be negative; thus, careful clinical evaluation and darkfield examination are often essential.
2. The RPR and VDRL tests are extremely sensitive for secondary syphilis; both tests are nonspecific, thus they should be confirmed by a treponemal test.
3. In tertiary syphilis the nontreponemal tests are negative in 30% of cases. A treponemal test should be ordered together with an RPR or VDRL in all cases of suspected tertiary syphilis.
4. Currently, there are no good serologic tests to confirm congenital syphilis or neurosyphilis.
5. Falling titers of nontreponemal antibodies are useful in confirming successful therapy.

Background

In lesions of primary syphilis, darkfield microscopy of wet-mounted exudate specimens usually reveals motile spirochetes. Darkfield diagnosis should be used in early primary syphilis because antibody detection tests may be negative. Darkfield examination has high specificity in typical penile and vulvar lesions, but in oral or rectal mucosal lesions nonpathogenic spirochetes may be detected. In these latter lesions, clinical judgment and serologic tests must be relied on for diagnosis.

Serologic tests are the main laboratory tool for diagnosing all more advanced stages of syphilis. They are useful in monitoring treatment in all stages. Two types of antibodies may be detected. Nontreponemal antibodies are autoantibodies directed against host tissue cardiolipin antigens. These antibodies develop in other conditions as well as syphilis. Treponemal antibodies react with the treponemes specifically. Both nontreponemal and treponemal antibodies begin to appear in the serum 4 to 6 weeks from the date of infection and up to 3 weeks after the appearance of a primary chancre. Positive nontreponemal antibody tests must be confirmed with a treponemal antibody test. If the latter test is negative, the nontreponemal antibody test is regarded as a biological false positive. There is one exception: in some cases of early primary syphilis the nontreponemal antibody test may become positive before the treponemal antibody test. Darkfield examination is helpful in this situation.

Syphilis Tests

Nontreponemal Antibody Tests

Nontreponemal antibody tests are used in the diagnosis and treatment follow-up of syphilis. The VDRL and the RPR tests are the most frequently used nontreponemal antibody tests. The VDRL utilizes a cardiolipin-lecithin-cholesterol antigen and is performed as either a qualitative or a quantitative test. Qualitative test results are reported as nonreactive, weakly reactive, and reactive. Reactive specimens are diluted and the VDRL is repeated to give a quantitative result. Serum specimens that react undiluted only are reported as reactive, 1:1. The RPR is basically a modified VDRL test, but is more rapidly performed. Test results are reported as reactive or nonreactive and samples may also be quantitated by diluting samples. Unfortunately, neonatal umbilical cord blood and cerebrospinal fluid (CSF) samples cannot be tested by the RPR.

Nontreponemal antibody tests are recommended by the Centers for Disease Control (CDC) for syphilis screening; however, two problems exist. First, these tests may be nonreactive in cases of early primary syphilis and become negative in up to one third of cases of late latent and tertiary syphilis. Second, biological false positives can occur.

The incidence of biological false positives varies from 1% to 15% of all the positive VDRL tests, depending on the population tested. Usually the VDRL titer will be less than 1:8 in nonsyphilitic individuals. There are two types of biological false positives. An acute biological false positive appears and returns to nonreactive status within 6 months; this course occurs in patients with acute infections, including bacterial pneumonias and renal infections. Chronic biological false positivity persists longer than 6 months. Five conditions are associated with a relatively high incidence of chronic biological false positivity: lepromatous leprosy, drug addiction, pregnancy, collagen vascular diseases (especially systemic lupus erythematosus), and hypergammaglobulinemia. Aged individuals have an increased incidence of biological false positivity.

The quantitative titer results of nontreponemal antibody tests are helpful both in diagnosis and when following a course of treatment. A fourfold fall in titer (which should occur by 3 months) indicates adequate treatment in primary or secondary syphilis. Treatment of latent or tertiary syphilis causes a slower titer decline, and up to 40% of patients with late latent syphilis may fail to show titer decline. Furthermore, up to 50% of patients with late syphilis may still have a positive VDRL at 2 years. These individuals are called "serofast," but are considered to have been successfully treated.

Treponemal Antibody Tests

Treponemal antibody tests detect specific treponemal antibodies. Unlike nontreponemal antibodies, these antibodies nearly always persist for life, even in successfully treated patients.

Fluorescent Treponemal Antibody Absorption Test. The fluorescent treponemal antibody-absorption test (FTA-Abs) uses an indirect fluorescence method with a pathogenic treponeme as the antigen. A sorbent is used to absorb nonspecific antibodies, which are directed against nonpathogenic treponemal antigens, in the patient serum. The intensity of fluorescence compared with control slides is reported as reactive, equivocal, and nonreactive. Equivocal reports represent weak, but definite, fluorescence. In patients with equivocal serum results, a second serum sample should be evaluated.

Microhemagglutination Assay for _Treponema pallidum_ Antibodies. The MHA-TP detects antibodies that agglutinate erythrocytes sensitized with _Treponema pallidum_ antigens. This test has largely replaced the FTA-Abs because of ease of performance. An absorption step is again used to remove nonpathogenic treponemal antibodies. Results are reported as reactive, weakly reactive, or nonreactive. Inconclusive MHA-TP results may sometimes occur and these tests should be repeated on a second sample 1 to 3 weeks later.

Use. Treponemal tests should not be used as screening tests for syphilis. This recommendation is made by the CDC for several reasons. First, treponemal antibody tests are more expensive. Second, treponemal antibody tests are positive in individuals who have been successfully treated in the past. Third, and most importantly, as many as 2% of the general population may have false-positive FTA-Abs and MHA-TP test results. This is likely due to incomplete removal of antibodies to nonpathogenic treponemes during the absorption step in the test procedure. A 0.5% to 1.5% false-positive rate is unacceptably high for a widely used screening test to detect a low incidence disease if there is no follow-up confirmatory test. Treponemal antibody tests should be reserved for distinguishing between a biological false positive and syphilis and for confirming a clinical suspicion of late latent or tertiary syphilis when the nontreponemal antibody test is negative. They should not be ordered in patients with suspected very early syphilis who have negative nontreponemal antibody test results. Rather, these patients should undergo darkfield microscopy, repeated nontreponemal antibody testing, and an evaluation for nonsyphilitic causes of their disease. Treponemal antibody tests are not useful in evaluating the success of therapy because they remain positive following treatment for syphilis.

False-positive treponemal antibody tests may occur in systemic lupus erythematosus, herpes simplex infections, pregnancy, Lyme disease, and some normal individuals for unexplained reasons. Since all treponemes are immunologically

Table 5.1 Recommendations for the Use of Diagnostic Tests for Syphilis.*

Group	Initial Test	Follow-up
Patients with primary syphilis	Darkfield exam (RPR ancillary test; repeat if negative)	VDRL (or RPR) titer for following treatment response
Patients with secondary syphilis	RPR† (may use darkfield for rapid diagnosis of condylomata)	VDRL (or RPR) titer for following treatment response
Selected asymptomatic persons (all pregnant women, contacts of syphilitic individuals, high-risk groups)	RPR†	VDRL (or RPR) titer for following treatment response
Patients with tertiary syphilis	RPR and MHA-TP	VDRL (or RPR) titer for following treatment response
Patients with early and late syphilis confirmed	VDRL (or RPR) titer 3, 6, and 12 months after treatment	Re-treat if titer does not fall appropriately‡ or if titer has increased after initial fall
Seropositive persons with neurologic findings	CSF cell count, VDRL, and protein determination	Treatment for neurosyphilis if CSF-VDRL is positive and/or cell count is elevated; even if CSF findings are normal, consider treating seropositive patients with neurologic findings indicative of active disease
Patient follow-up after treatment for neurosyphilis	CSF cell count 1½, 3, and 6 months after treatment	Re-treat if abnormal at 3 months; repeat CSF cell count at 12 and 24 months if normal at 6 months
Infants whose mothers have untreated syphilis	NA	Treat regardless of serology; VDRL titer for follow-up

* Reproduced, with permission, form G. Hart, Syphilis tests in diagnostic and therapeutic decision making. *Ann Intern Med.* 1986;104:368-376.
† A positive RPR (or other nontreponemal test) should be confirmed with MHA-TP.
‡ In primary and secondary syphilis, a fourfold fall in titer should occur within 3 months. Decline is slower in latent or tertiary disease.

---

similar, patients infected with nonsyphilitic treponemes (eg, yaws, pinta) will also have positive treponemal antibody test results. Nontreponemal antibody tests will also be positive in diseases caused by these latter treponemes.

Congenital Syphilis
Congenital syphilis is readily diagnosed when the typical signs of rhinitis, hepatomegaly, rash, anemia, and osteochondritis are present in an infant of a mother who has positive serologic tests for syphilis. A problem arises in serology-positive but normal-appearing neonates born of mothers with syphilis who may or may not have been adequately treated. The infant's positive serology may represent active syphilitic infection or passive transfer of syphilis-related antibodies. Rising VDRL titers in a neonate indicate congenital syphilis, because if a positive

Table 5.2 Sensitivity of Serologic Tests in the Four Stages of Syphilis.*

Stage	% Sensitivity			
	RPR	VDRL	MHA-TP	FTA-Abs
Primary	86	80	82	98
Secondary	100	100	100	100
Early latent	99	96	100	100
Late latent or tertiary	73	71	94	96

* Adapted, with permission, from S. A. Larsen and L. L. Bradford, Serodiagnosis of syphilis. In: N. R. Rose, H. Friedman, and J. L. Fahey, eds. *Manual of Clinical Laboratory Immunology*. Washington, DC: American Society for Microbiology; 1986:425-343.

VDRL is secondary to passive transfer of the mother's IgG antibodies, the titer will decline sharply during the infant's first 2 to 3 months of life. Another diagnostic dilemma presents when a mother acquires syphilis late in pregnancy, giving birth to an infant with a negative serologic test for syphilis but one who might eventually develop clinical syphilis. Neonates whose mothers have syphilis should be treated even if they are asymptomatic at birth, especially when adequate follow-up of newborn infants is questionable, because treatment is relatively safe, and the risk of congenital syphilis manifesting in infants of mothers with primary or secondary syphilis is high (about 90%). Infants suspected of having neurosyphilis should be treated more vigorously because high levels of antibiotic therapy are required to achieve therapeutic levels across the blood-brain barrier.

Neurosyphilis

Neurosyphilis, when considered as a diagnosis due to appropriate symptoms, necessitates an examination of the CSF. Tests should include a spinal fluid protein, white blood cell (WBC) count, and VDRL. Patients with neurosyphilis usually, but not always, have an elevated protein concentration and an increased WBC count. The CSF-VDRL is positive in only 60% of patients with neurosyphilis, and there are no treponemal antibody tests on CSF that are recommended by the CDC, largely because there is a high false-positive rate for treponemal antibody tests in the CSF of patients with a positive serum treponemal antibody test. Thus, in any patient with symptoms of central nervous system disease of obscure origin and positive serum serology, a trial of antisyphilis therapy should be strongly considered even if all spinal fluid findings are normal. A routine VDRL on CSF from asymptomatic patients with positive serum syphilis tests is to be discouraged, as the yield of positive tests is vanishingly small. In patients treated for neurosyphilis with abnormalities in the CSF, follow-up should be monitored using CSF cell counts, which should return to normal in 3 to 12 months. Following successful treatment of neurosyphilis, quantitative CSF-VDRL titers usually decline gradually; as a rule, the test usually remains positive at low titers for several years after therapy. The elevated protein concentration falls with the VDRL.

Summary

Tables 5.1 and 5.2 summarize the recommendations for use of diagnostic tests and the sensitivity of serologic tests for syphilis, respectively.

References

Hart G. Syphilis tests in diagnostic and therapeutic decision making. *Ann Intern Med.* 1986;104:368-376.

Larsen SA, Bradford LL. Serodiagnosis of syphilis. In: Rose NR, Friedman H, Fahey JL, eds. *Manual of Clinical Laboratory Immunology.* 3rd ed. Washington, DC: American Society for Microbiology; 1986:425-434.

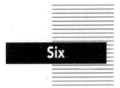

Six

Therapeutic Drug Monitoring

Key Points

1. Therapeutic ranges are well established for some but not all classes of drugs. Target ranges may be utilized for drugs with poorly defined therapeutic ranges.
2. Therapeutic drug monitoring (TDM) is most effective when a drug has a narrow or well-defined therapeutic range.
3. TDM can establish patient noncompliance, identify individual variation in drug utilization or metabolism, point out changes caused by disease or physiological state, and define drug interactions.

Background

TDM, by establishing serum or plasma concentrations of a specific medication, can help a clinician define the optimal clinical response of a patient to medication. It is hoped that each patient will reach a stable blood concentration of medication that can be monitored over the time the drug is administered in an attempt to prevent underutilization and therefore ineffectiveness of the drug, or overutilization with the risk of toxicity or unwanted side effects.

TDM is a laboratory specialty—related to but different from clinical toxicology. Clinical toxicology attempts to identify and semiquantitate a wide range of toxic drugs and compounds that a patient has inadvertently consumed or knowingly abused. TDM helps to define and optimize clinical response by using serum or plasma concentrations of drugs, and helps to minimize toxic effects. Many of the same laboratory instruments and procedures for testing are utilized for both TDM and toxicology tests.

TDM has been part of clinical laboratory medicine for more than 50 years. In the 1920s physicians monitored blood bromide concentrations to aid in differentiating bromide-induced psychosis from psychosis attributable to other causes. During World War II, the search for antimalarial drugs yielded improvements in drug quantitation techniques and led to the development of the first accurate analytical instruments. The first studies correlating drug concentrations in blood with therapeutic efficacy were published in the 1950s. It was not until the mid-1960s, however, that TDM in its current form was born. Gas liquid chromatography was utilized systematically for the first time to measure anticonvulsant drug concentrations as physicians searched for ways not only to select appropriate anticonvulsant medication for particular patients but also to maximize effectiveness and minimize toxicity.

The development of high-pressure liquid chromatography and early immunoassay techniques in the 1970s reduced the complexity of the technology. Radioimmunoassay techniques, which permitted quantitation of drug concentrations in a very small volume of serum or plasma, enzyme-multiplied immunoassay techniques, and fluorescence polarization immunoassay techniques were developed in the 1980s. Recent introduction of the cloned enzyme donor immunoassay promises to again upgrade the methodology of TDM.

Therapeutic Drug Monitoring Applications

For TDM to be an effective and optimal clinical tool, a number of conditions must be met. The drug measured must meet four criteria: it should have a reasonable or narrow therapeutic range; it should be able to be used over a period of time; it should have potentially toxic side effects in overdose or at too-high concentrations; and it should have minimal therapeutic effects if dosage and blood levels are too low. For drugs such as anticonvulsants, therapeutic ranges are reasonably well defined and correlate extremely well with seizure control and toxicity; minimum therapeutic concentrations have been established and toxic concentrations for these drugs are reasonably well understood. Consequently, between the minimum effective concentration and minimum toxic concentration a "therapeutic range" is established. Similar situations are true for aminoglycoside antibiotics and some cardiac (antiarrhythmic) drugs.

For other medications, such as antidepressants, some benzodiazepines (antianxiety drugs), and some neuroleptics (antipsychotics), target concentrations are probably more appropriate than are therapeutic concentrations. Target concentrations are those that are most often present in patients who respond to the drug. Obtaining a target concentration in a particular patient does not ensure that clinical response will in fact occur, because many patients fail to respond to some drugs (eg, antidepressants). Difficulties in establishing adequate doses while simultaneously controlling side effects and determining a clinical end point make the use of target concentrations important. Failure to achieve a target concentration means that the patient has not received an adequate clinical trial of that drug, not necessarily that the drug has failed.

TDM can be most beneficial in identifying and compensating for individual variations in drug metabolism and utilization. Interindividual differences in absorption, distribution, and metabolism of many medications are highly variable and may approach 30-fold differences for certain drugs. While the vast majority of patients treated with a particular medication will have levels near or within the therapeutic range, a significant percentage of patients in any population will be genetically either fast or slow drug metabolizers. Fast metabolizers require significantly higher doses to achieve adequate serum concentrations, while slow metabolizers may become toxic at relatively modest doses. Metabolism of one drug can be affected by the presence of another. Anticonvulsants or barbiturates can stimulate metabolism so that patients who are not genetically fast metabolizers appear to be so. Conversely, metabolism of some drugs such as tricyclic antidepressants can be blocked by coadministration of neuroleptic medications, making patients appear to be slow metabolizers who otherwise would not be.

TDM can assist the clinician in identifying noncompliance. Patients who have chronic diseases or conditions requiring polypharmacy may not take medications as prescribed, either knowingly or inadvertently. The elderly are particularly prone to difficulties when they are prescribed several medications, each with a different schedule of administration. Apparent noncompliance can also occur due to drug interactions that cause alterations in absorption and metabolism of medications.

Altered drug utilization can occur in chronic disease states. Acute or chronic uremia can dramatically decrease urinary excretion of drugs; renal failure can alter protein-binding characteristics of drugs that may be bound to albumin. In this situation, the ratio of free drug to total drug may also increase to the point that free drug concentrations are high enough to produce clinically evident drug toxicity even though total serum concentrations are within therapeutic ranges. Hepatic disease can extensively alter a patient's response to drugs by impairing or enhancing metabolic capacity.

TDM can also be useful in patients with altered or unusual physiological status. Children tend to metabolize drugs more quickly than adults, while the elderly tend to have reduced metabolism and reduced renal clearance. Pregnancy, puberty, and even chronic cycles of dieting can alter drug utilization and metabolism, yielding unusual clinical results that can at least be identified if not rectified through measurement of serum concentrations.

Guidelines for Therapeutic Drug Monitoring

For TDM to be optimally effective, all information relevant to a patient's pharmacological condition should be available to both the clinician and the laboratory.

Patient information, including age, weight, concurrent prescribed and over-the-counter medications, total daily dosage of drugs, and clinical history, may all be necessary to interpret TDM information. As mentioned, wide individual variability can exist in a patient's utilization of drugs as a direct consequence of multiple drug therapy, age, weight, genetic factors, and medical status.

Critical time intervals must also be observed. The time at which the last dose of drug was administered and the time at which the blood specimen was drawn may be essential, particularly for antibiotics where peak and trough concentrations are necessary to interpret TDM data.

The clinical status of the patient, while well known to the treating physician, may also be important to laboratory personnel when they are faced with unusual or abnormal findings. Concurrent medications can not only alter metabolism and disposition of drugs in patients but may also interfere with various analytical procedures. Cross-reactions in immunologic procedures and outright interference in chromatographic procedures may make interpretation of TDM data impossible if the laboratory is not aware of concurrent medications being administered.

Analysis of TDM data must always be correlated with the clinical status of the patient. Clinicians should be concerned more with optimal concentrations for individual patients than with the therapeutic ranges published by the laboratory. The optimal concentration is defined as that concentration which provides a desired therapeutic response in a particular patient. Therapeutic ranges or target ranges should serve only as guidelines. It is possible that particular patients will exhibit desired therapeutic effects with plasma concentrations well below the target or therapeutic range, while others require levels above those usually considered optimal and may, without adverse effects, exhibit levels that would be toxic in other patients. Some patients will not achieve the desired therapeutic effect even when plasma concentrations are elevated into the toxic range. For these patients we must admit that our present knowledge concerning free drug concentrations and transport and binding phenomena is incomplete. Advances in these areas will aid our patients.

References

Gerson B. *Essentials of Therapeutic Drug Monitoring.* New York, NY: Igaku-Shoin Medical Publishers Inc; 1983.

Pribor HC, Morrell G, Scherr GH. *Drug Monitoring and Pharmacokinetic Data.* Park Forest South, Ill: Pathotox Publishers Inc; 1980.

Taylor WJ, Diers-Caviness MH. *A Textbook for the Clinical Application of Therapeutic Drug Monitoring.* Irving, Tex: Abbott Laboratories, Diagnostics Division; 1986.

Taylor WJ, Finn AL. *Individualizing Drug Therapy: Practical Applications of Drug Monitoring, I.* New York, NY: Gross, Townsend, Frank Inc; 1981.

Wong SHY. *Therapeutic Drug Monitoring and Toxicology by Liquid Chromatography.* New York, NY: Marcel Dekker Inc; 1985.

Seven

Toxicology and Substance Abuse Testing

Key Points

1. A "positive" drug screen does not necessarily mean that a toxic level of drug is present in a patient in an emergency department.
2. A "positive" drug screen from a patient in a medical or psychiatric setting should be considered presumptive until confirmed by appropriate alternate analytical methodology.
3. A "negative" drug screen does not necessarily mean that a particular drug or class of drugs is not present or has not been taken by a patient. The limitations of particular drug screening methodology must be taken into account when interpreting drug screen reports.
4. When a particular drug or toxin is present or highly suspected, quantitative analysis of at least two specimens drawn several hours apart provides more useful information than drug screens.
5. A "negative" drug screen can best be interpreted as "drugs tested for are not detectable by the methods used with reliability or are not present in concentrations consistent with toxic symptoms."

Background

Some clinicians may argue that the toxicology laboratory contributes little to the care of acutely poisoned patients because therapy must be initiated immediately and laboratory data therefore cannot be available in a time frame useful to the clinician. While it is clear a patient who has ingested a toxic substance or taken an overdose of an illegal drug must be treated promptly, therapy is usually supportive since few substances have specific therapies available. A prompt, reliable positive report of a toxic or abused drug may only minimally alter a poisoned patient's therapy; however, such positive results may avert the need for other more expensive and time-consuming diagnostic tests. A negative report may suggest that other diagnoses must be considered to ensure proper patient care. The possibility that drugs or analytes not routinely tested for are present must also be considered and appropriate alternate testing initiated by the clinician if other drugs are suspected.

The advent of rapid, relatively broad-spectrum drug detection by immunologic procedures has added dramatically to the laboratory's ability to provide preliminary drug screening results within minutes of receiving a urine specimen. Therefore, the toxicology laboratory can now be a useful resource when managing a poisoned or overdosed patient. Many physicians still have the misconception that a toxicology screen will detect and identify any of the hundreds of drugs available and thousands of toxins that might be ingested. Even the most technically advanced laboratories suffer under financial considerations or personnel and time constraints that make such a complete screening prohibitive, even if it were possible.

Drug Screens and Testing

The toxicology laboratory, usually part of the clinical chemistry section, is asked to perform drug screening/testing on specimens received from many areas of the hospital. While the original mission of the clinical toxicology laboratory was to aid in the diagnosis of acute poisoning, the laboratory's expertise has expanded to include therapeutic drug monitoring, screening of drugs subject to abuse, and forensic toxicology. While the laboratory techniques are similar for these different missions, other constraints applied are quite different. Analytical methods, time requirements, the type of medical-legal proof needed to ascertain the origin of the specimen, and the type of specimen required all may differ.

Drug screens are among the most frequently and inappropriately ordered laboratory tests because of false expectations by the clinician utilizing the results. A toxicology screen should be ordered when a patient has symptoms and signs of true overdose or poisoning and is brought to an emergency department. To be useful and cost-effective, the screen should provide results within a very short time (minutes or hours, not days), should exclude drugs that occur at less than toxic concentration, should identify or rule out overdoses of common over-the-counter medications such as acetaminophen or salicylate, antihistamines, or decongestants, should identify those substances where quantitation is critical to management such as antidepressant medications, and should help determine a patient's prognosis.

When ordering a drug screen, it is important for the clinician to recognize that only selected groups of drugs are tested for in the majority of toxicology screens. Opiates, benzodiazepines, cocaine and its metabolites, amphetamines, barbiturates, tricyclic antidepressants (but not often other antidepressants), and phencyclidine (PCP) are usually included in a typical toxicology screen. These screens will identify high or toxic concentrations but will not discriminate illegal substances (opiates originating from morphine or heroin) from legitimate medication (opiates originating from codeine in prescription pain medications). Other classes of drugs, including phenothiazines, antiarrhythmics, antibiotics, and heavy metals, are not included in the typical "drug screen."

Most laboratories utilize urine as the initial test fluid, but the results may differ when blood is tested from the same patient. For example, a urine screen may fail to identify small concentrations of benzodiazepines, while blood drawn from the same patient at the same time may yield positive results because of fluid concentration differences and different laboratory methods used for blood and urine screening.

Sometimes a drug screen appears to contradict a clinical diagnosis or history. A urine screen requested on a patient for PCP overdose may be reported as negative even though the patient clearly appears to have taken PCP and even admits to its use. This can occur because the urine screen has limited sensitivity for this particular drug in all but those cases where a large dose was taken or when the time between ingestion and obtaining the specimen is short.

Despite very strong evidence for use or abuse of drugs, toxicology screens can be negative because structural analogues, so-called designer drugs that exert similar biological effects, may have been ingested but are not detected by the screens.

In those cases where a true inclusive drug screen is required, the physician should be as specific as possible and provide a list of possible drugs/medications involved. Long-term medications used by the patient and those that have been administered to the patient in the emergency department should also be listed. Inclusive drug screens often require reference laboratory expertise and so will increase turnaround time.

Analytical Techniques

The most widely used analytical techniques in the toxicology laboratory fall into two categories: chromatographic and immunologic.

Chromatographic Techniques

Chromatographic techniques, which rely on physical extraction and separation of analytes from interfering substances and the biological matrix, are the oldest. They are still widely used because of their ability to identify and quantitate an extraordinarily wide range of analytes and toxins. Chromatography can be further divided into thin-layer chromatography, gas chromatography, and high-pressure liquid chromatography.

Thin-layer chromatography, such as in the commonly used Toxi-Lab® (Toxi-Lab Inc, Irvine, Calif) commercial system, is a relatively simple qualitative analytical technique. A thin layer of inorganic substance such as silica or aluminum oxide is applied to a glass plate as a sorbent. A liquid solvent system is then placed at the base of the plate where an extract containing the drugs to be separated and identified is located. As the solvent climbs the plate by capillary action, the analytes begin to migrate upward. Separation occurs because absorption or partition of the analytes varies as the mobile solvent moves across the stationary sorbent phase. The plate is then dried and developed by any of a number of chemical techniques. Each individual compound has a particular migration pattern and identification scheme. This technique, while simple and inexpensive, is highly dependent on the technician's analytical skill and practice. It can detect a very wide range of compounds but sensitivity is usually limited to high or toxic concentrations in urine.

Gas chromatography is more sophisticated than thin-layer chromatography and can be used for both qualitative and quantitative identification. The liquid or solid specimen, which has been extracted from its biological matrix in organic solvent, is injected into the chromatographic column, which consists of a solid sorbent phase coated with an organic phase. The specimen is vaporized by heat and carried through the column by inert carrier gas. Interaction between the analytes and the sorbent material within the column causes each analyte to migrate at a different rate. As specimens emerge from the column, the detector recognizes the presence of each compound and graphically plots its emergence as a function of time. Concentrations are relative to detection signal, and thus quantitation is possible. Modern capillary gas chromatographic columns are capable of separating literally hundreds of compounds simultaneously but at the expense of time. Such separations require careful extraction of the analytes from the biological matrix or tissue samples, and chromatographic times can exceed 2 hours. Sensitivity is usually higher than with other methods.

High-pressure liquid chromatography is similar in many ways to gas chromatography, except that it is not restricted to volatile compounds and utilizes a liquid mobile phase rather than a gaseous one. Sensitivity is similar to gas chromatography, but the array of compounds that can be detected at any one time is usually limited to a single drug class.

Immunologic Techniques

The most commonly used screening techniques in the laboratory today utilize immunologic methods. Originally, radioimmunoassay was used because of its high sensitivity and ability to provide quantitative analyses. Most radioimmunoassays have been replaced by nonradiometric immunoassays, including the enzyme multiplied immunoassay technique and fluorescence polarization immunoassay, which were developed originally for quantitative analysis of therapeutic drugs and have now been applied extensively to substances of abuse. These techniques are less sensitive than radioimmunoassay and much easier to use than chromatographic techniques, but their use is limited to individual classes of drugs occurring at toxic concentrations. Like all immunoassays, they cannot detect all of the drugs within a class, ie, all opiates and metabolites, with the same level of certainty, and cannot distinguish between abused drugs and prescription drugs in the categories. Cross-reactivity may cause difficulty. For example, very high doses of over-the-counter antihistamines or therapeutic doses of ranitidine can yield signals equivalent to those obtained with amphetamine abuse.

Positive tests using immunoassay methodology should always be confirmed with another technique whenever medical-legal decisions or significant treatment decisions will be based on the result. Legally defensible results require the use of an enzyme multiplied immunoassay technique or other immunoassay technique such as radioimmunoassay or fluorescence polarization immunoassay, followed by gas chromatographic analysis or gas chromatography with mass spectrometry confirmation.

Summary

The toxicology laboratory can be most useful to the emergency department physician when used appropriately to assist in diagnosis and management of poisoned or overdosed patients. The emergency department physician must be cognizant of the limitations of the test results to maximize utility without error.

References

Bryson PD. *Comprehensive Review in Toxicology.* 2nd ed. Rockville, Md: Aspen Publishers Inc; 1989.

Casarett LJ, Doull J. *Toxicology: The Basic Science of Poisons.* 3rd ed. New York, NY: Macmillan Publishing Co; 1986.

Goldfrank LR, Flomenbaum NE, Lewin NA, et al. *Goldfrank's Toxicologic Emergencies.* 4th ed. East Norwalk, Conn: Appleton & Lange; 1990.

McEvoy GK, ed. *AHFS Drug Information.* Bethesda, Md: American Society of Hospital Pharmacists Inc; 1990.

Skoutakis VA. *Clinical Toxicology of Drugs: Principles and Practice.* Philadelphia, Pa: Lea & Febiger; 1982.

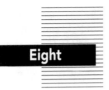
Pregnancy: Related Tests

Key Points

1. The laboratory cannot measure pregnancy; it can only measure phenomena associated with pregnancy, such as human chorionic gonadotropin (HCG). The clinician confirms pregnancy with physical examination or ultrasound.
2. Rising or falling levels of HCG, measured quantitatively in serum, are far more informative and reliable than urine measurements, which are at best semiquantitative.
3. Assays are now readily available that are truly specific for ßHCG with negligible interference (corollary: assays not specific for the epitopes [antigenic sites] of the beta chain of HCG should be abandoned).
4. The half-life of HCG is brief, such that a fully infarcted tubal implantation may be a persisting threat of hemorrhage even after measurable HCG has vanished.

Background

The first signs of intrauterine pregnancy (breast fullness, urinary frequency, nausea, and vomiting) are usually not noticed until 5 or 6 weeks after the last normal menstrual period. Definitive findings on examination take at least as long to become apparent. Therefore, the detection of HCG in serum or urine is useful as presumptive evidence of early pregnancy.

HCG is a glycoprotein composed of two subunits, alpha and beta. HCG is produced by the placental trophoblast shortly after implantation. The alpha subunits of luteinizing hormone (LH), thyroid-stimulating hormone (TSH), follicle-stimulating hormone (FSH), and HCG are identical, but their beta subunits are partially different. Today, immunoassays for ßHCG in urine and serum should be used exclusively because they are specific for the unique binding sites of the ßHCG subunit.

ßHCG in serum or urine is expressed as international units (IU). In normal, nonpregnant women ßHCG is not detectable in serum or urine by even the most sensitive assay procedures. Serum ßHCG first can be detected by immunoassay 24 to 48 hours after implantation, and peak serum and urine levels are usually reached by 60 to 80 days after the last normal menstrual period. There is considerable intraindividual variation in the production and excretion of HCG, but a continually rising level is the norm during the first trimester. The range for the 60- to 80-day period is 7000 to 22,000 IU/d. Following this peak a plateau is reached by 120 days, which is maintained with gradual drop-off thereafter.

Immunoassays for HCG were introduced in the early 1960s and have now completely replaced the older bioassays as routine laboratory tests for pregnancy. There is considerable variation in the sensitivities of the various commercially available immunoassays that use an antibody specific for ßHCG. The overall sensitivity and specificity of these tests is comparable with that of quantitative serum immunoassay, described below. Several rapid and sensitive colorimetric "slide" tests and other office tests have been developed that are as rapid and as easy to perform as the latex test tube tests, with a similar sensitivity. These are suitable for most clinical purposes and can detect HCG elevation on or before the first day of expected menses (ie, 14 days after implantation). Hybritech Inc (San Diego, Calif) has produced an effective serum or urine ßHCG test using an Immuno Concentrator (ICON^TM), a disposable testing device. The ICON^TM is packaged as a small plastic cup with a membrane in the center. The membrane contains three zones: a test zone, a positive zone, and a negative zone. ßHCG reacts with a monoclonal antibody bound to the membrane in the zones. A second antibody labeled with an enzyme is added to the ICON^TM and a color develops if ßHCG is present. The other two zones serve as a positive and negative control. The HCG ICON^TM can detect 20 IU/L of HCG greater than 99% of the time. This level would detect pregnancy at about 1 week after implantation. Abbott Labs Inc (Chicago, Ill) has developed a similar product that displays a (+) if the test is positive and a (-) if negative. These tests use five drops of urine and take only 5 minutes to perform.

Although they are not essential for the routine laboratory detection of pregnancy, quantitative immunoassays for ßHCG have definite advantages. Their great sensitivity (beta subunit, 5 IU/L) makes them ideal for detection of very early pregnancy. They are also used in patients with suspected threatened abortion or ectopic pregnancy, and, critically, in the detection and follow-up evaluation of HCG-producing tumors (trophoblastic disease, testicular tumors, and certain nonendocrine tumors). Immunoassays can be performed on serum or urine. HCG results from different manufacturer kits can vary by 50% depending on which World Health Organization standard is used. Caution: Some assays do not measure the free beta chain but only the intact HCG; others may "see" either form.

As with any diagnostic tests, assays for ßHCG in serum or urine may be falsely positive or negative. False-negative results in viable intrauterine pregnancy are now truly rare. False-negative results may occur in patients experiencing ectopic pregnancy or spontaneous abortion, or in the second or third trimester of a normal pregnancy as a result of the short half-life and decrease in output. Very dilute urine may cause falsely low levels.

Exogenous HCG administration and neoplastic HCG production cause non-pregnancy false-positive results, although in a general hospital population this is rare. The beta-subunit reagent greatly reduces the chance of a false-positive reaction, but the assay may pick up very low level physiological fluctuations in HCG unrelated to pregnancy.

Most ectopic pregnancies can be detected by these sensitive tests, although physicians still rely on clinical features plus ultrasound of the pelvis for the diagnosis of ectopic pregnancy. Lower than expected or declining levels of ßHCG may be indicative of spontaneous abortion, so in this situation the more sensitive quantitative HCG assays are preferable. However, they should not be used without clinical correlation.

Quantitative assays for serum ßHCG are preferred in patients with trophoblastic disease. They may have markedly elevated serum or urine HCG levels, but the levels may be low if the tumor does not express the marker. Hence, tests with the best sensitivity are preferred. Tumors may produce free beta subunits not detected if only the whole HCG is measured. Levels of ßHCG in serum should decline if the patient has been adequately treated. Ectopic HCG production by nonendocrine tumors can also be documented. Multiple gestation pregnancies can produce high levels of ßHCG closer to the range produced by some tumors.

Tests to Monitor Pregnancy

Biochemical studies can be used to augment the clinical monitoring of complicated high-risk pregnancies (eg, women with diabetes, hypertension).

Alpha-Fetoprotein

Alpha-fetoprotein (AFP), a fetal serum protein marker, appears in the amniotic fluid in the presence of certain fetal deformities. Open neural tube defects, abdominal wall defects, and congenital nephrotic syndrome are suggested by increased levels. Normally, the amniotic fluid AFP reaches the maximum of 15 mg/L at 16 weeks and then falls progressively until term. Elevations of amniotic fluid AFP, when compared with gestational age-matched controls, are highly suggestive of an abnormal fetus. Accurate assessment of gestational age is imperative for proper interpretation. Previous delivery of an affected child is one indication for such a study in a subsequent pregnancy. Ultrasonographic imaging can detect and/or confirm many of these gross abnormalities. It can also estimate gestational age and rule out multiple fetuses as the cause of the AFP elevation. Elevations in the amniotic fluid levels of AFP are reflected also in the maternal serum, and most obstetricians are now screening pregnant women by measuring AFP in their serum at 16 to 20 weeks' gestation. Maternal serum AFP values greater than two and a half multiples of the median deserve further investigation for the possibility of neural tube defect. A false-positive result, which may lead to an unwarranted termination of a normal pregnancy, is an undesirable side effect of such testing. The predictive value and cost-benefit ratio is enhanced in areas of the world where the prevalence for neural tube defects is greater than in the United States. Low maternal AFP values have been reported in association with fetal trisomy 21.

Surfactant

Surfactant level measurements may help determine whether a third trimester fetus is not growing well secondary to maternal problems (eg, reduced blood flow to the placenta). A better outcome for the fetus might be accomplished by elective delivery before 40 weeks' gestation. One would prefer to deliver an infant early only if the surfactant system of the fetal lungs has matured to the point that the infant will not develop hyaline membrane disease. Between 35 and 37 weeks' gestation, the chemical composition of "surfactant" in fetal lung changes rapidly to include a large amount of lecithin (phosphatidylcholine). This raises the concentration of amniotic fluid lecithin as a consequence, and it is used as an indication that fetal lungs are mature enough to support life.

A variety of techniques exist to estimate the amount of lecithin in amniotic fluid either alone or as a ratio with sphingomyelin. These techniques range from chromatography and fluorescence polarization to a simple shake test. The latter is an observation of the stability of bubbles in a shaken tube of amniotic fluid. Although all techniques have problems, thin-layer chromatography remains the method of choice for predicting maturity. A lecithin-sphingomyelin ratio greater than 2:1 implies a mature fetal lung. A ratio less than 2:1 indicates significant risk for the development of hyaline membrane disease. In the experience of most investigators, infants of diabetic mothers may develop respiratory distress even with an apparently adequate ratio. Lecithin, when present in amniotic fluid, essentially assures the presence of a mature surfactant system.

Estriol

Estriol in pregnancy is produced by fetal adrenal, liver, and placenta. Levels in the maternal urine (normalized to creatinine excretion) reflect the integrity of multiorgan fetal biochemical pathways. When correlated with reference ranges for each week of gestation, estriol measurements supplement information obtained from the physical examination, ultrasound, and other methods of monitoring high-risk fetuses. Any compromise of the fetoplacental unit, be it of fetal or maternal origin, will reduce urine estriol values. Low estriol values, except when related to cirrhosis or renal failure in the mother, suggest compromise to the fetus. Other maternal factors may be measured (eg, placental lactogen, pregnanediol, prolactin), but data supporting their usefulness in monitoring fetal status are less clear. Measurement of estriol level is rarely done.

References

Deutchman M. The problematic first-trimester pregnancy. *Am Fam Physician*. 1989; 39:185-198.

Dubin SB. Assessment of fetal lung maturity: in search of the holy grail. *Clin Chem*. 1990;36:1867-1869.

Rugg JA, Rigl CT, Leung K, et al. Radial partition immunoassay applied to automated quantification of human chorionic gonadotropin with use of two monoclonal antibodies. *Clin Chem*. 1986;32:1844-1848.

Steier JA, Bergsjo P, Myking O. Human chorionic gonadotropin in maternal plasma after induced abortion, spontaneous abortion, and removed ectopic pregnancy. *Obstet Gynecol.* 1984;64:391-394.

Wilcox AJ, Weinberg CR, O'Conner JF, et al. Incidence of early loss of pregnancy. *N Engl J Med.* 1988;319:189-194.

Nine

Tumor Biomarkers

Key Points

1. Tumor biomarkers are either produced by the tumor cells themselves, or are related to host response to the tumor.
2. The markers are usually detected in serum or urine, or are immunologically located in thin-cut tumor tissue slices on glass slides.
3. Tumor markers are not used as screening tests, but are useful to establish a baseline and then monitor for both tumor progression and treatment effectiveness.

Background

Roughly 500,000 US deaths each year are related to cancer. As treatments become increasingly effective, early cancer detection and postcancer surveillance become correspondingly important.

Tumor marker substances are either tumor-specific (produced by the tumor cells themselves) or tumor-associated (related to host response to the tumor) (Table 9.1). They can be present and assayed for in body fluids such as blood and urine, or immunoassays can be applied to a thin slice of tumor on a microscopic slide to determine tumor cell characteristics and hopefully tumor diagnosis.

The ideal tumor marker would be both sensitive (no false negatives) and specific (no false positives), and its levels would rise in serum parallel to tumor burden. If it were also inexpensive, practical, and reproducible, it would indeed be an effective screening tool. Not suprisingly, no tumor biomarkers have been found that fulfill all these criteria.

None of the biomarkers discussed below are used as screening tools, nor should they be because as screens they are neither sensitive nor specific enough. Rather, their utility lies in establishing a baseline value of the marker in question

Table 9.1 Tumor Markers and Associated Tumors.

Marker	Tumor Association
PSA	Prostatic adenocarcinoma
PAP	Prostatic adenocarcinoma, especially metastic
CEA	Colorectal adenocarcinoma and breast carcinoma
AFP	Selected germ cell tumors of gonads, hepatocellular carcinoma
βHCG	Choriocarcinoma of gonads and uterus
ALP	Metastases to bone
VMA	Neuroblastoma, pheochromocytoma
Bence Jones proteins	Multiple myeloma
5-HIAA	Carcinoids
Calcinonin	Medullary carcinoma of thyroid

at the time a tissue diagnosis is made by a pathologist. The marker can then be used to evaluate effectiveness of therapy (by seeing dropping serum levels of the marker) and as an early predictor of tumor recurrence (when serum levels rise over a period of time), often before clinical symptoms or signs present themselves.

Assays and Their Interpretation

Prostate-Specific Antigen
Prostate-specific antigen (PSA) is a tumor-specific marker elaborated by prostatic adenocarcinoma cells. PSA may be detected in serum of patients with prostatic adenocarcinoma, and reliably is present when tumor has advanced beyond the prostate. This test is often ordered when a man has a palpable prostatic nodule. It can be used on tumor tissue in the histology laboratory to help establish whether a metastic focus originated in the prostate. Sensitivity and specificity in this setting exceed 95%.

Prostatic-Fraction Acid Phosphatase
Prostatic-fraction acid phosphatase (PAP) is a tumor-associated marker that is usually within normal limits in the absence of benign prostatic hyperplasia (BPH) or adenocarcinoma, usually normal or slightly elevated when BPH exists or adenocarcinoma is confined to the prostate, but very elevated in the serum of patients when prostatic adenocarcinoma has extended outside the gland or is metastatic, for instance, to bone. Because levels can rise due to digital examination, blood should be drawn before or several days after the manual palpation of the prostate.

Carcinoembryonic Antigen
Carcinoembryonic antigen (CEA) is produced both by early embryonic tissue and as a result of gene activation by certain tumors. Although normally elaborat-

ed in small amounts by normal gastrointestinal (GI) mucosal cells, sharp elevations of CEA are seen in 60% to 65% of patients with colorectal adenocarcinomas (higher values with higher stage disease) and in roughly half of patients with metastasizing breast carcinomas. Values can also rise in the presence of lung, pancreas, and other GI tumors. False-positive elevations (usually of modest degree) are seen in heavy smokers and persons with inflammatory bowel disease, hepatic disease, or infections.

Alpha-Fetoprotein

Alpha-fetoprotein (AFP) is present prenatally and in the first year of life, synthesized by fetal yolk sac, liver, and GI tract. Serum half-life is 6 days. High levels in nonpregnant adults usually indicate serious disease. AFP is associated with germ cell tumors (most specifically endodermal sinus tumor) of the testis or ovary, and is present in 70% of patients with hepatocellular carcinomas. False-positive elevations are seen with hepatic regeneration (due to viral or traumatic injury), inflammatory bowel disease, and pregnancy (both maternal and fetal levels may be elevated).

Beta Subunit Human Chorionic Gonadotropin

Beta subunit human chorionic gonadotropin (ßHCG) is produced in the placenta by syncytiocytotrophoblastic cells. Serum half-life is 30 hours. Levels are raised therefore during pregnancy and in choriocarcinoma of the testis and ovary/uterus. Very small amounts of the substance can be detected by radioimmunoassay, and levels seem related to tumor volume.

Alkaline Phosphatase

Alkaline phosphatase (ALP) elevations, though nonspecific, can suggest metastases to bone in the appropriate clinical setting.

Vanillylmandelic Acid and Homovanillic Acid

Vanillylmandelic acid (VMA) and homovanillic acid (HVA) are associated with neuroblastoma because they are breakdown products released in the urine from catecholamines produced by the tumor. Some foods, such as chocolate, coffee, tea, tomatoes, bananas, and vanilla, give false-positive results. VMA is also associated with pheochromocytoma.

Bence Jones Proteins and Monoclonal Immunoglobulins

Bence Jones proteins (urine) and monoclonal immunoglobulins (blood) are associated with multiple myeloma 50% and 95% of the time, respectively.

5-Hydroxyindoleacetic Acid

5-Hydroxyindoleacetic acid (5-HIAA) is a metabolic by-product of 5-hydroxytryptamine commonly secreted by carcinoid tumors.

Calcitonin

Calcitonin is associated with medullary carcinoma of the thyroid.

Summary

This chapter touches on tumor markers used routinely. Many more (CA125 [epithelial ovarian neoplasms], CA19-9 [pancreatic adenocarcinomas], ferritin [head and neck and hematogenous malignant neoplasms]) have been reported and have varying utility. T and B cell markers in malignant lymphomas are used to further define the malignant process. Estrogen and progesterone receptors in breast carcinomas are used to help guide therapy as well as predict prognosis. Do not forget that these same substances can also be used effectively in other clinical settings, ie, amniotic fluid AFP for detection of neural-tube defects in fetuses in utero, and ßHCG for pregnancy testing.

References

Humphrey PA. The role of tumor markers in early detection of cancer. *Semin Surg Oncol.* 1989;5:186-193.

Kelly WM. Tumor markers: a review. *Radiography.* 1988;54:14-17.

Rainwater LM. Prostate-specific antigen testing in untreated and treated prostatic adenocarcinoma. *Mayo Clin Proc.* 1990;65:1118-1126.

Torosian MH. The clinical usefulness and limitations of tumor markers. *Surg Gynecol Obstet.* 1988;166:567-579.

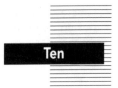

Ten

Myocardial Injury: Laboratory Tests

Key Points

1. Elevation of creatine kinase–MB (CK-MB) does not exclusively connote classic infarction, because nonischemic diseases also produce myofiber necrosis with elevated markers.
2. The test for CK-MB has great predictive value for accurately diagnosing acute myocardial infarction: a positive result is strong evidence for acute myocardial infarction, whereas a series of negative results rules out a myocardial infarction having occurred within the study period and up to 12 hours prior to the baseline.
3. When serum CK-MB is present, an isoenzyme pattern positive for increased lactate dehydrogenase–1 (LD-1) corroborates the diagnosis of myocardial infarction.
4. When serum CK-MB is present but the isoenzyme pattern is negative for LD, the results may be interpreted in various ways. The findings suggest that myocardial damage is limited but that a small amount of myocardial necrosis is present.
5. A pattern of elevated total CK or LD levels in the absence of an isoenzyme pattern positive for CK-MB or elevated LD-1 generally indicates that the elevated total CK or LD is not of cardiac origin.
6. Increased total LD with an isoenzyme pattern positive for increased LD-1 in the absence of CK-MB is compatible with a myocardial infarct occurring 2 or more days prior to the study. Other disorders should be excluded, including acute renal infarct, megaloblastic anemia, and hemolytic anemia.
7. When a laboratory evaluation is performed more than 48 hours after the onset of myocardial infarction, the results are often equivocal. However, analysis of both total LD and LD isoenzymes still can yield information that is diagnostic in some cases.

8. Laboratory criteria (all not necessarily present simultaneously) for diagnosing acute myocardial infarction include: (a) increased serum CK, (b) the presence of serum CK-MB, (c) increased total serum LD, and (d) the presence of an increased LD-1/total LD or an LD flip.

Background

The clinical diagnosis of acute myocardial infarction is based on three parameters: assessment of the patient's history to document characteristic chest pain; the results of a physical examination to detect arrhythmias, congestive heart failure, or cardiogenic shock; and an electrocardiogram. For many patients, this analysis leads to a firm diagnosis. However, many patients have an atypical history and/or nondiagnostic electrocardiogram. For these patients, laboratory evaluation can be an important aid in establishing the diagnosis. Even when the diagnosis of myocardial infarction is virtually certain on clinical grounds alone, a laboratory evaluation is usually performed for confirmation.

A laboratory evaluation of myocardial infarction involves serum measurement of molecules that are highly concentrated in myocardial cells but that are subsequently released into the extracellular spaces with infarction/ischemia and cell membrane damage, and then are released into the circulation where they can be measured in a serum sample. These molecules include myoglobin, myosin components, and certain enzymes. A typical laboratory evaluation is limited to tests for serum enzymes, which include CK, LD, and aspartate aminotransferase (AST). Although many of the enzyme molecules are degraded in the heart, enough molecules reach the blood intact so that serum enzyme levels become elevated for a few days and up to 2 weeks after a myocardial infarct. In experimental animals, as little as 1 g of necrotic myocardium can be detected by changes in serum enzymes. The magnitude and duration of elevations in serum enzyme levels are roughly proportional to the size of an acute myocardial infarct; however, determining the exact size of an infarct from serum enzyme analysis is problematic. Myocardial ischemia without necrosis, as in angina pectoris, generally does not cause elevations of serum enzyme levels.

Measurements can be made of total enzyme and isoenzymes (Figure 10.1, Table 10.1). Although analysis of isoenzymes provides more precise information, none of the tests are completely specific for myocardial infarction. Therefore, the results of the tests must be interpreted in relation to other information available. The pattern of change in serum levels of the enzymes occurring after acute myocardial infarction follows.

Specimen Information and Test Interpretation

To perform a proper laboratory evaluation of suspected acute myocardial infarction, serial blood samples should be obtained to identify any transient increases in enzyme levels. Serial sampling of the blood can be accomplished successfully by obtaining blood samples on admission and every 8 to 12 hours thereafter for 2 days. The typical "cardiac panel" measures total CK, CK-MB (isoenzymes), total

Figure 10.1 Pattern of Changes in Serum Enzymes With Acute Myocardial Infarction (MI).*

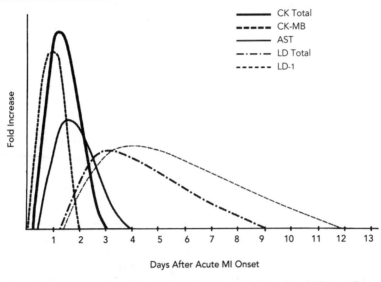

* Adapted, with permission, from R. Ravel, *Clinical Laboratory Medicine*. 5th ed. Chicago, Ill: Year Book Medical Publishers; 1989:325.

LD, and LD isoenzymes. Opinions differ about the optimal use of serum enzyme analysis. One approach relies primarily on the analysis of CK isoenzymes and reserves the analysis of LD isoenzymes for equivocal cases or cases where the suspected myocardial infarction began over 24 to 48 hours before admission. Another approach routinely uses analysis of both CK and LD isoenzymes. The latter approach is based on the concept that the two tests provide complementary information, thereby enhancing the overall diagnostic capability of serum-enzyme analysis.

Creatine Kinase

CK, called creatine phosphokinase in the old nomenclature, catalyzes the reversible phosphorylation of creatine by adenosine triphosphate. CK is highly concentrated in myocardium, skeletal muscle, and brain. Although small amounts of CK exist in many other tissues, virtually no CK is present in liver or erythrocytes. Normal serum CK activity is derived largely from routine skeletal muscle degradation. Normal serum CK varies with sex, race, muscle mass, and physical conditioning, giving rise to a broad reference or "normal" range (eg, 12 to 191 U/L). Values in the upper third of the reference range may be abnormal for a small, lightly muscled person, while a very high CK may be "normal" for an athlete after a marathon. CK values of women are normally two thirds of those in men.

After an acute myocardial infarct, the activity of serum CK begins to rise within 6 hours, peaks at 24 hours, and returns to normal within 3 to 4 days. Peak levels of activity may reach values 5 to 10 times greater than normal. Serum CK

Table 10.1 Average Time (Range) of Enzyme Titer Rise Following Myocardial Infarction.*

Iso/Enzyme	Begins to Rise	Peaks	Returns to Normal
CK (sensitive)	4-6 h (2-8 h)	24 h (12-36 h) Values 5-10 x nl	3-4 d (1.5-10 d)
CK-MB (specific)	4 h (2-12 h)	18 h (12-24 h) Present if >5% of total CK	2 d (1.2-3 d)
AST	8 h (2-36 h)	24-48 h (24-48 h)	4 d (3-7 d)
LD	24 h (12-48 h)	3 d (2-4 d) Values 2-3 x nl	8-9 d (7-18 d)
LD-1	24 h (12-48 h)	3 d (1-5 d) LD flip	12 d (7-16 d)

nl = normal test value
* Adapted, with permission, from R. Ravel, *Clinical Laboratory Medicine*. 5th ed. Chicago, Ill: Year Book Medical Publishers; 1989:325.

increases in virtually all cases (nearly 100%) of myocardial infarction and, therefore, is the most sensitive test for detecting acute myocardial infarction. When serum CK fails to increase within the time frame described above, the diagnosis of acute myocardial infarction is excluded in those cases where onset occurred close to the time of hospital admission. However, increased serum CK is not very specific for myocardial infarction because a wide variety of conditions are associated with it, including myocarditis, cardiac contusion, cardiac surgery or catheterization, cerebrovascular accidents, head injuries, encephalitis, delirium tremens, hepatic coma, uremic coma, epileptic attacks, myositis, alcoholic myopathy, muscular dystrophy, surgery involving skeletal muscle, and extreme muscle exertion. In addition, hyperkalemia, hypothyroidism, and hyperthyroidism are associated with elevated levels of CK because of the effects these disorders have on skeletal muscle. Intramuscular injections cause a mild increase in total CK. Other conditions that occasionally are associated with elevated levels of CK are pulmonary disorders, including pulmonary edema and infarction, and carcinomatosis. For reasons unknown, healthy newborns have elevated levels of CK for the first 3 days of life.

Creatine Kinase Isoenzymes

The CK molecule is a dimer composed of either, or both, of two subunits: M (muscle-type) or B (brain-type). Consequently, there are three CK isoenzymes: BB, MB, and MM. CK-BB is found predominantly in brain and lung with lesser amounts in smooth muscle (eg, uterus, gastrointestinal tract). CK-MM occurs in skeletal muscle and myocardium, whereas CK-MB is found predominantly in myocardium and in trace amounts in skeletal muscle and other tissues. The tissues that are major sources of CK and the proportions of CK isoenzymes found in them are as follows: myocardium, 60% MM and 40% MB; skeletal muscle, 98% MM and 2% MB; and brain, 90% BB and 10% MM. Techniques for fractionation of isoenzymes include column chromatography, electrophoresis, immunoinhibition, and enzyme immunoassays. The immunoassays are superior to the other procedures because of their enhanced sensitivity and effective quantitation of the isoenzymes. However, electrophoresis permits visualization of the different CK isoenzymes. Sera rarely contain variant CK molecules, such as macro-CK (a complex of the BB isoenzyme and alpha globulin) and mitochondrial CK. These variant enzymes can produce false-positive results for CK-MB, particularly when immunoinhibition assays are employed. The newer enzyme immunoassays have corrected this problem.

Normal serum CK is composed almost entirely of CK-MM, and elevations over normal are due to skeletal muscle disorders. The accumulation of CK-BB in serum is uncommon but may occur in postpartum patients, and with severe shock, biliary atresia, and carcinomatosis. Smooth muscle is the most likely source of CK-BB in these situations. Paradoxically, with brain lesions the levels of serum CK-MM increase but those of serum CK-BB do not.

Because CK-MB is found almost exclusively in myocardium, the presence of CK-MB in serum is highly specific for myocardial damage. Following myocardial infarction, CK-MM and CK-MB are released into circulation and mixed with the CK-MM normally present. The presence, not the amount, of CK-MB in the serum is more useful for diagnostic purposes. However, quantitative analysis can provide useful information, since the percentage of CK-MB is generally greater than 5% of the total CK in cases of acute myocardial infarction, whereas smaller amounts of CK-MB may occur with other conditions.

CK-MB appears in serum about 4 hours after the onset of an acute myocardial infarct, peaks at 18 hours, and disappears after 2 days, 1 day sooner than the time it takes for levels of total serum CK to return to normal. During this time, serum CK-MB is present in virtually all patients with myocardial infarction. Therefore, the diagnosis of myocardial infarction can be excluded when serum CK-MB is absent during the first 48 hours after the onset of chest pain. Conversely, measurements of serum CK-MB at 48 hours after the onset of chest pain or later are unreliable for either establishing or excluding a diagnosis of myocardial infarction. When serum CK-MB is detected more than 2 to 3 days after the onset of a clinical episode, either the original infarct has extended or a new infarct has developed. Accelerated release of CK-MB and early peaking of serum CK-MB indicate successful coronary reperfusion in patients receiving thrombolytic therapy for a coronary occlusion occurring with an acute myocardial infarction.

The presence of CK-MB in serum is a sensitive and specific marker for acute myocardial infarction, having excellent predictive value. However, the presence of CK-MB is not specific solely for myocardial infarction because it can be found in the sera of patients with other conditions, such as myocarditis, cardiac contusions, cardiac catheterization, electroshock cardioversion, and cardiac surgery. However, the level of CK-MB is minimally elevated (<5% of total) in the absence of a myocardial infarction. Some patients with a clinical diagnosis of severe angina pectoris or coronary insufficiency have small but significant amounts of serum CK-MB and slight increases in serum total CK. These findings raise the question of whether ischemia occurring without infarction can elevate serum CK levels. Clinicopathological studies suggest that patients with severe angina pectoris often have small, patchy areas of myocardial necrosis that likely are responsible for the elevated levels of serum CK. When disorders involving skeletal muscle lead to marked increases in total CK, a small amount of CK-MB may be found in serum along with large amounts of CK-MM. In these instances, serum CK-MB is usually less than 5% of total serum CK. However, when injured skeletal muscle is actively regenerating, the level of CK-MB may be significantly elevated due to altered expression of isoenzymes in the regenerating muscle. This factor explains why increased CK-MB occurs with increased total CK in early stages of muscular dystrophy. Serum CK-MB also may be found in the blood for several days after extreme physical exertion, such as occurs in marathon runners, and this change also appears to be related to the repair of injured muscle.

Lactate Dehydrogenase

LD catalyzes the reversible oxidation of lactate to pyruvate. LD is found in cardiac muscle, skeletal muscle, liver, lung, kidney, and erythrocytes and their bone marrow precursors. The level of LD is greatly influenced by accidental hemolysis of blood samples, so quality control must be exercised to avoid this problem. A typical reference range for serum LD level is 83 to 200 U/L, but the reference range varies according to the assay system employed.

LD is localized in cell organelles rather than cytosol and escapes more slowly than CK from necrotic cells. LD activity is evident in serum about 24 hours after the onset of an acute myocardial infarct, peaks at approximately 3 days, and returns to baseline values within 8 to 9 days. This activity is increased in more than 90% of patients who have had a myocardial infarction, and the levels peak usually at two to three times the normal values.

Because of the widespread distribution of LD, elevated levels of LD occur in a variety of conditions, making the measurement of total LD a nonspecific test for myocardial infarction. Elevations are seen in myocarditis, pericarditis, cardiac surgery, shock, congestive heart failure, liver disease, pulmonary infarction, hypoxemia, carcinomatosis, hypothyroidism, delirium tremens, skeletal muscle injury (including muscular dystrophy), megaloblastic anemia, hemolytic anemia, leukemias, and myeloproliferative diseases.

Lactate Dehydrogenase Isoenzymes

More specific information regarding myocardial infarction can be obtained by analyzing LD isoenzymes. Each LD molecule has four subunits of the H or M type. Five LD isoenzymes are readily identified by electrophoresis: LD-1 (composed of four H subunits [H4]) and LD-2 (H3M) are present mainly in myocardium, kidney, and erythrocytes. LD-3 (H2M2) is found mainly in lung. LD-4 (HM3) and LD-5 (M4) are present primarily in skeletal muscle and liver. Normal activity of serum LD derives principally from erythrocytes and is composed predominantly of LD-2 with smaller amounts of LD-1 (LD-1 to LD-2 ratio of approximately 2:3).

An increase predominantly in LD-4 and LD-5 indicates hepatocellular necrosis or skeletal muscle damage. Injury to skeletal muscle causes greater increases in levels of LD, particularly of LD-5, than does hepatocellular necrosis. Pulmonary embolization usually causes an increase in LD-3, although increases in any of the other isoenzymes or no changes at all may occur. Nonselective increases in all of the isoenzymes occur in cases of shock, congestive heart failure, and carcinomatosis.

With myocardial infarction, there is a proportionally greater increase in LD-1 than in the other isoenzymes. This increase can be detected and monitored in several ways. When LD-1 increases to an extent sufficiently greater than LD-2, a level of serum LD-1 higher than that of LD-2 occurs along with reversal of the normal LD-1 to LD-2 ratio, a phenomenon known as the "LD flip." The significance of an LD flip is equivocal without a concurrent increase in total LD. LD-1 can be measured selectively after it is separated from the other isoenzymes by immunologic or chemical methods and the LD-1 to total LD ratio then determined. Typical reference values are 30 to 80 U/L for LD-1 and less than 40% for the LD-1 to total LD ratio.

The LD flip, which occurs after CK-MB is detected in serum, is detected in 80% of patients within 48 hours of onset of an acute myocardial infarction. Thereafter, the percentage of patients with an LD flip decreases to less than 50% by 7 days. The LD-1 level alone is more sensitive, but less specific, for myocardial infarction when compared with the LD flip. The most sensitive and specific marker is the LD-1 to total LD ratio. An increased LD-1 to total LD ratio is frequently seen in cases of acute myocardial infarction within 12 hours of onset, is positive in over 90% of patients within 48 hours, and persists for several days. However, tests for the LD isoenzymes are not specific for myocardial infarction; they also may be positive in cases of acute renal infarct, megaloblastic anemia, and hemolytic anemia.

Aspartate Aminotransferase

AST catalyzes a reversible reaction involving the interconversion of L-aspartate + α-ketoglutarate to oxaloacetate + L-glutamate. AST, known previously as serum glutamic-oxaloacetic transaminase (SGOT), occurs in many tissues, including myocardium, liver, skeletal muscle, kidney, pancreas, and lung. Levels of serum AST (normal range, 5-35 U/L) become elevated 8 to 12 hours after myocardial infarction, peak at 24 to 48 hours after infarction, and return to normal within 3 to 7 days.

An elevation in serum AST levels is a sensitive indicator for myocardial infarction, with over 90% of cases having positive results, but it has low specificity because serum AST levels are elevated in many conditions. An increase in AST is especially common with hepatocellular injury, including hepatic congestion and necrosis, conditions that often occur in patients with acute myocardial infarction. Measurement of AST is now regarded as a secondary test for myocardial infarction and is used only if the more specific tests are not available.

Recent Developments

In recent years, new approaches to assess myocardial damage have been suggested but not consistently adopted. Advocates of myosin light chains as markers for myocardial injury initially reported absolute specificity of this marker for myocardial origin. Further documentation of the marker and the opportunity to challenge these assertions has been stalled by lack of availability of the reagents. Consequently, the original work has not been corroborated. On the other hand, commercial production of the reagents for the isoforms of CK-MM and CK-MB are proliferating. These analytical approaches attempt to identify variants of the native CK isoenzymes, which differ by virtue of loss of a single lysine amino acid from the carboxy-terminal end of the enzyme, resulting in both electrophoretic and immunologically recognizable differences. The assays represent increased expense and difficulty and are not routinely recommended at this time because the major claim or advantage is a minimal shortening of the time to earliest diagnosis. This is not a proportionately valuable clinical gain to be sufficiently cost-effective.

Studies of troponin-T are generating sufficient evidence to anticipate that this marker, utilizing an antibody truly specific for a myocardial form of troponin, will provide the organ specificity to replace CK and LD as the primary marker of myocardial injury. Fulfillment of this promise awaits commercial production, which has been initiated. This marker has the advantage of appearing slightly earlier than CK, rising to a higher level, and remaining elevated for as long as 2 weeks after a transmural infarction. We await its development and availability with eagerness.

References

Galen RS. The enzyme diagnosis of myocardial infarction. *Hum Pathol.* 1975;6:141-155.

Katus HA. Enzyme linked immuno assay of cardiac troponin T for the detection of acute myocardial infarction in patients. *J Mol Cell Cardiol.* 1989;21:1349-1353.

Lee TH, Goldman L. Serum enzyme assays in the diagnosis of acute myocardial infarction: recommendations based on a quantitative analysis. *Ann Intern Med.* 1986;105:221-233.

Lott JA. Serum enzyme determinations in the diagnosis of acute myocardial infarction: an update. *Hum Pathol.* 1984;15:706-716.

Poliner LR, Buja LM, Parkey RW, et al. Clinicopathologic findings in 52 patients studied by technetium-99m stannous pyrophosphate myocardial scintigraphy. *Circulation.* 1979;59:257-267.

Ravel R. *Clinical Laboratory Medicine.* 5th ed. Chicago, Ill: Year Book Medical Publishers; 1989:320-328.

Warhol MJ, Seigel AJ, Evans WJ, et al. Skeletal muscle injury and repair in marathon runners after competition. *Am J Pathol.* 1985;118:331-339.

Weidner W. Laboratory diagnosis of acute myocardial infarct: usefulness of determination of lactate dehydrogenase (LDH)-1 level and of ratio of LDH-1 to total LDH. *Arch Pathol Lab Med.* 1982;106:375-377.

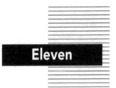

Eleven

Plasma Lipoproteins

Key Points

1. Triglycerides and cholesterol, the major lipids of the blood, are transported in lipoproteins. Very-low-density lipoprotein (VLDL) and low-density lipoprotein (LDL) are primarily responsible for the delivery of triglyceride and cholesterol, respectively, to peripheral tissues. High-density lipoprotein (HDL) is involved in the return transport of cholesterol to the liver for excretion.

2. Hyperlipidemia may result from primary and secondary disorders of lipoproteins. Primary hyperlipoproteinemias may reflect single gene defects or multifactorial disorders. The single gene defects are familial hypercholesterolemia, familial hyperlipidemia (familial combined hyperlipidemia), and familial dysbetalipoproteinemia (broad-ß disease). The multifactorial disorders are polygenic hypercholesterolemia and sporadic hypertriglyceridemia. The secondary hyperlipoproteinemias are associated with a wide variety of conditions.

3. Evaluation of a suspected lipid disorder is based on measurement of total cholesterol and triglycerides in blood. HDL cholesterol also can be easily measured. The amount of LDL cholesterol is then estimated by the Friedewald formula as follows:
   LDL cholesterol = total cholesterol − (HDL cholesterol + [triglyceride/5])

4. In general, the more cholesterol carried in LDL and the less carried in HDL the greater the risk of cardiovascular disease; conversely, the less cholesterol carried in LDL and the more carried in HDL, the lower the risk.

5. The National Cholesterol Education Program (NCEP) recommends screening for risk of cardiovascular disease using total serum cholesterol; decisions regarding therapy should be made on the basis of calculated LDL cholesterol levels. The NCEP's categories for total cholesterol are: desirable, lower than 5.15 mmol/L (200 mg/dL); borderline-high, 5.15 to 6.20 mmol/L (200-239 mg/dL); and high, 6.20 mmol/L (240 mg/dL) or higher.

Table 11.1 The Major Lipoprotein Groups.

Electrophoretic Migration	Density on Ultracentrifugation	Composition	Major Apoproteins
α	High density (HDL)	15% C, 5% TG, 30% PL, 50% P	AI, AII, C, D
β	Low density (LDL)	45% C, 10% TG 20% PL, 25% P	B-100
Pre-β	Very low density (VLDL)	15% C, 60% TG 15% PL, 10% P	B-100, C, E
Chylomicrons*	Extremely low density	5% C, 85% TG, 5% PL, 2% P	B-48, C, E

C = cholesterol; TG = triglyceride; PL = phospholipid; P = protein
* Do not migrate during electrophoresis.

Background

Disorders of blood lipids and lipoproteins are important clinically because of their association with accelerated atherosclerotic cardiovascular disease, particularly coronary heart disease. The major lipids of the blood are triglycerides and cholesterol. Because of their insolubility in an aqueous environment, these lipids are transported in lipoproteins that are soluble macromolecular complexes containing both lipid and protein. All lipoproteins are composed of triglyceride, cholesterol, phospholipid, and polypeptide (apoprotein) in proportions that are characteristic for each type. Apo(lipo)proteins contain moieties that bind selectively to different cell receptors, thereby initiating the cellular metabolism of the lipoproteins, an important function. Free fatty acids are bound to albumin when transported in the blood.

Lipoproteins can be readily separated and characterized by electrophoresis and, more quantitatively, by ultracentrifugation. Based on the different densities they exhibit when sedimented (floatation) during ultracentrifugation, lipoproteins are distinguished as HDLs, LDLs, VLDLs, and extremely low-density lipoproteins (the chylomicrons). Lipoproteins are classified further according to their electrophoretic mobility, being designated by the plasma protein fraction with which they migrate—alpha-lipoproteins, beta-lipoproteins, and prebeta-lipoproteins—except for the chylomicrons, which do not migrate but remain at the point of origin. The current nomenclature of the lipoproteins, their chemical compositions, and their major apoproteins appear in Table 11.1.

Lipoprotein metabolism can be summarized simply as follows. Chylomicrons are involved in the transport of exogenously derived lipids and the other lipoproteins are involved in the transport of endogenously derived lipids. VLDL is synthesized in the liver, with a portion of it being converted to LDL. VLDL and LDL are primarily responsible for the delivery of triglyceride and cholesterol, respectively, to peripheral tissues. HDL is involved in the return transport of cholesterol to the liver for excretion.

Table 11.2 The Hyperlipoproteinemias.*

Electrophoretic Lipoprotein Phenotype (Prevalence)	Elevated Lipoproteins	Plasma Cholesterol	Plasma Triglyceride	Appearance of Chilled Plasma	Primary Disorders	Secondary Disorders
Type I (rare)	Chylomicrons	Normal or slightly elevated	Markedly elevated	Creamy layer above clear or slightly turbid infranate	Familial lipoprotein lipase deficiency	SLE; not associated with atherosclerosis
Type IIa (moderately common)	LDL	Moderately elevated	Normal	Clear	Familial hypercholesterolemia; familial combined hyperlipidemia; polygenic hypercholesterolemia	Nephrotic syndrome; hypothyroidism
Type IIb (common)	LDL; VLDL	Moderately elevated	Slightly elevated	Slight to moderate turbidity	Familial combined hyperlipidemia; polygenic hypercholesterolemia (dietary excess)	Nephrotic syndrome; stress-induced
Type III (rare)	Broad β lipoprotein	Moderately elevated	Moderately to markedly elevated	Turbid or opaque layer above turbid infranate	Familial dysbetalipoproteinemia (broad β disease)	Hypothyroidism; monoclonal gammopathies
Type IV (common)	VLDL	Normal or slightly elevated	Moderately to markedly elevated	Turbid to frankly opaque	Familial (mild) Tangier disease	Diabetes mellitus; alcoholism; uremia; stress; oral contraceptives
Type V (fairly common)	Chylomicrons; VLDL	Moderately elevated	Markedly elevated	Creamy layer over turbid to opaque infranate	Familial combined hyperlipidemia	Alcoholism; oral contraceptives; diabetes mellitus

* Adapted, with permission, from R. J. Havel et al, Lipoproteins and lipid transport. In: P. K. Bondy and L. D. Rosenberg, eds. Metabolic Control and Disease. 8th ed. Philadelphia, Pa: WB Saunders Co; 1980:393–494.

Hyperlipidemia is an increase in blood lipids, ie, in triglyceride or cholesterol, or both. Hyperlipoproteinemia is an increase in the concentration of one or more of the blood lipoproteins, and is almost always accompanied by hyperlipidemia. These disorders of lipoproteins were once classified according to the various patterns obtained by lipoprotein electrophoresis. Later, a more precise classification system based on genetic analysis was derived. The electrophoretic patterns of lipoproteins are now recognized to represent different phenotypes, which include both primary and secondary disorders of lipoproteins. The classification system of hyperlipoproteinemias is outlined in Table 11.2.

Disease States

Primary Hyperlipoproteinemias

Single Gene Disorders. Familial hypercholesterolemia (type IIA, rarely type IIB) is a common autosomal-dominant disorder characterized by elevated levels of LDL cholesterol in the blood. The genetic defect in this disorder results in decreased activity of LDL receptors, leading to elevated levels of LDL in the plasma. Familial hypercholesterolemia manifests as premature coronary atherosclerosis, xanthomas of the skin and tendons, xanthelasma, and arcus corneae. Heterozygous subjects have elevated levels of cholesterol in their plasma from birth, but usually do not develop symptoms until early to middle adulthood. Homozygous subjects, who have much higher levels of cholesterol in their plasma than do heterozygotes, develop xanthomas within the first 6 years of life. Their disease progresses at an accelerated rate and they usually die from complications of coronary heart disease before 20 years of age.

Familial hypertriglyceridemia (type IV) is a common autosomal-dominant disorder characterized by elevated levels of VLDL triglyceride in the blood. Approximately 2 to 3 persons per 1000 are affected by this disorder. The findings in the peripheral blood often are accompanied by the clinical triad of obesity, hyperglycemia, and hyperinsulinemia. The disorder usually does not manifest until adulthood. Persons affected with the disorder usually have premature atherosclerosis; the exact relationship of the lipoprotein abnormality to the vascular disease process is not clear. Xanthomas are not characteristic of the disorder. During exacerbations of their disease, patients may have elevated levels of chylomicrons in the blood and a type V electrophoretic pattern.

Multiple lipoprotein-type hyperlipidemia, or familial combined hyperlipidemia (types IIA, IIB, IV or V), is an autosomal-dominant disorder characterized by elevated levels of cholesterol and/or triglycerides in the blood. An increase in the rate of hepatic secretion of VLDL has been implicated. As with familial hypertriglyceridemia, persons affected usually have premature atherosclerosis and do not develop xanthomas. This disorder is difficult to diagnose with current clinical and laboratory methods.

Familial dysbetalipoproteinemia, or broad-ß disease (type III), is a rare disorder characterized by elevated levels of both cholesterol and triglyceride (to approximately the same extent) in the blood and electrophoretic pattern characterized by a "floating ß" lipoprotein. These abnormal lipoproteins represent remnant-like particles that become more prevalent in the blood because of impaired uptake and metabolism of VLDL in the liver. The basic defect in familial dysbetalipoproteinema is an abnormally structured apoprotein E. Persons affected with the disorder present with tuberous and planar xanthomas and prematurely develop atherosclerosis. Hypothyroidism is known to markedly worsen the symptoms of the disorder.

Multifactorial Disorders. Polygenic hypercholesterolemia (type IIA or IIB) is characterized by elevated levels of LDL cholesterol in the blood. The cholesterol levels vary and are quite sensitive to different environmental factors, such as drugs, diet, alcohol consumption, obesity, and concurrent diseases. Of patients with primary hyperlipoproteinemia and elevated levels of blood cholesterol, 5% are estimated to have familial hypercholesterolemia, 10% to have multiple lipoprotein-type hyperlipidemia, and 85% to have polygenic hypercholesterolemia.

Sporadic hypertriglyceridemia is a disorder characterized by elevated levels of endogenous triglycerides in the blood with or without elevated levels of chylomicrons. The etiology of this disorder apparently is not genetic and it presumably occurs as a result of exogenous factors. Relatives of persons affected with the disorder usually have normal levels of triglyceride in the blood, a characteristic that distinguishes it from familial hypertriglyceridemia.

Secondary Hyperlipoproteinemias

Secondary hyperlipoproteinemias are associated with a variety of conditions. The pathogenic mechanism for some is quite clear, whereas for others it is obscure. Women who are in the third trimester of pregnancy or who have taken oral contraceptives may have elevated levels of VLDL cholesterol in the blood secondary to an estrogen-induced increase in hepatic secretion of VLDL. A variety of drugs, including thiazide diuretics, can produce hyperlipidemia. The nephrotic syndrome often is associated with elevated levels of cholesterol and triglycerides in the blood. The mechanisms in these cases involve a defect in the clearance of VLDL and LDL from the peripheral tissues or overproduction of lipoproteins in the liver in response to hypoalbuminemia. Extrahepatic biliary tract obstruction and primary biliary cirrhosis often are associated with elevated levels of cholesterol in the blood due to impairments in the biliary excretion of, and the enterohepatic circulation of, cholesterol.

Hypothyroidism often is associated with elevated levels of cholesterol in the blood, reflecting decreased metabolic activity, particularly in metabolizing LDL. Patients with Cushing's syndrome may have elevated levels of both cholesterol and triglyceride in the blood due to increased hepatic secretion of VLDL, which subsequently is converted to LDL. Uremic patients often have elevated levels of triglyceride in the blood due to decreased catabolism of VLDL secondary to a reduction in the activity of lipoprotein lipase.

Chronic consumption of large amounts of ethanol often leads to increased levels of triglyceride in the blood. Ethanol inhibits fatty acid oxidation and increases fatty acid synthesis in the liver. Some patients with a history of alcoholism can develop massive hyperlipidemia as a result of impaired catabolism of VLDL, in addition to the other effects ethanol has on lipid metabolism, and are at risk for developing pancreatitis.

Three forms of hypertriglyceridemia can develop in patients with diabetes mellitus. Diabetic patients who are deprived of insulin can develop a marked increase in the levels of triglycerides, chylomicrons, and VLDL in their blood. Diabetic patients with acute ketoacidosis frequently exhibit mild hyperlipidemia with elevated levels of VLDL, but not chylomicrons, in their blood. Even patients whose diabetes is well controlled may exhibit mildly to moderately elevated levels of VLDL triglyceride in their blood. Lipid abnormalities found in diabetic patients are mediated by the effects of insulin deficiency on lipid metabolism. With acute insulin deficiency, increased mobilization of free fatty acid from adipose tissue leads to increased secretion of VLDL in the liver. With chronic insulin deficiency, the activity of lipoprotein lipase decreases, leading to decreased clearance of chylomicrons and VLDL circulating in the blood. In cases of secondary hyperlipoproteinemia, it is important to document a patient's underlying disease because effective treatment of the primary condition usually corrects the hyperlipoproteinemia.

Assays and Their Interpretation

Evaluation of Suspected Lipid or Lipoprotein Disorders
Evaluation of suspected lipid or lipoprotein disorders begins with a complete and detailed history and physical examination.

Family History. Family history is particularly important to help distinguish primary from a secondary process and to assess the patient's risk for developing cardiovascular disease. A laboratory evaluation should include measurements of blood cholesterol and triglyceride. The clinical laboratory's instructions for the collection and transportation of specimens for lipid analysis must be strictly followed for accurate data.

Collection of Samples. Total cholesterol and triglyceride levels can be measured in serum or in plasma. Lipoprotein electrophoresis is best performed on plasma that preferably was obtained from blood anticoagulated with ethylenediaminetetraacetic acid (EDTA). However, because this procedure is not routinely performed, serum is used for screening in most laboratories. Specimens ideally should be transported and stored at 4°C. The serum cholesterol level is affected very little by food intake from a single meal, whereas levels of triglyceride and HDL cholesterol are significantly affected by food intake. Therefore, blood specimens for lipid screening are collected by venipuncture in the morning after overnight fasting of 12 to 14 hours, unless only serum cholesterol is to be measured. Patients to be evaluated should not have experienced a recent gain or loss of weight, or be taking any medications known to affect lipid metabolism. No alcoholic beverages or drugs of any kind should be ingested within 24 hours before the evaluation. Because any illness or prolonged bed rest can lead to lowering of serum cholesterol levels, evaluation should be performed on outpatients rather than inpatients. For patients with a recent myocardial infarction, an evaluation should be delayed 2 to 3 months to allow lipid levels in the blood to return to steady state.

Measurement of Blood Lipids. Total cholesterol can be measured by colorimetric and enzymatic methods, with the former recognized as the reference procedure. The total triglyceride level is measured using assays for the glycerol component. A concerted effort has been made to standardize these assays using national norms and to improve the precision since risk assessment is based on relatively small changes in lipid levels. Values from a given laboratory should be corrected to account for factors unique to the assays employed. For instance, plasma values are slightly lower than serum values for cholesterol (3%) and triglyceride (2%-4%).

A useful adjunct in screening for lipoprotein abnormalities is visual inspection of serum or plasma. Turbidity or lactescence of a fresh specimen suggests an elevated triglyceride level. The specimen should be refrigerated overnight and reexamined. A creamy layer at the top of the refrigerated specimen indicates increased chylomicrons, and lactescence of the infranate indicates increased VLDL. Both abnormalities can be present, indicating elevated levels of both exogenous and endogenous triglycerides. An elevated cholesterol level does not cause turbidity or lactescence of plasma.

To measure the cholesterol contained in different lipoproteins, the lipoproteins must first be separated by ultracentrifugation. This procedure is generally performed only in reference laboratories. However, HDL cholesterol is now more easily measured and is frequently tested. To measure HDL cholesterol, other lipoproteins (the apoprotein B–containing lipoproteins) are separated using a variety of procedures, such as polyanion-divalent cation precipitation, and HDL cholesterol is analyzed in the remaining fraction. Once the HDL cholesterol is measured, LDL cholesterol can then be estimated by the Friedewald formula, as follows:

LDL cholesterol = total cholesterol - (HDL cholesterol + [triglyceride/5])

Triglyceride/5 is an estimate of VLDL cholesterol from the ratio of triglyceride to cholesterol in VLDL. A recent report suggests that triglyceride/6 rather than triglyceride/5 gives a more accurate estimate of LDL cholesterol; however, triglyceride/5 is the current standard. The estimate of VLDL becomes inaccurate when the triglyceride level is greater than 10.35 mmol/L (400 mg/dL).

Screening for Arteriosclerosis Risk

Screening for arteriosclerosis risk is important becuse a strongly positive correlation exists between the LDL level and risk for atherosclerotic disease. Because serum cholesterol is composed mainly of LDL, which is difficult to measure, total cholesterol is used as a substitute for LDL in the initial screening for lipid disorders. An inverse relationship also exists between HDL level and the risk for atherosclerosis. LDL and HDL levels therefore are independent risk factors: In general, the less cholesterol carried in LDL and the more in HDL, the lower the risk of cardiovascular disease. There also is an inverse relationship between HDL and triglyceride levels such that elevated triglyceride levels tend to be associated with low HDL levels. However, triglyceride levels alone do not have strong predictive value for atherosclerosis.

Common problems in screening for lipid disorders have involved documenting the tests most appropriate for screening and determining optimal "normal" values. Epidemiological studies, such as the Framingham study, have established lipid lev-

Table 11.3 Relative Risk of Coronary Heart Disease Based on Laboratory Parameters.*

Relative Risk[†]	Total Serum Cholesterol, mmol/L (mg/dL)	HDL Cholesterol mmol/L (mg/dL)		Total Cholesterol/ HDL Cholesterol Ratio		LDL Cholesterol/ HDL Cholesterol Ratio	
		Male	Female	Male	Female	Male	Female
1/2 Average	3.90 (150)	1.55 (60)	1.80 (70)	3.4	3.3	1	1.5
Average	5.80 (225)	1.15 (45)	1.40 (55)	5	4.4	3.5	3.2
2x Average	6.70 (260)	0.65 (25)	0.90 (35)	10	7	6.3	5
3x Average	7.75 (300)	–	–	24	11	8	6.1

* Adapted from Ravel.
† Based primarily on data from the Framingham Coronary Disease Study.

els associated with the relative risk for atherosclerotic disease in a given population, influenced by the prevalence of this disease in the population (Table 11.3).

Previous recommendations for proper screening of atherosclerotic disease have included age- and sex-related normal values. However, the most authoritative standards currently in use were put forward in 1988 by an expert panel of the NCEP of the National Institutes of Health (NIH). The NCEP recommends that screening be performed using total serum cholesterol and that decisions regarding therapy be made on the basis of calculated LDL cholesterol levels (Table 11.4).

The cutoff points are applied uniformly to adult men and women over 20 years of age. The recommendations are based on epidemiological evidence indicating that the risk for atherosclerotic disease increases steadily as cholesterol increases in the blood, particularly when cholesterol reaches levels above 5.15 mmol/L (200 mg/dL). Patients with cholesterol levels of 5.15 mmol/L (200 mg/dL) or greater should have the value confirmed by repeating the test. Analysis of lipoprotein is recommended for patients with high levels of blood cholesterol and for those with borderline-high levels of blood cholesterol who are at increased risk because of established coronary heart disease or the presence of two other risk factors (ie, male sex, family history of premature coronary heart disease, history of cigarette smoking, hypertension, low level of HDL cholesterol (below 0.90 mmol/L [35 mg/dL]), diabetes mellitus, personal history of cardiovascular disease, or severe obesity). Dietary and/or drug therapy is then based on the level of LDL cholesterol.

There is less consensus about the use of HDL cholesterol for screening and risk assessment. The metabolism of HDL is complex and the mechanism responsible for the protective effect of high levels of HDL has not been adequately defined. However, HDL values are known to be age- and sex-dependent. Total HDL is composed of two major subfractions, HDL-2 and HDL-3, and several minor ones. The protective effect of high levels of HDL is mediated primarily by the level of HDL-2. Exercise and moderate alcohol consumption increase the level of total HDL and, based on the most recent evidence, both also increase the level of HDL-2. The ratio of total cholesterol or LDL cholesterol to HDL

Table 11.4 Criteria of the National Cholesterol Education Program for Identification and Treatment of Patients With Lipid Disorders.*

Category	Total Cholesterol	LDL Cholesterol
Desirable	<5.15 mmol/L (200 mg/dL)	<3.36 mmol/L (130 mg/dL)
Borderline-High	5.15-6.18 mmol/L (200-239 mg/dL)	3.36-4.11 mmol/L (130-159 mg/dL)
High	≥6.20 mmol/L (240 mg/dL)	≥4.14 mmol/L (160mg/dL)

* Patients were classified according to their total cholesterol and treatment was based on the level of LDL cholesterol.

cholesterol provides an index of the joint contributions of the different lipid fractions. However, this ratio should be used with caution in screening for atherosclerotic disease because it may not adequately reflect the independent contributions of the different lipid fractions. Problems with accurately measuring small changes in HDL cholesterol levels and then reproducing the results also complicate the issue. In the NCEP scheme, HDL is not used as a primary parameter; however, a confirmed low level of HDL cholesterol (below 0.90 mmol/L [35 mg/dL]) is considered a major risk factor in assessing risk for coronary heart disease, since the most recent evidence indicates a low HDL level is an independent predictor of disease.

According to an NIH Consensus Conference, a fasting triglyceride value of 2.82 mmol/L (250 mg/dL) represents the upper limit of normal values for adults, while fasting values of 5.66 mmol/L (500 mg/dL) are definitely abnormal.

Analysis of Apoprotein Levels

Analysis of apoprotein levels may provide more precise information about prognosis than the measurement of blood lipids. In particular, low apoprotein A1 (a major component of HDL), high apoprotein B (a major component of LDL), and the apoprotein A1 to apoprotein B ratio are strong predictors of coronary heart disease. The risk for coronary heart disease also is associated with high levels of apolipoprotein(a) in conjunction with lipoprotein(a), a quantitatively minor lipoprotein that appears to promote thrombosis. Assays of apolipoprotein are not yet used routinely in the clinical setting.

Summary

Proper evaluation of a suspected lipid disorder is based on accurate measurements of cholesterol and triglyceride levels in the blood. A lipid disorder can confidently be ruled out if the levels of triglyceride and cholesterol are normal and the sample remains clear after refrigeration. When a primary lipid disorder is suspected, other family members should be evaluated. When a secondary lipid disorder is suspected, an accurate history, a thorough physical examination, and the appropriate laboratory tests will delineate the underlying disease process. Appropriate screening of patients with lipid disorders for risk of cardiovascular disease is based on measurement of total cholesterol and, when indicated, an analysis of the lipoprotein profile is used for treatment decisions. The Lipid Research Clinics Coronary Primary Prevention Trial has provided the strongest evidence that lowering of serum cholesterol levels decreases the risk for coronary heart disease. In this trial, there was a 2% reduction in the risk for coronary heart disease with every 1% reduction in blood cholesterol for hypercholesterolemic subjects.

References

Castelli WP, Garrison RJ, Wilson PWF, et al (The Framingham Study). Incidence of coronary heart disease and lipoprotein cholesterol levels. *JAMA*. 1986;256:2835.

DeLong DM, DeLong ER, Wood PD, et al. A comparison of methods for the estimation of plasma low- and very low-density lipoproteins. *JAMA*. 1986;256:2372-2377.

Durrington PN, Ishola M, Hunt L, et al. Apolipoprotein(a), AI, and B and parental history in men with early onset ischemic heart disease. *Lancet*. 1988;1:1070-1073.

The Expert Panel. Report of the National Cholesterol Education Program Expert Panel on detection, evaluation, and treatment of high blood cholesterol in adults. *Arch Intern Med*. 1988;148:36-69.

Goldstein JL, Brown MS. Familial hypercholesterolemia. In: Stanbury JB, Wyngaarden JB, Fredrickson DS, et al, eds. *The Metabolic Basis of Inherited Disease*. 5th ed. New York, NY: McGraw-Hill Inc; 1983:672-712.

Havel RJ, Goldstein JL, Brown MS. Lipoproteins and lipid transport. In: Bondy PK, Rosenberg LD, eds. *Metabolic Control and Disease*. 8th ed. Philadelphia, Pa: WB Saunders Co; 1980:393-494.

Hoeg JM, Gregg RE, Brewer HB Jr. An approach to the management of hyperlipoproteinemia. *JAMA*. 1986;255:512-521.

Kottke BA, Zindmeister AR, Holmes DR Jr, et al. Apolipoproteins and coronary artery disease. *Mayo Clin Proc*. 1986;61:313-320.

Lipid Research Clinics Program. The Lipid Research Clinics Coronary Primary Prevention Trial results: I and II. *JAMA*. 1984;251:351-374.

Ravel R. *Clinical Laboratory Medicine*. Chicago, Ill: Year Book Medical Publishers; 1989:357-368.

Rifai N. Lipoproteins and apolipoproteins. *Arch Pathol Lab Med*. 1986;110:694-701.

Rimm R, Giovannucci EL, Willett WC, et al. Prospective study of alcohol consumption and risk of coronary disease in men. *Lancet*. 1991;338:464-468.

Stampfer MJ, Sacks FM, Salvini S, et al. A prospective study of cholesterol, apolipoproteins, and the risk of myocardial infarction. *N Engl J Med*. 1991;325:373-381.

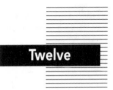

Twelve

Cerebrospinal Fluid

Key Points

1. Cerebrospinal fluid (CSF) is an important body fluid specimen when central nervous system disease arises. It should be examined grossly, microscopically, chemically, and for cellular content.
2. Central nervous system syphilis must always be confirmed by examination of CSF for evidence of antibody production.

Background

CSF is produced by a combination of active transport and ultrafiltration of plasma. After formation in the choroid plexuses of the ventricles and other sites, it exits the ventricular system through the foramina of Luschka and Magendie, circulates over the surface of the cerebral hemispheres and downward over the spinal cord and nerve roots, and is resorbed primarily by arachnoid villi in the dural sinuses. CSF may be examined after lumbar puncture for total and differential cell counts, various chemical determinations (usually total protein and glucose), and microbiological studies including direct examination and cultural isolation of organisms. In addition to these studies, the physician who performs a lumbar puncture can make important observations regarding pressure, color, and consistency (Table 12.1).

Lumbar puncture allows the collection of CSF for analysis. The technique originated with Quincke in 1891. It is indicated in patients who are suspected of having a variety of neurologic conditions—meningitis and other inflammatory disorders of the central nervous system, subarachnoid hemorrhage and other local vascular disturbances, leukemia and other tumors—and as a technique to introduce drugs or radiographic contrast material. Lumbar puncture carries a mortality of 0.3% if the patient has papilledema. In addition, there is some mor-

Table 12.1 Cerebrospinal Fluid Findings.

Disorder	Opening Pressure, mm Hg	Color	Clarity	Total Cell Count, No. of Cells/μL
Normal	70-180	Colorless	Clear	0-5
Bacterial meningitis	200-750+	Faint xan-thochromia	Opalescent or purulent	500-20,000
Tuberculous meningitis	150-750+	Faint xan-thochromia	Opalescent	25-500
Aseptic meningitis	130-750+	May be xan-thochromic	Clear, cloudy or turbid	5-5000
Neurosyphilis	Normal to 300	Colorless	Clear	10-150
Viral meningo-encephalitis	Normal to 450	Colorless	Clear	10-150
Traumatic puncture	Normal or low	Colorless supernatant	Variably bloody; with clot	Variable
Cerebral thrombosis	Normal to 200	Colorless	Clear	0-10
Cerebral hemorrhage	100-1100	Xanthochromic supernatant	Bloody	Variable
Subarachnoid hemorrhage	110-700+	Xanthochromic supernatant	Uniformly bloody	Variable
Brain tumor	150-800+	Occasional xanthochromia	Clear	Normal to 25
Spinal cord tumor	Normal or low	Colorless or xanthochromic	Clear; with clot	Normal to 100
Multiple sclerosis	Normal	Colorless	Clear	Normal to 40

* Increases by approximately 0.01 g/L (1 mg/dL) per year after age 40.

bidity associated with the procedure, primarily postpuncture headache resulting from leakage of CSF out of the subarachnoid space. Precipitation of cerebellar tonsillar herniation in patients with increased intracranial pressure, introduction of infectious agents, or progression of paralysis in patients with spinal cord tumors are more serious complications. Therefore, a lumbar puncture should not be considered an innocuous procedure, and any patient who lacks a clear indication for the examination of CSF should not be subjected to it. Lumbar puncture may be performed as an emergency procedure when a patient is suspected of having meningitis, central nervous system leukemia, or a subarachnoid hemorrhage. Otherwise, lumbar punctures are best scheduled routinely early in the morning when most of the hospital's consultative and support facilities are available. Computed tomographic (CT) or magnetic resonance imaging (MRI) scan of the

Differential Cell Count	Protein g/L (mg/dL)	Glucose mmol/L (mg/dL)	Remarks
Mononuclear cells only	0.15-0.45 (15-45)*	2.8-4.4 (50-80)	—
Neutrophilic pleocytosis	0.50-15.0 (50-1500)	0-2.5 (0-45)	Direct smears and cultures needed
Lymphocytic pleocytosis	0.45-5.0 (45-500)	0-2.5 (0-45)	Direct smears and cultures needed
Mixed or lymphocytic pleocytosis	0.20-2.0+ (20-200+)	Usually normal	Marked changes with brain abscess; note normal glucose
Lymphocytic pleocytosis	0.45-1.5 (45-150)	Usually normal	May vary with activity of disease
Lymphocytic pleocytosis	0.15-1.1 (15-110)	2.8-6.1 (50-110)	Typically, normal glucose values
Erythrocytes predominate	Normal	Normal	Usually less blood in each tube collected
Usually mononuclear	Normal to 1.0 (100)	2.8-5.5 (50-100)	Changes are usually unremarkable
Erythrocytic or mixed pleocytosis	0.20-20.0 (20-2000)	2.8-5.5 (50-100)	Pleocytosis with nonbloody fluids
Erythrocytes predominate	0.20-10.0 (20-1000)	2.8-5.5 (50-100)	Xanthochromia depends on time of puncture
Lymphocytic pleocytosis	0.20-5.0 (20-500)	2.8-5.5+ (50-100+)	Variable findings depending on location
Lymphocytic pleocytosis	0.35-35.0 (35-3500)	2.8-5.5 (50-100)	Usually partial or complete block
Lymphocytic pleocytosis	Normal to 1.30 (130)	2.8-5.0 (50-90)	Immunologic protein tests useful

head should be performed prior to lumbar puncture if an intracranial mass lesion or increased intracranial pressure is suspected. Two or three milliliters of CSF are collected in each of three or four sterile tubes. It is customary to submit a separate tube for each laboratory procedure: cell counts, including what cell types are present, chemistry determinations, and microbiology studies.

Visual Interpretation of Cerebrospinal Fluid

After the clinician has noted the CSF pressure and has considered the condition associated with that pressure, the fluid itself should be assessed visually, noting the presence of blood, and its color, clarity, and clotting potential. Normal CSF is crys-

Table 12.2 Characteristics Distinguishing Traumatic Lumbar Puncture From Subarachnoid Hemorrhage.

Traumatic Lumbar Puncture	Subarachnoid Hemorrhage
Progressively less blood in tubes as collected	Uniformly bloody in all tubes as collected
CSF usually clots on standing	CSF does not clot on standing
Xanthochromia absent	Xanthochromia may be present

tal clear and colorless. Pathological colorations are best appreciated by observing a sample of CSF against a white background and beside a tube of distilled water.

Blood
The presence of blood within CSF may color the fluid red, pink, yellow, or grossly bloody. It is important to distinguish a traumatic puncture from subarachnoid hemorrhage (Table 12.2). Observation of fluid collected sequentially in three separate tubes helps aid in this distinction.

Color
Any specimen of CSF that is not colorless should be centrifuged so a cell button will form. Normally, the resultant supernatant is colorless. A pale pink to pale orange color in the supernatant is termed xanthochromia. Rapid lysis of erythrocytes in the CSF occurs within 1 to 4 hours after these cells enter the subarachnoid space. Because CSF is isosmotic with plasma, the absence in CSF of certain plasma proteins that protect the erythrocytic membrane is postulated as the cause of this lysis. Xanthochromia may appear if normal CSF is not examined within 1 hour of collection.

Orange xanthochromia, usually due to oxyhemoglobin in CSF, is seen in 90% of patients with a subarachnoid hemorrhage, appearing from 2 to 4 hours following the hemorrhage. The typical yellow xanthochromia of bilirubin appears in CSF if the hemorrhage has occurred more than 12 hours before lumbar puncture. Yellow xanthochromia also occurs with increased CSF protein levels and with conjugated or unconjugated hyperbilirubinemia. Other substances that may cause pigmentation of CSF are methemoglobin, melanin pigment in metastatic malignant melanoma, contamination with thimerosal (Merthiolate), and carotene. Xanthochromia occurring in a CSF sample whose total protein content is less than 1.5 g/L and in the absence of jaundice or hypercarotenemia, indicates previous bleeding into the CSF or into adjacent brain or spinal cord tissue.

Clarity
Normal CSF is crystal clear when compared with a tube of distilled water; any turbidity is abnormal. Turbid fluid may result from the presence of erythrocytes (at least 400 cells/µL), leukocytes (at least 200 cells/µL), microorganisms, radiographic contrast material, or epidural fat. If these substances are present, CSF may appear opalescent, milky, or frankly purulent. Usually the degree of turbidity reflects the amount of abnormal substance present. A slight opalescence typically is associated with tuberculous meningitis.

CSF that contains cells in numbers less than those needed to produce turbidity can be detected by the Tyndall effect. Observations of such specimens in direct sunlight viewed against a darker background reveal a characteristic "snowy" or "sparkling" appearance when the specimen tube is lightly tapped.

Clotting

Normal CSF, with very low fibrinogen levels, does not clot. Clotting may occur after a traumatic puncture, with markedly elevated CSF protein levels (usually >10 g/L and often in association with Froin's syndrome [see "Chemistry Determinations" below] or severe meningeal inflammation), or in tuberculous meningitis. Tuberculous meningitis is often associated with the formation of a web-like clot called a pellicle, which appears after the fluid has been refrigerated overnight.

Laboratory Tests

Laboratory tests provide data on cell counts and which cell types are present, chemistry assays (especially protein and glucose), and microbiology.

Cell Counts and Cytology

An erythrocyte count and total and differential leukocyte counts may be performed on CSF. Because of the fragility of these cells in CSF, cell counts must be performed within 1 hour after collection. Normal CSF contains less than five mononuclear leukocytes per microliter. The presence of any number of granulocytes is generally considered to be abnormal. Newborn infants may have normal CSF total leukocyte counts up to 18 to 20 mononuclear cells per microliter. Lymphocytes, monocytes, and other mononuclear cells, such as pia arachnoid cells and ependymal cells, may be identified in CSF. Neutrophilic and eosinophilic leukocytes in the CSF are always abnormal. Erythrocyte counts of the CSF are usually performed to provide a correction figure for the measured protein level. Cytologic centrifugation, microporous membrane filtration, and immunofluorescent techniques aid in the identification of cells in CSF.

A pathological increase in the number of CSF leukocytes is a pleocytosis. Any form of meningeal irritation or inflammation can produce this and the degree will usually reflect the type, duration, and intensity of the causative process. The most common cellular reactions in CSF are neutrophilic, lymphocytic, eosinophilic, and mixed pleocytoses.

A neutrophilic pleocytosis is usually due to meningitis caused by pyogenic microorganisms. Such meningitis may result in CSF leukocyte counts of 1000 to 20,000 cells per microliter, with 90% neutrophils. Rarer causes are early tuberculous or fungal meningitis, early meningovascular syphilis, primary amebic meningoencephalitis, aseptic meningitis, reactions to central nervous system hemorrhage or infarction, repeated lumbar punctures or foreign materials within the subarachnoid space, chronic granulocytic leukemia involving the central nervous system, and chemical meningitis.

A lymphocytic pleocytosis is a predominance of lymphocytes, usually with some plasma cells, in the CSF. Infectious causes of a lymphocytic pleocytosis are viral and syphilitic meningoencephalitis, tuberculous and fungal meningitis, parasitic central nervous system disease, subacute sclerosing panencephalitis, partially treated bacterial meningitis, and bacterial meningitis due to unusual organisms (eg, *Leptospira, Listeria*). Noninfectious causes include multiple sclerosis and other demyelinating disorders, chemical meningitis, sarcoidosis, and vasculitis.

An eosinophilic pleocytosis can occur with any of the infectious disorders responsible for a neutrophilic or a lymphocytic pleocytosis, but it occurs most commonly with central nervous system parasitic diseases or coccidioidomycosis. In addition, rabies vaccination, intrathecal injections of foreign material or protein, bronchial asthma and other allergic disorders, and central nervous system lymphocytic leukemia can be causes.

A mixed pleocytosis shows a variety of cells—neutrophils, lymphocytes, plasma cells, monocytes, and pia arachnoid mesothelial cells. Disorders causing such a mixed population are tuberculous and fungal meningitis, chronic or atypical bacterial meningitis, aseptic meningitis, various types of meningoencephalitis, demyelinating disorders, and ruptured brain abscess.

In addition to these types of pleocytoses, abnormal cells may appear in CSF. Leukemic leukocytes or other neoplastic cells, fungal organisms (especially *Cryptococcus neoformans*), amebae (in association with primary amebic meningoencephalitis), or Mollaret cells (associated with a particular form of recurrent meningitis) can be seen.

Chemistry Determinations

Protein. Protein is always present in CSF, due to a combination of transport across the blood/CSF barrier and synthesis within the central nervous system. The CSF protein concentration varies with age, with normal concentrations of 0.2 to 0.5 g/L in persons 10 to 40 years old and higher concentrations in infants under 3 months of age and in elderly persons. Cisternal and ventricular CSF has a lower total protein concentration than lumbar fluid. Three types of protein determinations are available in most clinical laboratories: semiquantitative "screening" tests (eg, Pándy's test); quantitative turbidometric, colorimetric, or spectrophotometric tests; and complex "fractionation" tests (eg, electrophoresis). In the vast majority of cases, quantitation of the protein concentration is sufficient.

Abnormal CSF total protein concentrations may signify clinical disease. Decreased concentrations are associated with several disorders, the most important of which is leakage of CSF (eg, previous lumbar puncture, CSF rhinorrhea). An increased concentration of CSF protein is the single most important abnormality of this fluid indicating disease. The concentration of CSF protein may be increased following a traumatic lumbar puncture or with any lesions causing injury to cerebral tissue or the blood-brain barrier, increased permeability of the blood/CSF barrier, obstruction to CSF circulation, or increased synthesis of protein in the central nervous system. Conditions commonly associated with increased levels are the meningitides or meningoencephalitides, polyneuritis, brain abscess or parameningeal infections, subarachnoid or intracerebral hemorrhage, degenerative central nervous system diseases, aseptic meningeal reactions, brain and spinal cord tumors, diabetic neuropathy, and various intoxication states. Most of these diseases and conditions are also associated with CSF pleocytosis. Multiple sclerosis, cerebrovascular thrombosis, subdural hematoma, and viral meningoencephalitis are usually associated with only slightly elevated protein concentrations (<1.0 g/L).

Two specific groups of CSF findings are worthy of note. Albuminocytological dissociation is the presence of an increased CSF protein concentration and a normal or nearly normal fluid total cell count. This condition classically is seen with the Guillain-Barré syndrome, but it may also be seen with brain tumors, multiple sclerosis, cerebrovascular thrombosis, subarachnoid block, neurovascular syphilis, polyneuritis, or chronic infections of the central nervous system. Froin's syndrome is the term for CSF changes associated with complete subarachnoid block at or below the level of the foramen magnum. These findings include markedly increased total protein concentrations (often >10 g/L), xanthochromia, moderate pleocytosis, and spontaneous clotting.

The major indication for fractionation measurements of the protein in CSF is multiple sclerosis. Most clinical laboratories are able to concentrate and electrophoretically separate CSF proteins in the same way as serum or urine. This type of electrophoresis does not reveal oligoclonal bands. All of the serum protein fractions, plus an additional "prealbumin" fraction, are demonstrable in CSF. Immunologic measurements of CSF albumin and IgG are also available and are used with serum values to calculate an IgG synthesis rate, which presently is the best test for detecting central nervous system immunoglobulin production. In multiple sclerosis, there is often an increase in CSF IgG levels with prominent oligoclonal IgG bands as the result of an increased immunoglobulin production in areas of demyelination. The increase is variable and multiple determinations on the same patient are frequently necessary. Patients with infectious and degenerative disorders of the central nervous system also may have increased CSF IgG concentrations. Other demyelinating disorders aside from multiple sclerosis may also produce oligoclonal bands of IgG CSF. Nonetheless, 75% to 95% of patients with multiple sclerosis eventually demonstrate these findings. Determination of CSF myelin basic protein is helpful in monitoring the degree of activity of multiple sclerosis or other diseases that destroy myelin.

Glucose. CSF glucose is derived solely from plasma, and its concentration varies with the blood concentration. Normally the CSF glucose concentration is 60% to 80% of the blood concentration. It appears in the CSF by active transport and passive diffusion. Because there is a transport maximum, if the blood glucose concentration is very high (≥44.4 mmol/L [800 mg/dL]), the CSF concentration may be only 30% to 40% of this value. Passive diffusion responds rather slowly to changes in blood glucose concentrations. Changes in the blood glucose level can take 1 to 3 hours to appear as changes in the CSF level. CSF and blood glucose levels should always be obtained simultaneously, if possible, and should be performed at least 3 hours after oral or parenteral intake of glucose-bearing substances, if feasible.

The main pathological finding is a CSF glucose concentration that is lower than normal (ie, <2.2 mmol/L [40 mg/dL]). This situation is termed hypoglycorrhachia and is seen in systemic hypoglycemia, bacterial, fungal, or tuberculous meningitis, meningeal irritation due to neoplasms, subarachnoid hemorrhage, central nervous system involvement by sarcoidosis, some viral meningoencephalitis, and other disorders. Hypoglycorrhachia results from impaired glucose transport and/or increased glucose utilization by central nervous system tissues, leukocytes, or microorganisms. Hypoglycorrhachia is seen in approximately 50% of patients with bacterial meningitis and, if severe, CSF glucose may be unmeasurably low. A few patients with bacterial meningitis have persistent hypoglycorrhachia for up to 10 days following adequate treatment and clinical improvement. An elevated CSF glucose concentration is evidence only of hyperglycemia occurring from 1 to 4 hours prior to lumbar puncture. Testing for CSF glucose is not a reliable means of differentiating CSF rhinorrhea (or otorrhea) from serous drainages. Testing of these drainage fluids for chloride concentrations is probably more accurate.

Chloride. Chloride levels, once a routine determination, are now rarely performed. Many different enzymes have been measured, but none of these measurements have provided specific results referable to a particular disease.

Calcium. Calcium levels parallel those of serum ionized calcium (see Chapter 23).

Electrolyte, pH, pCO_2, and pO_2. These measurements are rare and are indicated in cases of coma or traumatic brain injury.

Glutamine. Glutamine levels have been shown to correlate with the degree of hepatic encephalopathy. Newer methods for measuring blood ammonia levels, however, are easier to perform. Lactic acid levels have been used in the evaluation of meningitis, but their value is controversial.

C-Reactive Protein. C-reactive protein may be useful in distinguishing between bacterial and other forms of meningitis (elevated in bacterial infection). The exact degree of usefulness of this test awaits further clarification. Some investigators have found that the determination of adenosine deaminase is a useful procedure to predict the presence of tuberculous meningitis. This enzyme is produced by T lymphocytes, and thus might be an indicator of any process characterized by cell-mediated immunity. The clinical usefulness of this procedure has not yet been clarified. Should the situation arise where any of these uncommonly performed tests is indicated, it is imperative to consult with the clinical laboratory before lumbar puncture is performed, to ascertain the feasibility of the desired tests.

Microbiological Techniques

Useful microbiological techniques include direct examination of CSF, cultural isolation and identification of any microorganisms present, and identification of antigens by latex particle agglutination (or other immunologic techniques). Examination of a Gram's-stained smear of CSF is the single best test for rapid diagnosis of bacterial meningitis. The sensitivity of this test is reported as 70% to 90%. Staining artifacts and nonviable bacteria can cause false-positive results. The value of this test as a rapid diagnostic procedure, with the therapeutic and prognostic implications of delayed treatment, cannot be overemphasized. Positive identification of microorganisms, however, rests on cultural isolation. If few organisms are present, it may be necessary to centrifuge the fluid and examine the sediment, especially in suspected cases of bacterial meningitis when the cell count is low or when the fluid is not very turbid. If tuberculous meningitis is suspected, one must centrifuge a relatively large volume of CSF and examine the sediment with acid-fast stains. If a pellicle is present within the CSF specimen, it should be carefully examined by direct smear and culture for mycobacteria. The most commonly performed CSF serologic test for syphilis is the VDRL.

In cases of fungal meningitis due to *Cryptococcus neoformans*, a suspension of india ink and CSF may reveal the typical budding, heavily encapsulated microorganisms in approximately 50% of cases. More specialized fungal stains, fungal cultures, and cryptococcal antigen determination are necessary to identify the other patients. Recognition of primary amebic meningoencephalitis can be lifesaving. Patients with this rapidly fatal disease often have motile trophozoites in their CSF which can be seen by direct microscopic examination of a wet mount of the fluid. They may also be seen on Giemsa-stained smears of CSF.

When microbiological studies of CSF from patients with unusual infections are necessary, it is always wise to consult with the clinical microbiology laboratory before lumbar puncture is performed. This will ensure that the appropriate volume of fluid is obtained, that there is no undue delay in processing the specimen, and that appropriate direct examinations and cultures are performed. The most common errors are improper plating of specimens at night and refrigerating specimens of CSF overnight before plating. It is better to wake up a consultant in microbiology at home than to needlessly waste a CSF specimen by incorrect technique.

References

Carozcio JT, Kochwa S, Sacks H, et al. Quantitative cerebrospinal fluid IgG measurements as a marker of disease activity in multiple sclerosis. *Arch Neurol.* 1986;43:1129.

Daniel TM. New approaches to the rapid diagnosis of tuberculous meningitis. *J Infect Dis.* 1987;155:599.

Davis LE, Schmitt JW. Clinical significance of cerebrospinal fluid tests for neurosyphilis. *Ann Neurol.* 1989;25:50.

Gondos B. Millipore filter vs. cytocentrifuge for evaluation of cerebrospinal fluid. *Arch Pathol Lab Med.* 1986;110:687.

Hayward RA, Dye RK. Are polymorphonuclear leukocytes an abnormal finding in cerebrospinal fluid? Results from 225 normal cerebrospinal fluid specimens. *Arch Intern Med.* 1988;148:1623.

Krieg AF, Kjeldsberg CR. Cerebrospinal fluids and other body fluids. In: Henry JB, ed. *Clinical Diagnosis and Management by Laboratory Methods.* 18th ed. Philadelphia, Pa: WB Saunders Co; 1991:445-457.

Livingston AE. The spinal tap. *Ann Intern Med.* 1986;105:464.

Thirteen

Synovial Fluid

Key Points

Synovial fluid examination is indicated to:
1. distinguish between inflammatory, noninflammatory, and hemorrhagic arthritides when other tests are nonconfirmatory.
2. establish the diagnosis of gout vs pseudogout.
3. obtain fluid for culture in septic arthritis.

Background

Joint spaces normally contain small amounts of fluid consisting of a plasma ultra-filtrate that includes hyaluronic acid. Hyaluronic acid, a high-molecular-weight glycosaminoglycan secreted by synovial-lining cells, imparts a relatively high vis-cosity to the synovial fluid. Because the characteristics of synovial fluid change in various diseases, joint aspiration and fluid analysis may aid considerably in making a diagnosis. The three indications for synovial fluid analysis are (1) to distinguish between noninflammatory and inflammatory joint disease (see groups I and IV vs II and III in Table 13.1), (2) to detect and identify crystals in crystal-induced joint disease, and (3) to detect and identify infectious agents in septic arthritis.

Synovial Fluid Examination

First, grossly examine freshly aspirated joint fluid and examine a wet coverslipped slide preparation under the microscope for crystals and cells. If crystals are present they should be examined by compensated polarized light microscopy so the type of crystal can be specifically identified. Finally, one should determine the white blood cell concentration. When indicated, Gram's stain and culture should be performed.

Table 13.1 Differential Diagnosis by Joint Fluid Groups. *

Group I (Noninflammatory)	Group II (Inflammatory)	Group III (Septic)	Group IV (Hemorrhagic)
Osteoporosis	Rheumatoid arthritis	Bacterial infections	Hemophilia or other hemorrhagic diathesis
Trauma†	Acute crystal-induced synovitis (gout & pseudogout)		Trauma with or without fracture
Osteochondritis dissecans	Reiter's syndrome		Neuropathic arthropathy
Osteochondromatosis	Ankylosing spondylitis		Pigmented villonodular synovitis
Neuropathic arthropathy†	Psoriatic arthritis		Synovioma
Subsiding or early inflammation	Arthritis accompanying ulcerative colitis and regional enteritis		Hemangioma and other benign neoplasms
Hypertrophic osteoarthropathy	Rheumatic fever‡		
Pigmented villonodular synovitis†	Systemic lupus erythematosus‡		
	Progressive systemic sclerosis (scleroderma)‡		

* Adapted from R. Gatter and H. R. Schumacher, *A Practical Handbook of Joint Fluid Analysis.* 2nd ed. Philadelphia, Pa: Lea & Febiger; 1991.
† May be hemorrhagic.
‡ Groups I or II.

Examination of synovial fluid permits classification of joint disease into four general categories, as seen in Table 13.1. If blood is present in the fluid, consider a diagnosis from group IV in that table. Other findings one would expect when examining joint fluid from normal and diseased joints are given in Table 13.2.

Gross Examination

Gross examination of synovial fluid includes evaluation of volume, clarity/turbidity, color, and viscosity. Grossly detectable blood indicates hemorrhagic arthritis and a red blood cell count adds little to the gross observation. The normal amount of synovial fluid varies with different joints. For example, a volume of fluid greater than 3.5 mL is abnormal for the knee. Viscosity is best determined by slowly expressing the fluid a drop at a time from the syringe after removal of the needle. A drop stringing 5 cm or more is indicative of high viscosity, such as is found in normal and noninflammatory (group I) fluids. Decreased viscosity is related to decreased synthesis of synovial fluid hyaluronic acid, synthesis of abnormally short hyaluronic acid chains, and/or dilution as may occur in acute trauma.

Light Microscopic Examination

Light microscopic examination of a wet preparation for crystals and white blood cell counts and differentials must be performed on synovial fluid that has been anticoagulated with either sodium (not lithium) heparin or ethylenediaminetetraacetic acid (EDTA). Other anticoagulants will produce crystalline artifacts. The more intense the joint inflammation, the higher the total cell count and the greater the percentage of neutrophils. Bacterial arthritis should be the first diagnostic consideration when the total cell count approaches 100,000 cells/μL and

Table 13.2 Examination of Joint Fluid.*

Measure	Normal	Group I (Noninflammatory)	Group II (Inflammatory)	Group III (Septic)
Gross examination				
Volume (mL) (knee)	< 3.5	> 3.5	> 3.5	> 3.5
Clarity	Transparent	Transparent	Translucent-opaque	Opaque
Color	Clear	Yellow	Yellow to opalescent	Yellow to green
Viscosity	Very high	High	Low	Variable
WBC, x 10^9/L (per cu mm)	< 0.2 (200)	0.2-2.0 (200-2000)	2.0-100 (2000-100,000)	> 50 (50,000); usually > 100 (100,000)[†]
Polymorphonuclear leukocytes (%)	< 0.25 (25)	< 0.25 (25)	> 0.50 (50)	> 0.75 (75)[†]
Culture	Negative	Negative	Negative	Often positive

* Adapted from R. Gatter and H. R. Schumacher, *A Practical Handbook of Joint Fluid Analysis.* 2nd ed. Philadelphia, Pa: Lea & Febiger; 1991.
† Lower with infections caused by partially treated or low-virulence organisms.

there is a shift to the left (or an increase in immature neutrophilic forms) on the smear. Fluid should be sent to the microbiology laboratory for culture in any suspected infectious arthritis.

Compensated Polarized Light Microscopic Examination

Compensated polarized light microscopic examination of a wet preparation of synovial fluid permits detection of microcrystals. This technique accurately distinguishes the strongly negative birefringence of monosodium urate needles found in gout from the weakly positive birefringence of the rods and rhomboid crystals of calcium pyrophosphate found in pseudogout. This distinction requires a good microscope and a microscopist knowledgeable in its use. The physician should be certain that this study is done properly in the laboratory in which the sample is analyzed, because the decision as to whether the patient has gout or pseudogout, and thus what treatment should be undertaken, depends on this analysis.

Other analyses of synovial fluid such as protein, glucose, complement, and a mucin clot test, although used by some, are presently believed to be of limited value.

References

Gatter R, Schumacher HR. *A Practical Handbook of Joint Fluid Analysis.* 2nd ed. Philadelphia, Pa: Lea & Febiger; 1984.

Hasselbacher P. Arthrocentesis and synovial fluid analysis. In: Schumacher HR Jr, ed. *Primer on the Rheumatic Diseases.* 9th ed. Atlanta, Ga: Arthritis Foundation; 1988.

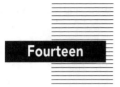

Fourteen

Connective Tissue Disease Tests

Key Points

1. A fluorescent antinuclear antibody (ANA) test should be ordered in all cases of a suspected connective tissue disease; it is most sensitive for systemic lupus erythematosus (SLE) and mixed connective tissue disease.
2. The presence of deoxyribonucleic acid (DNA) and/or Sm antibodies strongly indicates the presence of SLE.
3. High titers of rheumatoid factors suggest rheumatoid arthritis, but a positive rheumatoid factor test is neither sensitive nor specific for rheumatoid arthritis.
4. Tests for complement levels are useful in the diagnosis and follow-up of SLE, a limited number of immune complex–mediated diseases, and in suspected congenital deficiencies (a rare occurrence).

Background

The connective tissue diseases manifest autoimmune tissue injury, specifically to joints, skin, subcutaneous tissue, and various internal organs. They are systemic diseases with overlapping clinical symptoms and signs. Many of the laboratory tests used to diagnose these diseases depend on identifying autoantibodies that develop in the patient (some of which have pathogenetic significance), which are useful markers for the disease. Included in this category of diseases are SLE, rheumatoid arthritis, scleroderma, Sjögren's syndrome, polymyositis-dermato-myositis, and mixed connective tissue disease.

Antinuclear Antibody Tests

Four commonly utilized tests in the diagnosis of connective tissue diseases are the fluorescent ANA test, the anti–double-stranded DNA (dsDNA) test, the LE cell prep, and the tests for antibodies to various saline extractable nuclear antigens (ENAs).

Fluorescence Test for Antinuclear Antibodies

The fluorescent ANA test is positive in at least 95% of patients with SLE. Although this test is sensitive for SLE and is therefore a useful screening test, it is not specific.

About 5% of normal individuals have low titers of these antibodies. The incidence increases with age such that nearly 15% of people over age 60 years have the antibody. The fluorescent ANA test is also positive in a much lower incidence of diverse diseases, but is often positive in a number of other connective tissue diseases, including Sjögren's syndrome (60%-70% of patients), scleroderma (60%-70%), rheumatoid arthritis (30%-40%), and polymyositis (20%-30%). Antibodies to many nuclear proteins—histones, proteins associated with small nuclear ribonucleic acids (RNAs) (UI-RNP and Sm antigen), dsDNA, nucleolar proteins, and centromeric proteins—may produce a positive ANA test result. It is important to understand the overlapping of test results in different connective tissue diseases so that the most precise diagnosis can be made.

The pattern of nuclear fluorescence suggests the type of antibody present in the patient's serum. For instance, dsDNA antibodies may produce a nuclear circumferential or "peripheral" pattern, whereas antibodies to antigens in the nucleolus occur in 60% of patients with scleroderma and appear as a nucleolar fluorescence pattern in the ANA test. This latter pattern also occurs in a low percent of patients with SLE. A homogeneous nuclear fluorescence reflects antibodies to histones but may also occur in patients with dsDNA antibodies. Speckled nuclear fluorescence reflects antibodies to UI-RNP or Sm antigens as well as to other nuclear antigens and is always present in mixed connective tissue disease. Centromere antibodies produce a distinct pattern of 23 paired dots per nucleus and are present in 60% of patients with the CREST syndrome, a form of scleroderma with a more favorable prognosis. In patients with SLE, the most common ANA patterns are homogeneous or speckled. Indeed, because of the multiplicity of autoantibodies present in these patients, combinations of patterns are frequent.

Antibodies to Double-Stranded DNA

Antibodies to dsDNA have a high specificity for SLE. In addition, high levels of anti-dsDNA correlate with active lupus nephritis, and disease remissions are associated with a fall in antibody levels. It should be noted that dsDNA antibodies are often referred to simply as DNA antibodies. However, antibodies to single-stranded DNA occur widely in other collagen vascular diseases. Thus, the laboratory test must distinguish between dsDNA and single-stranded DNA antibodies. The most common test for dsDNA antibodies uses indirect immunofluorescence and the organism *Crithidia luciliae*, a blood flagellate, as the source of antigen. The organism's kinetoplast is a cytoplasmic organelle containing large amounts of dsDNA that binds dsDNA antibodies in the patient's serum. Utilizing the *Crithidia luciliae* assay, 50% to 60% of patients with SLE are positive for anti-dsDNA. Normal individuals and patients with other collagen-vascular diseases are almost always negative. Occasionally, an elevated level of histone

Table 14.1 Autoantibody Test Usage Summary.

Antinuclear Antibody
+   High titers suggest SLE, scleroderma, or mixed connective tissue disease (MCTD). Low titers occur in some SLE patients, particularly in less active stages of their disease, are common in other connective tissue diseases, and occur in 5% of normal individuals.

Anti-dsDNA
+   Highly suggestive of SLE and indicates probable active nephritis.
-        Negative in 40%-50% of patients with SLE.

LE Cell Test
+   May help confirm clinical diagnosis of SLE, but not diagnostic of SLE.
-        May be negative in 30% or more of patients with SLE.

Anti–Extractable Nuclear Antigens
  Anti–UI-RNP
+   Present in >95% MCTD, 40% of SLE.
-        Rules out MCTD.
  Anti-Sm
+   Present in 25%-30% of patients with SLE; rare in other connective tissue diseases. Thus, high specificity but poor sensitivity for SLE.
  Anti–SS-B
+   Suggestive of Sjögren's syndrome (present in 60% of cases of primary Sjögren's), but also present in 15% of patients with SLE.
  Anti–SS-A
+   Present in 70% of patients with subacute cutaneous lupus erythematosus, 60%-70% of patients with Sjögren's syndrome, and 20%-30% of patients with SLE. High incidence in infants with neonatal lupus and congenital heart block (and in their mothers).

---

antibodies will give a false-positive dsDNA test by the *Crithidia* assay. In addition to being present in many SLE patients, histone antibodies also occur in high titer in nearly all patients with drug-induced SLE. However, in contrast to classical SLE, in drug-induced SLE dsDNA antibodies are absent. Thus, in suspected drug-induced LEs with a positive ANA, histone and dsDNA antibody tests should be ordered.

LE Bodies and LE Cells
ANAs specific for histones are responsible for LE bodies and LE cells. A positive LE cell test occurs in 50% to 70% of SLE patients with active disease. A positive test may be present in other diseases such as rheumatoid arthritis, but the incidence is much less frequent. The LE cell preparation is much less sensitive than the ANA test and more time-consuming, and many experts consider it unnecessary if a fluorescent ANA test is available.

Antibodies to Extractable Nuclear Antigens
Detection of antibodies to various ENAs is of clinical utility, especially those to UI-RNP (often referred to simply as RNP), Sm, SS-B (sometimes referred to as La), and SS-A (Ro). Antibodies to these antigens are often determined by the Ouchterlony double-immunodiffusion techniques, although enzyme immunoassays are becoming more widely used. The sensitivity of these latter tests is greater, and thus it is likely the specificity is somewhat less. The significance of antibodies to ENAs is summarized in Table 14.1.

Antiphospholipid (Cardiolipin) Antibodies

About 15% of patients with SLE have positive nontreponemal antibody tests, indicating that they have antibodies to cardiolipin antigens. Measurement of cardiolipin antibodies with a more sensitive technique (enzyme immunoassays) has allowed the detection of these antibodies in over 60% of SLE patients. The antibodies react with negatively charged phospholipids and are related to the "lupus anticoagulant," which may cause a prolonged partial thromboplastin time. The presence of antiphospholipid antibodies of the IgG (and/or perhaps IgA) class correlates with three "cardiolipin antibody" syndromes: thrombocytopenia, recurrent abortion, and unexplained thrombotic states (the in vitro anticoagulant activities notwithstanding). Thus, antiphospholipid antibodies are a useful marker for these three syndromes, although it is not yet clear what their role is in causing disease. A significant problem involves the standardization of both the lupus anticoagulant and immunoenzyme tests. Nevertheless, if reliable laboratories perform both tests, the enzyme immunoassay is the more sensitive test for antiphospholipid antibodies, and a positive lupus anticoagulant test is the one more likely to predict presence or development of a cardiolipin antibody syndrome.

Rheumatoid Factors

Rheumatoid factors are antibodies specific for the Fc portion of IgG. Rheumatoid factors may belong to any immunoglobulin class or isotype. They are present in the serum of 60% to 85% of patients with rheumatoid arthritis, 10% of children with juvenile rheumatoid arthritis, over 90% of patients with mixed cryoglobulinemia and Sjögren's syndrome, 20% to 50% of patients with SLE, 25% of patients with scleroderma and dermatomyositis, but only 10% of patients with psoriatic arthritis, ankylosing spondylitis, and arthritis associated with enteritis syndromes. Patients with acute septic arthritis and osteoarthritis have rheumatoid factors in an incidence no higher than the normal population. Very high titers of rheumatoid factor have a high predictive value for rheumatoid arthritis.

The stimulus for rheumatoid factor production is chronic antigenic stimulation. Patients with extensive prophylactic immunizations, repeated blood transfusions, or chronic infections such as subacute bacterial endocarditis, leprosy, kala azar, or viral hepatitis often develop rheumatoid factors. When the infection clears, rheumatoid factors disappear from the serum. Rheumatoid factors are present in 5% of the normal population, and usually in low titers. Up to 36% of aged individuals may have low titer rheumatoid factors.

The most common rheumatoid factor test utilizes human gamma globulin–coated latex particles as the antigen. This test is used as a screening test, and serial dilutions of serum are made to quantitate the amount of antibody present. The latex agglutination test is considered positive when a positive reaction occurs at a serum dilution of 1:160 or higher. A rate nephelometric test for rheumatoid factor utilizing aggregated human gamma globulin as the antigen is performed in many centers. Values are expressed in international units per milliliter, and normal values are less than 30 IU/mL.

Table 14.2 Levels of Complement in Aquired Human Diseases.*

Disease	C4	C3
Bacterial endocarditis with nephritis	↓	↓
Systematic lupus erythematosus	↓	↓
Rheumatoid arthritis without vasculitis, serum	N,↑	N,↑
Acute poststreptococcal glomerulonephritis	N,↓†	↓
Hereditary angioedema	↓	N

* N indicates the test value remains constant within the normal limit; ↓, the test value is lower during the disease process; and ↑, the test value is higher during the disease process.
† Early in the disease; usually normal when patient first seen.

Complement

The most useful procedures for quantitative analysis of individual complement components are rate nephelometry and radial immunodiffusion. For most clinical applications, only C3 and C4 levels need be measured. With these tests, one can evaluate consumption of components of either the classical (C4, C3 both decreased) or the alternate (only C3 decreased) pathways.

Total hemolytic complement (CH50) is the assay that measures the ability of fresh serum to lyse sheep red blood cells coated with rabbit antibody to the red blood cells. The presence of all of the complement components of the classical pathway is required to lyse the antibody-coated sheep erythrocytes. Total hemolytic complement is an excellent screening test to detect a genetic deficiency of any of the complement components of the classical pathway.

Complement levels may be elevated in acute inflammatory conditions, including a number of arthritic diseases, among them rheumatoid arthritis. In such conditions complement is an "acute phase reactant" carrying the same significance as an elevated sedimentation rate.

Complement may be decreased because of either increased consumption or decreased rate of synthesis. Table 14.2 lists various diseases in which C3 and C4 abnormalities are present; in these diseases complement levels are helpful in making a diagnosis. When both early- and late-acting components are depressed, the classical pathway of complement activation is operative. When early component C4 is normal but C3 level is low, the alternate pathway may have been triggered. Detection of complement in body fluids other than blood is generally not useful.

The absence of C1 esterase inhibitor (C1inh), associated with hereditary angioedema, allows uncontrolled C1 esterase activation with the generation of a kinin-like plasma activity. Approximately 15% of patients with hereditary angioedema have normal or increased serum levels of C1inh by immunochemical measurements, but their C1inh is functionally inactive. Screening for this disease is best achieved by assessing C3 and C4 levels. C4 levels are decreased during both acute attacks and symptom-free periods. C3 and the later-acting complement components are little affected by the activation of C1 and are usually normal. Thus, a low C4 level and a normal C3 level are compatible with the diagnosis of hereditary angioedema. A functional assay for C1inh is available in reference laboratories to confirm the diagnosis.

References

Linker JB, Williams RC. Tests for detection of rheumatoid factors. In: Rose NR, Friedman H, Fahey JL, eds. *Manual of Clinical Laboratory Immunology*. 3rd ed. Washington, DC: American Association for Microbiology; 1986:759-761.

Mackworth-Young C, et al. Antiphospholipid antibodies: more than just a disease marker? *Immunol Today*. 1990;11:60-65.

Ruddy S. Complement. In: Rose NR, Friedman H, Fahey JL, eds. *Manual of Clinical Laboratory Immunology*. 3rd ed. Washington, DC: American Association for Microbiology; 1986:175-184.

Tan EM, Chan EKL, Sullivan KF, et al. Short analytical review; antinuclear antibodies (ANAs): diagnostically specific immune markers and clues toward the understanding of systemic autoimmunity. *Clin Immunol Immunopathol*. 1988;47:121-141.

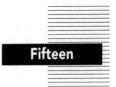

Fifteen

Intestinal Malabsorption Tests

Key Points

1. Malabsorption can result from intrinsic defects of the small intestine, loss of bile salts, or decreased secretion of enzymes from the exocrine pancreas.
2. The presence or absence of malabsorption can be detected by a fecal fat determination.
3. The D-xylose absorption test is an important general test of jejunal function.
4. Terminal ileal function analysis utilizes the Schilling test.
5. Small intestinal biopsy allows for both histologic diagnosis and specific histochemical determinations.

Background

The gastrointestinal (GI) tract functions by breaking down ingested food into small simple constituents that can be absorbed along with fluids, vitamins, and minerals. The waste products of this process are consolidated for elimination from the body. To understand the abnormalities of absorption, focused in the small intestine, normal absorption mechanisms need to be reviewed.

The major carbohydrates in the diet are starch and disaccharides. The more complex carbohydrates are broken down to oligosaccharides and disaccharides in the stomach and duodenum by salivary and pancreatic amylases. The small oligosaccharides and disaccharides are hydrolyzed into their absorbable component monosaccharides by oligosaccharidases and disaccharidases, which are present on the surface of the small intestinal microvilli.

Proteins come from both dietary and intraluminal sources contained in GI secretions and cells sloughed from the GI tract. Hydrolysis of protein begins with gastric pepsin and continues with pancreatic trypsin, chymotrypsin, and carboxypeptidase, resulting in three to six amino acid oligopeptides and lesser amounts of free amino acids. Peptidases present on the small intestinal microvilli hydrolyze the oligopeptides to tripeptides, dipeptides, and free amino acids. All three forms are transported into the intestinal cells where the remaining peptides are broken down to free amino acids.

Most dietary fat is in the form of long-chain triglycerides. Small quantities of other lipids include cholesterol, biliary lethicin, phospholipids, and fat-soluble vitamins (A, D, E, and K). Lipolysis begins in the stomach where churning produces emulsification, and oral and gastric lipase releases monoglycerides and fatty acids. In the duodenum at pH 6.5, the liberated fatty acids ionize and stimulate the release of cholecystokinin and pancreozymin (CCK-PZ) from endocrine cells in the small bowel. The CCK-PZ stimulates the pancreas to produce an enzyme-rich secretion and the gallbladder to contract, sending bile salts into the duodenum. The long-chain triglycerides form a finer emulsion that allows pancreatic lipase to hydrolyze them to monoglycerides and fatty acids. They become surrounded by bile salts and form water-soluble micelles. The lipids leave the core of the micelles by becoming soluble in the cell membrane of the small intestinal microvillus. Inside the intestinal epithelial cells the monoglycerides and fatty acids are resynthesized into long-chain triglycerides and are incorporated into chylomicrons that are transported away via the lymphatic system. The bile salts are reabsorbed in the terminal ileum and returned to the liver. The bile salt pool can recirculate via this enterohepatic circulation several times with each meal.

Eight to nine liters of fluid, with electrolytes, are presented daily to the GI tract. Most of this fluid is reabsorbed in the small intestine, particularly the proximal jejunum. About 1 to 1.5 L of fluid enter the colon, and all except 100 to 150 mL that are excreted in the feces are reabsorbed.

Most nutrients along with iron, other minerals, water, and electrolytes are absorbed in the proximal small bowel. The remainder of the small intestine is a lesser absorptive site. Bile acids and vitamin B_{12} are selectively absorbed in the distal ileum.

Malabsorption occurs when there is an abnormality in any of the following steps involved with the digestive process: (1) intraluminal digestion of food particles; eg, a lack of pancreatic enzymes or bile salts can prevent food from being broken down to an absorbable form; (2) mucosal digestion within epithelial cells where nutrients are absorbed and processed for transport; eg, Crohn's disease or celiac sprue results in insufficient cell surface area or insufficient lactase; (3) during transport out of the epithelial cells into the portal, systemic, or lymphatic circulations; eg, lymphatic duct obstruction or lymph node disease secondary to lymphoma or tuberculosis can block chylomicrons from entering the lymphatic circulation; and (4) multiple mechanisms, eg, where various different steps can be involved by such diseases as diabetes mellitus, giardiasis, acquired immunodeficiency syndrome (AIDS), or endocrinopathies such as hyperthyroidism.

Workup of Intestinal Absorptive Function Abnormalities

If the diagnosis of malabsorption is considered in a patient, the history and physical examination are important in evaluating suspected or known intestinal or pancreatic disease. The earliest signs of malabsorption may be subtle and nonspecific and include malaise, failure to maintain body weight, or an increase in stool frequency or volume. The physical examination at this point may be unremarkable. Only in more advanced malabsorptive states do the classic findings of abdominal distention with passage of large, greasy, foul-smelling stools ensue. Extraintestinal symptoms and signs such as pallor, bone pain, skin rashes, and purpura also are late findings.

The history will disclose information about conditions associated with malabsorption, such as alcohol abuse, recurrent pancreatitis, biliary obstruction, medications, possible exposure to parasites during travel, risk factors for HIV infection, sensitivity to certain foods, recurrent peptic ulcer disease, previous gastrointestinal surgery, and the presence of other systemic diseases such as diabetes mellitus.

Numerous tests are available for evaluating a patient suspected of having malabsorption secondary to intestinal or pancreatic disease. It is not necessary to run all of these tests for any given patient; only those tests that have the greatest possibility of a positive result should be utilized. For example, clues such as abdominal pain and a possible abdominal inflammatory mass are suggestive of Crohn's disease. Excess flatus, abdominal cramps, and watery diarrhea may suggest selective carbohydrate malabsorption since unabsorbed carbohydrates pass into the colon and are broken down and converted by the colonic bacteria to carbon dioxide, hydrogen, and short-chain fatty acids, which cause osmotic retention of fluid as well as gaseous distention. A history of peptic ulcer surgery suggests the possibility of a blind intestinal loop prone to have bacterial overgrowth.

Since each stage in the absorptive process is associated with a group of disease entities, it would be valuable if there was a test that would not only confirm malabsorption, but also associate it with the appropriate phase of digestion (eg, intraluminal, mucosal, or transport). Unfortunately, such a test does not exist. Consequently, it is necessary to perform a series of tests in an attempt to answer the questions. Most of the tests available give information about overall absorptive function, and if abnormal suggest several causes.

Fecal Fat

Fecal fat determination is a general test, sensitive for detecting malabsorption.

Microscopic Examination. Microscopic examination of the stool for fat and undigested muscle fibers is a simple and rapid method that will detect moderate to severe malabsorption, but is not sensitive enough to detect mild steatorrhea. It is performed on a glass slide by mixing a small amount of stool with several drops of glacial acetic acid and several drops of Sudan III stain in 95% alcohol. The mixture is coverslipped, gently heated to boiling, and then examined microscopically. If only a few fat droplets are present, the test is negative. If there are many fat droplets as well as undigested muscle particles, the test is considered positive and a quantitative stool fat determination should be considered.

Quantitative Stool Fat Determination. Quantitative stool fat determination, although inconvenient to the patient and distasteful to laboratory personnel, measures fat in a 72-hour stool sample and is the definitive test for steatorrhea. It should be one of the first tests considered in a patient suspected of having malabsorption. A normal individual will lose 1 to 3 g of fecal fat per day, even if there is no fat in the diet, from desquamated intestinal epithelial cells and intestinal bacterial lipids. To standardize test results, an adult patient should be placed on a diet that limits fat intake to between 60 and 100 g per day. On this diet, the normal individual will lose 3 to 5 g of fecal fat per day with 7 g the upper limit of normal. Loss greater than 7 g of fecal fat per day is considered abnormal.

Fecal fat determination does not define a specific cause for the malabsorption; the cause of the steatorrhea might be pancreatic, intestinal, or hepatobiliary. It is necessary to test further to delineate the site of the lesion responsible. Remember that there must be almost complete loss of exocrine pancreatic function before steatorrhea due to lack of pancreatic enzymes is evident.

D-Xylose Absorption Test

The D-xylose absorption test of jejunal function is a general test performed by giving an oral dose of D-xylose after overnight fasting and then measuring the 5-hour urinary excretion of the compound. D-xylose is a 5-carbon sugar that is absorbed in the small intestine, particularly the jejunum. It is poorly metabolized and greater than 20% of the dose of D-xylose should be excreted in the urine over 5 hours. Excretion is impaired in patients with renal failure or ascites. The test can cause diarrhea.

If the D-xylose test is abnormal, indicating upper small intestinal disease, then tests for bacterial overgrowth or peroral mucosal biopsy are possible depending on patient history or physical findings. If the D-xylose test is normal, then tests of real or relative bile salt deficiency, terminal ileal disease, or pancreatic function would be indicated depending on patient findings.

Bacterial Overgrowth Tests

The best bacterial overgrowth tests rely on the expired metabolic products of carbohydrates acted on by intestinal bacteria.

Hydrogen Breath Test. This test measures expired hydrogen and is based on several observations of normal individuals: (1) hydrogen is not produced by any cells in the body, (2) virtually no hydrogen is produced in the small intestine, and (3) hydrogen is produced by colonic bacteria from fermentation of carbohydrates. If carbohydrates are completely absorbed by the small intestine, then hydrogen will not be produced. However, hydrogen will be produced in the small intestine if there is small intestinal bacterial overgrowth acting on the carbohydrate before it can be absorbed. Hydrogen will also be produced if carbohydrates reach the colon because of small intestinal disease limiting absorption or if there is a specific disaccharide deficiency. After a normally easily absorbable carbohydrate such as glucose or lactose is given orally, an early peak of hydrogen production measured in expired air suggests small intestinal bacterial overgrowth, while a late peak of hydrogen suggests the carbohydrate has traveled all the way to the colon and is more indicative of diffuse small intestinal disease or a specific disaccharide deficiency.

Cholyl-^{14}C-Glycine Breath Test. This test uses ^{14}C-labeled conjugated bile salt given orally. If the bile salt enterohepatic circulation is intact, then almost no

$^{14}CO_2$ will be excreted by the lungs. If there is bacterial overgrowth in the small intestine, the bile salts are deconjugated by the bacteria and large amounts of $^{14}CO_2$ are absorbed through the intestine and are excreted by the lungs. Similarly, if there is ileal dysfunction, the bile salts pass into the colon where fecal bacteria cause release of $^{14}CO_2$, which can be absorbed and excreted by the lungs. The breath test will not differentiate between these two disease entities. However, simultaneous analysis of fecal bile salts in the stool helps separate them, since fecal bile salts will be low with bacterial overgrowth but high in bile salt malabsorption due to ileal dysfunction.

The ^{14}C-D-Xylose Breath Test. This test uses ^{14}C-D-xylose given orally, but instead of measuring the xylose absorption, the test measures expired $^{14}CO_2$, which will be produced and absorbed if bacteria are present in the small intestine. The test has the advantage that since D-xylose is absorbed in the proximal small intestine, terminal small bowel resections do not affect the results and there is very little to be metabolized by colonic bacteria, in contrast to the cholyl-^{14}C-glycine breath test. The results of this test may show small intestinal bacterial overgrowth even more reliably than culture.

Jejunal Culture. This procedure involves a small tube that is either swallowed and positioned in the jejunum or placed in the jejunum directly by endoscopy. If 10^5 or more aerobic or anaerobic organisms per milliliter are cultured, then the diagnosis of bacterial overgrowth is made.

Peroral Mucosal Biopsy
Peroral mucosal biopsy of the small intestine has expanded the scope of diagnostic gastroenterology. The histological features of many diseases are widely known. Some diseases (eg, celiac sprue, Whipple's disease, or eosinophilic gastroenteritis) have morphological changes that are relatively specific; other diseases have less-specific changes. Histochemical demonstration of certain enzymes (especially oligosaccharidases, disaccharidases, and oligopeptidases) within the brush border of intestinal cells can be performed on the same biopsy tissue taken for a morphological diagnosis. Fluid aspirated during endoscopy can be examined for *Giardia*, a parasite causing malabsorption.

Bile Salt Absorption
Bile salt absorption can be tested by the cholyl-^{14}C-glycine breath test already discussed. It has been utilized to identify patients who do not reabsorb bile salts adequately. Unfortunately, it does not differentiate between this condition and small intestinal bacterial overgrowth without measuring the fecal bile salts.

Terminal Ileal Function
Terminal ileal function analysis utilizes the Schilling test. Vitamin B_{12} absorption involves the binding of the vitamin by gastric intrinsic factor and transport of the vitamin B_{12}–intrinsic factor complex through the proximal small bowel to specific binding sites in the terminal ileum where absorption occurs. The Schilling test is performed by giving an oral dose of radioactive vitamin B_{12} along with an intramuscular injection of nonlabeled vitamin B_{12} to ensure saturation of

the plasma- and liver-binding sites. The amount of radiolabeled vitamin B_{12} excreted in the urine is measured. An adequate test depends on a fasting state, good renal function with maintenance of an adequate urine flow and a complete 24-hour urine collection. Normal individuals excrete more than 7% of the radio-labeled vitamin B_{12} in the urine in 24 hours. Decreased absorption (<7% excretion/24 hours) occurs if the terminal ileum is diseased (eg, Crohn's disease or lymphoma) or surgically bypassed or resected. However, test results can also be low due to lack of intrinsic factor (pernicious anemia or gastric resection), small intestinal bacterial overgrowth (bacterial metabolism of the vitamin), or pancreatic insufficiency (loss of pancreatic proteases in the duodenum, which are essential for the vitamin B_{12} to bind to intrinsic factor). These disorders can be differentiated by retesting the patient to see if various administered therapies correct the abnormal results (intrinsic factor for pernicious anemia, antibiotics for small intestinal bacterial overgrowth, replacement enzymes for pancreatic insufficiency). If none of these substances corrects the test, it confirms the presence of ileal disease.

Pancreatic Function Tests
Pancreatic function tests are also discussed in the chapter on the exocrine pancreas (Chapter 18). Low levels of pancreatic enzymes from the exocrine pancreas cause malabsorption, which must be separated from small bowel disease.

Secretin Stimulation Test. This test utilizes the hormone secretin, given intravenously (1 U/kg body weight), which causes the pancreas to increase flow of pancreatic juice and bicarbonate. The patient is required to have duodenal intubation, well positioned, and the rate of flow of pancreatic juice as well as the bicarbonate concentration is measured. Occasionally CCK-PZ, hormones that stimulate pancreatic enzyme secretion, are also given with the secretin, in which case the pancreatic enzymes are also measured. This test is one of the most sensitive tests of pancreatic insufficiency and may show diminished flow of bicarbonate and enzymes if as little as 75% of the pancreas is involved by disease and thus may be positive before steatorrhea due to loss of exocrine pancreas is present. The test has a sensitivity of 95%.

Lundl Test Meal. This test includes a liquid meal containing fat, protein, and carbohydrate, given orally. The meal, in turn, stimulates endogenous CCK-PZ release, which increases pancreatic enzyme production. The patient has duodenal intubation and the collected pancreatic juice is analyzed for pancreatic flow and enzyme production (trypsin is the enzyme measured).

Bentiromide Test. The bentiromide (N-benzoyl-L-tyrosyl-p-aminobenzoic acid) test utilizes bentiromide, which is split by pancreatic chymotrypsin so that the p-aminobenzoic acid (PABA) is absorbed by the small intestine, conjugated in the liver, and excreted in the urine. The concentration of PABA in the urine is an indirect measure of chymotrypsin activity in the small intestine. PABA excretion is reduced in severe pancreatic insufficiency when 95% or more of the pancreas is abnormal. Test results will also be abnormal if there is small intestinal disease interfering with absorption, liver disease interfering with metabolism, or renal disease interfering with excretion. The test is usually run in conjunction with the

D-xylose test to ascertain the absorptive capacity of the small intestine. Measurement of plasma PABA increases the accuracy of the test.

Blood Tests

A number of blood tests can be run that reflect impaired absorption of specific nutritional substances such as calcium, magnesium, iron, albumin, fat-soluble vitamins A, D, E, and K, folate, and vitamin B_{12}. Peripheral blood smears may show abnormal red blood cell morphology secondary to iron and folate deficiencies. A prothrombin time may be prolonged due to a lack of vitamin K.

Lactase Deficiency

Lactase deficiency causes abdominal cramps, distention, and diarrhea after ingestion of lactose or milk products. Acquired lactase deficiency is the most common disorder of carbohydrate absorption in humans. Congenital lactase deficiency is a rare disorder in which lactase levels are low at birth. Tests of lactase deficiency include:

Lactose Tolerance Test. Lactose is given orally and timed; sequential blood samples to measure serum lactose levels are obtained. A flat lactose tolerance curve (no absorption) indicates either defective transport across the intestinal mucosal membrane or a deficiency of the enzyme lactase. Development of diarrhea, cramps, and abdominal distention during the test indicates a lactase deficiency. To exclude defective monosaccharide transport, a glucose tolerance test is run; if this is also flat, indicating no absorption, there is defective intestinal transport rather than a lactase deficiency, in which case the glucose tolerance test would be normal.

Lactose Hydrogen Breath Test. As described, hydrogen is produced by bacterial metabolism of carbohydrate, and is absorbed and excreted by the lungs. An oral dose of lactose is given, which will not be absorbed if there is a lactase deficiency. The lactose can then be acted on by the colonic bacteria to produce breath hydrogen, which can be measured. It does not require use of radioactive labels.

Small Intestinal Biopsy. It is possible to directly measure the amount of lactase present in the small intestinal mucosa by tissue analysis of a biopsy specimen from the small intestinal mucosa.

Radiological Studies

A plain film of the abdomen might show calcifications in the region of the pancreas indicating chronic pancreatitis. Barium contrast studies of small intestine might show primary disease of the small intestine, such as Crohn's disease, diverticula, postsurgical changes, and diffuse changes of celiac sprue. Ultrasonography and computed tomographic scan are of value in inflammatory, ductal, and mass lesions, particularly involving the pancreas and liver.

References

Greenberger NJ. *Gastrointestinal Disorders: A Pathophysiologic Approach.* 4th ed. Chicago, Ill: Year Book Medical Publishers Inc; 1989:121-143,256-263.

Heyworth MF, Wright TL. Maldigestion and malabsorption. In: Sleisenger MH, Fordtran JS, eds. *Gastrointestinal Disease: Pathophysiology, Diagnosis, Management.* 4th ed. Philadelphia, Pa: WB Saunders Co; 1989;263-282.

Powell LW, Piper DW. *Fundamentals of Gastroenterology.* 4th ed. Balgowiah, Australia: ADIS Health Science Press; 1984;31-102.

Shearman DJD, Finlayson NDC, eds. *Diseases of the Gastrointestinal Tract and Liver.* 2nd ed. New York, NY: Churchill Livingstone Inc; 1989;359-401.

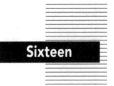

Sixteen

Gastric Secretion Tests

Key Points

1. Gastric acid output testing is useful when acid levels are very high, or very low to absent. Pentagastrin is the stimulating agent of choice. Endoscopy has replaced acid collection as the primary diagnostic tool.
2. Fasting serum gastrin levels vary inversely with gastric acid secretion. The hormone gastrin is the most powerful gastric acid stimulator known.
3. Administration of the hormone secretin stimulates gastrin production in patients with a gastrinoma but not in patients with other causes of hypergastrinemia.

Background

The stomach functions as a reservoir where food is mixed with gastric secretions, predominately hydrochloric acid and pepsin, breaking the food into small particles that are then propelled into the duodenum. Gastric secretion is influenced by neural, mechanical, and hormonal factors. Of these, the most important appear to be vagal nerve control and the hormone gastrin.

Currently, the most frequently used clinical tests of gastric function are measurement of gastric acid output and determination of serum gastrin levels.

Laboratory Tests of Gastric Secretion and Associated Diseases

Gastric Acid Output

Gastric acid output is measured less often today than in the past. Improved radiographic procedures and fiberoptic endoscopy plus realization of the overlap and imprecision of results have contributed to the decline in use. However, there are still clinical instances where knowledge of acid output is helpful: documenting very high acid output or very low or no acid output. Clinical research on effects of antisecretory agents demands gastric acid output measurement.

The gastric secretions are collected in a fasting patient who has had a properly positioned tube placed in the stomach with the fluid already present in the stomach aspirated and discarded. Collections of gastric juice are then obtained every 15 minutes. One hour is reserved for collection of basal acid output (BAO) and then a gastric secretory stimulant such as pentagastrin (a synthetic pentapeptide consisting of the C-terminal tetrapeptide of gastrin plus beta-alanine) or a histamine-like drug is administered and another hour of 15-minute collections determines the maximal acid output (MAO). Pentagastrin provides maximal stimulation and is therefore recommended.

Interpretation of acid output shows that the range of values for normal subjects is extremely broad and overlaps considerably with the values found with disease. There are definite age- and sex-related differences. Women generally have lower BAO and MAO levels than men. With increasing age there is a decline in the BAO and MAO levels, probably as the result of chronic gastritis and a diminution in the number of parietal cells. Most normal adults have a basal fasting secretory volume of 30 to 70 mL/h and a BAO in the range of 1 to 5 mEq/h. The average MAO in most reported studies of normal individuals is 20 mEq/h, with the upper limit of normal 40 mEq/h. Anacidity is defined as a failure of the pH of gastric secretion to fall below 6.0 during stimulated collection. Anacidity is considered an abnormal finding.

Gastric acid output analysis is frequently not helpful in either diagnosing or excluding peptic ulcer disease. Duodenal ulcer patients, as a group, show an increase in gastric secretion over normal individuals, whereas gastric ulcer patients have less gastric secretion than average. However, there is considerable overlap of both duodenal and gastric ulcer patients with normal values. There was some thought that before surgery for peptic ulcer disease, gastric analysis might be helpful in determining the optimal type of operation. There is currently considerable debate as to whether this is of any benefit. Gastric analysis has also been utilized to a minor extent in patients who have had an acid-reducing operation and who later develop symptoms that may indicate a recurrent ulcer. Patients with a recurrent ulcer show increased gastric secretion in response to pentagastrin stimulation; if there is no or very low acid output, then the symptoms are probably not related to a recurrent ulcer.

Hypoglycemia excites vagal nerve activity, which, in a normal individual, stimulates increased gastric acid output. Severing the vagus nerves to the stomach is one of the operations done to diminish gastric acid output. Following this type of operation, insulin can be utilized as a stimulus during gastric analysis to determine the completeness of the vagotomy, since denervated parietal cells should not respond to the vagal stimulus produced by hypoglycemia. This test is not frequently used, however.

Since patients with benign gastric ulcer always secrete some gastric acid, the finding of anacidity after stimulation in a patient with a gastric ulcer almost always indicates malignancy, specifically gastric carcinoma. Improved radiological techniques and fiberoptic gastroscopy with biopsy and cytology have made gastric analysis of less value. This is particularly true since, while anacidity virtually excludes the diagnosis of a benign ulcer, most patients with gastric carcinoma secrete some gastric acid.

The symptoms of the Zollinger-Ellison syndrome result from the effects of excess gastrin produced by an endocrine tumor, the gastrinoma, predominately found in the pancreas. While there is some overlap of gastric analysis between normal individuals and duodenal ulcer with Zollinger-Ellison syndrome patients, about half of the patients with Zollinger-Ellison syndrome have a BAO greater than 15 mEq/h and approximately two thirds have BAO levels greater than 10 mEq/h. Since patients with gastrinomas have continuous secretion of gastrin, they are secreting acid at a rate closer to maximal than normal. However, the BAO to MAO ratio usually does not distinguish gastrinoma patients from those with nongastrinoma peptic ulcers.

Reduced secretion of gastric acid is common in chronic gastritis. Generally, the more atrophy of the gastric mucosa, the more severe the hypoacidity. Patients with the most severe form of gastric atrophy, fundal atrophy, are usually anacidic. If there is, in addition, an absence of intrinsic factor secretion by the parietal cells, pernicious anemia results. Because there is no acid to initiate inhibition of gastrin secretion, adult patients with pernicious anemia will have elevated serum gastrin levels as well as anacidity.

Serum Gastrin Levels

Serum gastrin levels can be helpful. The hormone gastrin is a heterogeneous group of molecules produced by G cells present mainly in the gastric antrum, with a lesser number present in the duodenum and pancreatic islets. The predominate gastrin types produced are G-34 and G-17, the number referring to the number of amino acids present in the molecule. The G-17 molecule is a more powerful stimulus of gastric secretion than G-34, but the G-34 molecule remains in circulation longer, so the net effect on gastric secretion is similar between the two molecules.

Gastrin is the most powerful stimulus to gastric secretion that has been identified. Gastrin accounts for basal level gastric output with ongoing secretion regulated by a feedback mechanism where gastrin release is inhibited by the presence of acid.

The test is sensitive and readily available, and should be performed on a fasting patient. Fasting serum gastrin levels are inversely proportional to the rate of gastric acid secretion in normal individuals. The major indications for serum gastrin measurements are patients with possible Zollinger-Ellison syndrome or pernicious anemia.

Fasting serum gastrin levels are elevated more than five times the upper range of normal in patients with gastrinomas (Zollinger-Ellison syndrome). The high levels of gastrin stimulate excess acid production, which acidifies the upper small bowel and causes small bowel ulceration and diarrhea. Two thirds of these patients have sporadic gastrinomas despite no family history for it, and one third have associated multiple endocrine neoplasia syndrome. Other causes of hypergastrinemia with normal or increased gastric acid secretion (hyperchlorhydria) include renal failure (loss of degradation of gastrin by renal parenchyma), extensive small bowel resection, retained gastric antrum (antrum retained in the proximal bowel segment after gastrojejunostomy performed for acid reduction allows continuous gastrin secretion without acid inhibition), antral G cell hyperplasia/hypersensitivity (there may be only slightly elevated fasting gastrin levels but there is an excessive response to normal physiological stimuli of gastrin release), ordinary duodenal ulcer, gastric outlet obstruction (excess stimulation of retained food in antrum), and diabetes mellitus (increased responsiveness of G-cells). The reference range of fasting gastrin levels is 20 to 70 ng/L.

An important ancillary test utilizing the hormone secretin can be performed to help separate patients with gastrinoma from those with other causes of hypergastrinemia. Normally, secretin stimulates pancreatic secretion and inhibits gastrin release. However, in the case of a gastrinoma, secretin paradoxically causes an increase in gastrin secretion whereas in the other instances, secretin causes a fall in serum gastrin levels.

There are instances where hypergastrinemia is associated with decreased gastric secretion (hypochlorhydria or achlorhydria). Atrophic gastritis with achlorhydria (with or without pernicious anemia) is associated with hypergastrinemia (continuous secretion without acid inhibition). Other conditions with a similar mechanism of action include ordinary gastric ulcer, gastric carcinoma, postvagotomy, and drug-induction states.

References

Chopra S, May RJ, eds. Peptic ulcer disease. In: *Pathophysiology of Gastrointestinal Diseases.* Boston, Mass: Little, Brown & Co Inc; 1989:71-96.

Shearman DJD, Finlayson NDC, eds. *Diseases of the Gastrointestinal Tract and Liver.* 2nd ed. New York, NY: Churchill Livingstone Inc; 1989:201-254.

Feldman M. Gastric secretion in health and disease. In: Sleisenger MH, Fordtran JS, eds. *Gastrointestinal Disease: Pathophysiology, Diagnosis, Management.* 4th ed. Philadelphia, Pa: WB Saunders Co; 1989:713-734.

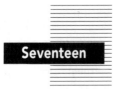
Liver Function Tests

Key Points

1. Elevation of bilirubin levels is specific for hepatobiliary dysfunction.
2. Transaminase enzyme elevations are most useful in determining hepatocellular damage.
3. Alkaline phosphatase (ALP) elevation is a sensitive indicator of biliary obstruction or infiltrative lesions of the liver.
4. Tests of synthetic and catabolic capability are of greatest value in determining prognosis.

Background

Many laboratory tests of liver function have been developed; few have survived to be used routinely. The liver function tests that have survived include those that measure liver excretion (eg, bilirubin), synthetic capability (eg, albumin, prothrombin time [PT]), release of enzymes from epithelial cells (eg, aminotransferases, ALP), and blood serology. An additional group of tests, useful as markers for specific hepatic diseases, includes viral serology, alpha$_1$-antitrypsin, antimitochondrial antibodies, and ceruloplasmin.

Tests Based on Excretion of Bile Pigments

Excretion of bilirubin in the bile requires production (largely from hemoglobin breakdown), transport in the plasma to the liver, uptake by hepatocytes, conjugation within the hepatocytes, and secretion across the canaliculus into the biliary system. A defect of any step can lead to abnormal bilirubin values and provide clues to the possible etiology of the liver abnormality.

Serum Bilirubin

Serum bilirubin is usually measured by reaction with diazotized sulfanilic acid to produce purple azobilirubin. When serum is mixed directly with this reagent only the water-soluble conjugated bilirubin and a small fraction of unconjugated bilirubin react promptly. This is termed direct-reacting or direct bilirubin. If the test is run with methyl alcohol added, the remaining nonpolar water-insoluble unconjugated bilirubin will also react, giving a value for total serum bilirubin (conjugated + unconjugated). Exposure of the serum sample to light results in the breakdown of bilirubin pigment and spuriously low values. Alternative methods for directly measuring the conjugated and unconjugated fractions of bilirubin include high pressure liquid chromatography and assays based on dry reagent chemistry on photographic film.

It has been established that there is no conjugated bilirubin present in normal serum. However, at any given time there is a small amount of unconjugated bilirubin that can react directly with the diazotized sulfanilic acid. The longer the direct reaction is allowed to proceed the greater the amount of bilirubin that will be in the direct fraction. As a result, the standard time limit for the direct reaction to continue is 1 minute by which time less than 30% of the total bilirubin will be direct reacting. If the percent of direct reacting bilirubin is greater than 30%, even if the total bilirubin is still within normal limits, there is an abnormal increase in the conjugated bilirubin fraction. Because the direct reaction shows a spurious fraction of apparent conjugated bilirubin occurring normally, the values for direct and indirect bilirubin obtained by the diazotized sulfanilic acid method do not correlate well with those obtained by the newer methods of direct measurement of conjugated and unconjugated bilirubin fractions, particularly at low total serum bilirubin concentrations. However, the diazotized sulfanilic acid method has been used for many decades, is cheaply and easily performed, can be automated, and is the method used by almost every routine clinical laboratory. There is a wealth of clinically correlated data associated with its use, so it is still the method of choice in the day-to-day practice of medicine.

One interesting outcome of the new methods is the recognition of a new bilirubin fraction, bilirubin delta, which is bilirubin tightly, covalently bound to albumin. This fraction, not present normally, seems to require the conjugating mechanism of the hepatocyte and rises with the total and conjugated fraction of bilirubin in hepatobiliary liver disease but falls at a slower rate than the other bilirubin fractions, having a half-life similar to albumin. It is not increased in unconjugated hyperbilirubinemias as seen with hemolysis or Gilbert's disease. Little is known about this fraction; however, it will account for the finding that if dry reagent chemistry or high-pressure liquid chromatography is utilized, the total bilirubin may not equal the conjugated plus the unconjugated fractions. The delta fraction accounts for the persistent slowly resolving jaundice sometimes observed following the resolution of active hepatobiliary disease. Therefore, it is important to know the methodology being used for the bilirubin determination. Clinical jaundice is usually detectable when the serum bilirubin level rises above 52 μmol/L (3 mg/dL).

Serum bilirubin is a highly specific test of hepatobiliary dysfunction (with the exception of hemolysis or impaired hemoglobin formation), but it is not a sensitive test of liver damage because the functional reserve of the liver is at least two to three times greater than the normal daily pigment load. The causes of a predominately unconjugated hyperbilirubinemia (conjugated bilirubin <20% of elevated level of total bilirubin) are limited to hemolysis, impaired hemoglobin formation, or hereditary diseases that are defects of bilirubin transport into the hepatocyte or defects of bilirubin conjugation (eg, Gilbert's syndrome or Crigler-Najjar syndrome). Conjugated hyperbilirubinemias can be caused by hereditary disease (eg, Dubin-Johnson syndrome), hepatocellular damage (eg, viral hepatitis or alcoholic damage), or extrahepatic or intrahepatic biliary obstruction.

Several clinical correlations are helpful. High serum bilirubin levels roughly parallel the histological severity of viral hepatitis and the length of disease. However, patients with fulminant hepatitis may die with only a small elevation of serum bilirubin because there is insufficient time for the bilirubin to rise. Glucose-6-phosphate dehydrogenase (G6PD)–deficient patients (predominately black) may have increased hemolysis during illness and bilirubin may be elevated out of proportion to the extent of liver damage. A serum bilirubin above 86 μmol/L (5 mg/dL) correlates with a poor prognosis in patients with acute alcoholic hepatitis.

Urine Bilirubin
Urine bilirubin (urine "bile"), from the conjugated fraction of bilirubin, is not present in urine of normal individuals by routine methods of measurement. Urine bilirubin is often tested as part of the routine "dipstick" urinalysis. A positive test for urine bilirubin confirms the presence of clinically suspected jaundice and attests to the presence of liver disease. Absence of urine bilirubin in the presence of jaundice strongly suggests unconjugated hyperbilirubinemia, as might be associated with hemolysis. Bilirubin may appear in the urine in the absence of overt jaundice and before the total serum bilirubin becomes elevated. This may provide a sensitive indication of early hepatitis or occult liver dysfunction. On the other hand, in resolving hepatitis, bilirubin may disappear from the urine before the total serum bilirubin returns to normal.

Phenazopyridine hydrochloride (Pyridium—a commonly used urinary tract analgesic agent) or large amounts of phenothiazine (an antihistaminic, sedative, anti–motion-sickness, and antiemetic agent) may give false-positive results. Allowing the urine to stand will result in loss of reactivity due to oxidation and/or hydrolysis and could produce a false-negative result.

Do not forget that unconjugated bilirubin is reversibly noncovalently bound to albumin in the circulation, and the coupling with albumin does not allow it to filter through the glomerular capillary. Likewise, delta bilirubin, which is tightly covalently bound to albumin, cannot be filtered in the urine. Hence, bilirubinuria primarily is a reflection of conjugated bilirubin.

Urine Urobilinogen
Urine urobilinogen is normally present in urine and may be detected by urine dipstick. With total obstruction of the extrahepatic biliary tract, bile does not reach the bowel and urobilinogen is not formed. As a result, urine urobilinogen falls below normal levels and is recorded as negative or trace on the dipstick. If there is only incomplete obstruction, the levels may not be decreased. Increased bilirubin loads (ie, hemolytic anemia) or hepatocellular injury may be associated

with abnormally high urine urobilinogen levels. Increased urine urobilinogen may be a sensitive indicator of mild hepatic damage in the absence of jaundice, as might occur with mild cirrhosis, metastatic carcinoma, or congestive heart failure.

Fecal Urobilinogen

Fecal urobilinogen is rarely measured because of practical considerations and because it closely parallels the information gained from the easily done urine urobilinogen. As might be expected, very low levels of fecal urobilinogen are associated with extrahepatic obstruction and high levels are associated with hemolysis. Broad-spectrum antibiotics may result in spuriously low fecal urobilinogen by suppressing intestinal bacteria, which convert bilirubin to urobilinogen.

Tests of Synthetic and Catabolic Capability

Prothrombin Time

The PT is not a sensitive index of liver disease because there is considerable hepatic reserve for its production. It also does not differentiate among various hepatocellular disorders.

The most important role of the PT is its prognostic value. A prolonged PT that fails to respond to vitamin K administration (required by most coagulation factors for synthesis in the liver) is the best early index of developing fulminant hepatic necrosis in patients with viral hepatitis or toxic or drug-induced hepatic injury. A chronic uncorrectable PT indicates extensive parenchymal damage and a poor long-term prognosis. A progressive shortening of the PT suggests an improving prognosis. The PT is also useful in assessing the relative safety of a liver biopsy or other surgical procedures.

Serum Albumin

Low serum albumin levels tend to correlate with the severity of hepatocellular dysfunction in both acute and chronic liver disease. Patients with cirrhosis who demonstrate a rise in serum albumin in response to therapy have a more favorable prognosis than those who fail to show a rise above 30 g/L. Significant hypoalbuminemia associated with an acute hepatic insult (eg, hepatitis) indicates extensive hepatic necrosis.

Enzyme Tests to Establish Hepatocellular Damage

Aspartate and Alanine Aminotransferases

Aspartate aminotransferase (AST) (formerly serum glutamic-oxaloacetic transaminase [SGOT]) and alanine aminotransferase (ALT) (formerly serum glutamate pyruvate transaminase [SGPT]) are the two major hepatocellular enzymes measured in serum. AST is found predominately in heart, liver, and skeletal muscle cells. Necrosis of these cells releases enzyme into the circulation where it is measured in increased amounts. ALT is found in many tissues but its concentration in tissues other than the liver is relatively low.

Increased AST and/or ALT levels are not specific for hepatobiliary disease. Both AST and ALT levels may also rise as a result of injury to heart or skeletal muscle. In nonhepatic injury, AST usually reaches higher relative levels than ALT. AST levels greater than 400 U/L usually indicate liver disease (or skeletal muscle injury, which may raise enzyme levels to 300-500 U/L). If due to heart disease, an AST level of 200 to 300 U/L is associated with such severe infarction that it is clinically and electrocardiographically obvious.

AST and ALT are sensitive indicators of liver cell damage from any cause. They represent the best early index of acute viral hepatitis and of recurrent activity during convalescence. They also provide a measure of continued hepatocyte damage in chronic hepatitis. Increased AST and, to a lesser extent, ALT levels are found in many patients with metastatic tumor to the liver, congestive hepatomegaly, granulomatous liver disease, and cirrhosis. Viral, drug, toxic, or ischemic injury give the highest values—often greater than 1000 U/L. In assessing obstructive liver disease vs parenchymal disease, levels as high as 400 U/L are found only rarely with biliary tract obstruction, and levels higher than 400 U/L usually indicate parenchymal disease. However, levels less than 300 U/L are of no help in separating these entities. The level of enzyme elevation has little prognostic value relating to outcome of the illness.

Alkaline Phosphatase

ALP is normally present in the serum, derived from bone, liver, and placenta. Bone is the major contributor, where the ALP comes from enzyme-rich osteoblasts; hence serum levels are much higher in children and adolescents than adults. Placental ALP is seen in the second half of pregnancy.

In the presence of known liver disease the ALP level is most useful in distinguishing biliary tract obstruction from hepatocellular injury. Serum ALP is a very sensitive indicator of both intrahepatic and extrahepatic cholestasis. Elevated enzyme levels may antedate the onset of jaundice and may persist after the resolution of the jaundice as the only evidence of continued partial biliary obstruction. ALP is often elevated in the absence of jaundice in patients with infiltrative diseases of the liver such as carcinoma, abscess, or granulomas. With obstruction and infiltrative lesions, the degree of elevation may be extreme (3- to 20-fold increase). Some of the highest levels of ALP are seen in patients with primary biliary cirrhosis. ALP levels are usually increased in patients with hepatocellular jaundice, but the increase is usually less than with obstruction (1- to 3-fold increase).

In summary, ALP is not specific for liver disease but is a sensitive indicator of biliary obstruction or infiltrative lesions of the liver. In the presence of jaundice, high levels suggest obstruction and low levels suggest hepatocellular injury. Low levels are a better diagnostic clue to lack of obstruction than high levels are to its presence.

Other enzyme studies are available in the laboratory that may supplement ALP determinations by distinguishing skeletal from hepatic origin of an elevated ALP. Leucine-aminopeptidase, and 5'-nucleotidase are not increased in bone growth or bone disorders, but may arise from the placenta. While a rise in one of these enzymes suggests that an increased ALP level is of hepatic origin, lack of a rise does not exclude the liver as the source of the increased ALP.

γ-Glutamyltransferase

γ-Glutamyltransferase (GGT) is a nonspecific enzyme that is present in numerous tissues but is a sensitive screen for liver disease, since it is elevated in many hepatic diseases. The enzyme is induced by a variety of drugs (eg, ethanol, phenobarbitol, phenytoin). Isolated elevations can suggest alcohol abuse and have been used to follow the course of alcoholic patients. If the ALP is elevated, but the GGT is normal, sources of the ALP other than liver are suggested. GGT is inhibited by gestational hormones so that it tends to remain normal in pregnant women despite the presence of hepatic disease.

Serum Serologic Studies

Serum serologic studies help define the viral hepatitides and primary biliary cirrhosis.

Hepatitis B Surface Antigen

Hepatitis B surface antigen (HBsAg) is first detected in the serum 1 to 10 weeks after exposure to the hepatitis B virus. The antigen persists for a variable period of time from weeks to several months. If the antigen persists beyond 6 months the patient is considered a chronic carrier, with or without chronic active liver disease. Many patients with hepatocellular carcinoma are chronic HBsAg carriers in regions of the world where hepatitis B is most prevalent.

Hepatitis B e Antigen

Hepatitis B e antigen (HBeAg) is typically detected 3 to 5 days after the appearance of HBsAg and persists for 2 to 6 weeks. Hepatitis B virus–specific deoxyribonucleic acid (DNA) polymerase activity appears in the serum at approximately the same time as HBeAg; HBeAg and hepatitis B virus-specific DNA polymerase are strongly associated with viral replication and infectivity.

Hepatitis C Antigen

Hepatitis C antigen (HCAg) circulates at very low levels and an assay is not available yet.

Antibody to Hepatitis B Surface Antigen

Antibody to surface antigen (anti-HBs) appears during convalescence 1 to 6 months after the loss of detectable HBsAg. It can persist for life but may disappear, leaving only anti-HBc. Anti-HBs is associated with recovery and the development of immunity. Failure to develop anti-HBs is associated with a chronic HBsAg carrier state. The antibody state determines what prophylactic measures need be taken on exposure to hepatitis B.

Antibody to Hepatitis B Core Antigen

Antibody to hepatitis B core antigen (anti-HBc) appears in the serum just prior to or simultaneously with the elevation of the serum aminotransferases. Antibody to core can persist for years and may represent the only evidence of previous hepatitis B infection. IgM anti-HBc may appear before IgG when HBsAg disappears and before antibody to surface antigen appears. Anti-HBc is almost always present in HBsAg carriers.

Antibody to Hepatitis B e Antigen

Antibody to hepatitis B e antigen (anti-HBe) appears after anti-HBc and is associated with disappearance of e antigen and lessening of infectivity.

Antibody to Hepatitis A Virus

Antibody to hepatitis A virus (anti-HAV) is helpful in the diagnosis of hepatitis only if a rising titer can be demonstrated between acute and convalescent sera or if IgM anti-HAV can be demonstrated in the acute sera by appropriate techniques. The appearance of anti-HAV coincides temporally with acute hepatocellular necrosis. Titers reach peak levels 2 to 3 months after the illness and fall gradually, but remain at detectable levels indefinitely. IgM anti-HAV appears transiently and usually becomes undetectable after 3 to 6 months.

Antibody to Hepatitis C Virus

Antibody to hepatitis C virus (anti-HCV) can be detected in 60% to 90% of cases of transfusion-associated hepatitis and in about 59% of cases of sporadic non-A non-B hepatitis. There is a delay of 1 to 3 months or even longer between the onset of acute hepatitis C until the antibody can be detected. This makes it difficult to use for early diagnosis of hepatitis C.

Anti–Smooth Muscle Antibodies

Anti–smooth muscle antibodies are found in less than 5% of normal persons. Up to 60% of patients with chronic active hepatitis of unknown origin and 10% to 15% of patients with biliary cirrhosis may demonstrate such antibodies. They may appear transiently in patients with acute viral hepatitis or infectious mononucleosis. Titers of 1:100 or above suggest progressive chronic active liver disease.

Antimitochondrial Antibodies

Antimitochondrial antibodies are found in less than 1% of normal persons but are present in up to 90% of patients with primary biliary cirrhosis and 25% of those with chronic active hepatitis or idiopathic cirrhosis. Titers greater than 1:160 are strongly suggestive of primary biliary cirrhosis. This test is useful in evaluating jaundice in that these antibodies are absent in early viral hepatitis, alcoholic cirrhosis, and extrahepatic biliary obstruction.

Serum Proteins

Specific serum proteins are easily assayed and can provide valuable data.

Alpha-Fetoprotein

Alpha-fetoprotein (AFP) is synthesized by tissue derived from endoderm and only small amounts are present in the serum of normal adults (25 µg/L). Increased levels may be present in a variety of non-neoplastic liver disorders, especially in the presence of active regeneration, but levels almost never exceed 500 µg/L. Levels above 1000 µg/L are suggestive of, and levels above 3000 µg/L are highly suggestive of, malignant hepatocellular carcinoma or germ cell tumor (yolk sac carcinoma). Less commonly, tumors of tissues other than hepatocyte (eg, pancreas or gallbladder) may produce AFP, but levels rarely exceed 1000 µg/L. Like other tumor markers it is more useful for therapy monitoring rather than establishing a diagnosis.

Alpha₁-Antitrypsin

Alpha$_1$-antitrypsin is a protease inhibitor found in normal serum. It comprises most of the alpha$_1$ globulin peak in a normal serum protein electrophoresis. Congenital deficiency of this enzyme is associated with cholestatic liver disease in infancy. Adults with alpha$_1$-antitrypsin deficiency most often present with precocious pulmonary emphysema, but chronic liver disease in adults or children may also be a manifestation of this congenital deficiency. There are a number of molecular forms of alpha$_1$-antitrypsin, and these may be separated by special electrophoretic techniques to produce a protease inhibitor phenotype. Phenotype MM is the normal pattern. The ZZ and, rarely, the MZ and SZ phenotypes are associated with disease. Low serum levels are associated with periportal, intracytoplasmic globules of the glycoprotein in hepatocytes on liver biopsy specimens.

Ceruloplasmin

Ceruloplasmin is a serum protein associated with copper transport. Low serum ceruloplasmin (<200 mg/L) occurs in 95% of patients with Wilson's disease, a disorder of copper storage associated with progressive liver damage. Once liver damage is advanced the ceruloplasmin may rise. Thus, a normal serum level in the presence of overt liver disease does not exclude this diagnosis; a low value provides strong evidence for the diagnosis.

References

Johnson PJ, McFarlane IG. *The Laboratory Investigation of Liver Disease.* Philadelphia, Pa: Baillière Tindall; 1989:11-47.

Kaplan MM. Diseases of the liver. In: Schiff L, Schiff ER, eds. *Laboratory Tests.* 6th ed. Philadelphia, Pa: JB Lippincott Co; 1987:219-260.

Shearman DJD, Finlayson NDC, eds. The liver: structure, function and clinical chemistry. *Diseases of the Gastrointestinal Tract and Liver.* 2nd ed. New York, NY: Churchill Livingstone Inc; 1989;605-638.

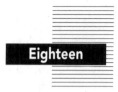

Eighteen

Exocrine Pancreas Tests

Key Points

1. Although the pancreas is one organ it possesses two separate functional units, the endocrine and the exocrine pancreas.
2. The primary marker of disease of the exocrine pancreas is amylase, but measurement of serum or urine levels is neither specific nor sensitive for pancreatic disease.
3. Amylase is widely found in tissues other than pancreas.
4. As markers of pancreatic injury, lipase corroborates amylase when both are elevated.
5. Initial assessment of serum and urine amylase, along with serum lipase, is recommended in evaluating patients for acute pancreatitis.

Background

Diseases that impair pancreatic function may cause obstruction to the flow of pancreatic secretions, with or without destruction of acinar-duct epithelium of the exocrine pancreas. Such processes may be reflected by a measurable change in the blood, urine, or serous fluid levels of pancreatic enzymes, such as amylase and lipase, and by abnormalities of exocrine pancreatic function, such as an abnormal secretin test result. The exocrine reserve capacity of this gland is great, so that as much as 90% of the pancreas may have to be destroyed before maldigestion or malabsorption occurs. The most sensitive tests of exocrine pancreatic function become abnormal only after functional loss of 75% of the pancreatic parenchyma. Furthermore, certain serious pancreatic diseases—principally chronic pancreatitis and pancreatic carcinoma—are usually not associated with any characteristic laboratory abnormalities. Finally, the most popular test of pancreatic function, serum amylase level, is a nonspecific indicator of pancreatic disease.

The exocrine pancreas is controlled primarily by hormonal mechanisms. Secretin, released in response to gastric acidity, stimulates the secretion of pancreatic juice rich in water and electrolytes. Gastric acid and certain nutrients in the duodenal and jejunal lumina stimulate release of cholecystokinin-pancreozymin, a hormone that causes the secretion of enzyme-rich pancreatic juice. Weaker stimuli for exocrine pancreatic secretion include gastrin, vagal activity, and bile salts.

Pancreatic secretions contain several important components. Bicarbonate is the electrolyte of primary physiological importance. Pancreatic bicarbonate neutralizes gastric acid and provides the optimum pH for pancreatic enzyme activity. Pancreatic enzymes are amylolytic, lipolytic, and proteolytic. All of these enzymes are important in the digestion and absorption of nutrients.

Exocrine Pancreas Function Tests

Amylase

The most commonly used laboratory test of pancreatic function measures the serum amylase level. This enzyme is an α-amylase (α-1,4-glucosidase), which randomly hydrolyzes the terminal α-1,4-glucosidic bonds of starch. Pancreas and salivary gland are the principal tissue sources of amylase, but the liver, kidney, heart, adipose tissue, muscle, and fallopian tubes all contribute lesser amounts. The amylase normally present in serum and urine comes from pancreas and salivary gland. Amylase has no known physiological function in serum. Increased serum amylase levels presumably result from pancreatic parenchymal damage with escape of pancreatic enzymes into the interstitial tissues and subsequent absorption through the veins and lymphatics. Normal adult serum amylase levels range from 0 to 200 U/L (depending on methods). Amylase appears in the serum of infants between 1 and 2 months of age, and its activity reaches low adult levels by 1 year.

Amylase in serum is cleared by the kidney through glomerular filtration, so loss of renal function results in elevations of the enzyme. Conversely, renal amylase clearance can accelerate with acute pancreatitis, causing a secondary rise in the levels of urine amylase. Values may remain elevated for 7 to 10 days even after the serum amylase is back within normal range. Normal urine amylase levels range from 0 to 300 U/L. The urine amylase to urine creatinine ratio utilizes accelerated clearance as a more sensitive marker for acute pancreatitis in nonazotemic patients, but it too is not infallible.

What is most needed in diagnosing acute pancreatitis is increased specificity, ie, we want to exclude disease with as much success as possible. The most specific test currently available is the ratio of amylase clearance to creatinine clearance, which requires serum and urine amylase and creatinine levels obtained simultaneously. It should be reserved for puzzling clinical cases, not ordered routinely.

$$\text{(Amylase Clearance/Creatinine Clearance) in \%} = 100 \times$$
$$\text{(Urine Amylase Concentration/Serum Amylase Concentration)} \times$$
$$\text{(Serum Creatinine/Urine Creatinine)}$$

The normal amylase to creatinine clearance ratio is less than 5%. This calculated ratio is beneficial in the setting of mild to moderate renal insufficiency and, though not perfect, can help to exclude other intra-abdominal emergencies in which the serum amylase is nonspecifically elevated.

Measurements of the activity of several isoenzymes of serum amylase, in addition to total serum amylase, are occasionally utilized, but they have proven to be of limited value. Occasionally, the amylase activity of ascitic fluid is measured. This measurement may differentiate a leaking pancreatic pseudocyst from non-pancreatic causes of ascites. Pleural fluid amylase may be elevated not only with acute and chronic pancreatitis, but also with carcinoma of the lung and esophageal perforation.

Lipase

Serum lipase elevation is present in 60% of patients with acute pancreatitis and tends to parallel serum amylase elevation, but it rises more slowly and persists longer. Until recently, measurement of serum lipase activity was a very time-consuming task; more rapid methods are now available. Theoretically, lipase is more specific than amylase for pancreatic disease because little lipase activity is found outside the pancreas and the intestinal mucosa. Lipase, however, is less sensitive than amylase for pancreatic disease. Both enzymes together have greater sensitivity than either alone. If both serum amylase and lipase levels are measured, approximately 85% of patients with acute pancreatitis will have abnormal results depending on case selection.

Secretin Test

The secretin test is the most sensitive measurement of the secretory reserve capacity of the exocrine pancreas. The test becomes abnormal only after more than 75% of exocrine function has been lost. The secretin test measures duodenal fluid components following pancreatic stimulation by intravenous secretin. An abnormal secretin test suggests that chronic pancreatic damage is present; the secretin test will not distinguish among causes of this damage. The test is difficult to perform and standardize, and is not widely used.

Other Tests

Other tests of exocrine pancreatic function are occasionally used. Measurements of chymotrypsin or "IRT"—immunoreactive trypsin of duodenal aspirates or feces (and recently serum)—are sometimes indicated. Screening tests for proteolytic activity in feces are also used. All of these tests are best reserved for the evaluation of pancreatic exocrine insufficiency, for example, with steatorrhea or cystic fibrosis.

Exocrine Pancreatic Disease

Acute Pancreatitis

The laboratory diagnosis of acute pancreatitis is subject to limitations. The following statements are generally valid. Usually, the serum amylase value becomes elevated 2 to 12 hours after the onset of acute pancreatitis, and values return to normal after 2 or 3 days. Values over five times the upper limit of normal are highly suggestive of acute pancreatitis. Approximately 75% of patients with acute pancreatitis have elevated serum amylase activity. There is no consistent clinical correlation between serum amylase values and the severity of the pancreatitis. If the serum amylase activity does not return to normal by 5 days, some complication of acute pancreatitis should be suspected. If there is a delay in obtaining the serum sample or if the patient has concurrent hypertriglyceridemia, the serum amylase level may be within normal limits despite the presence of acute pancreatitis.

The major disadvantage of serum amylase measurements in patients with acute pancreatitis is the relatively poor specificity of the test. The major diseases in the differential diagnosis of an elevated serum amylase activity plus abdominal pain are cholecystitis, perforated duodenal ulcer, strangulation or obstruction of the intestine, mesenteric thrombosis, and peritonitis. Elevations of serum amylase activity, likewise, can occur in patients with diseases not similar clinically to acute pancreatitis, such as diabetic ketoacidosis, infectious hepatitis, and mumps parotitis. The amylase to creatinine clearance ratio, already described, is the most specific routine test available to aid the diagnosis of acute pancreatitis.

Ancillary laboratory findings in acute pancreatitis are often very helpful. A leukocytosis of 15 to 20 x 10^9/L (15,000-20,000/μL) occurs frequently. Patients with severe disease may have an elevated hematocrit because retroperitoneal plasma loss produces hemoconcentration. Hyperglycemia may occur. Hypocalcemia occurs in one fourth of patients, who frequently have transient abnormalities of other liver function tests. The 15% to 20% of patients with concurrent hypertriglyceridemia often may have falsely normal or low serum amylase levels because of artefactual interference with amylase measurements.

Chronic Pancreatitis
Many patients with relapsing pancreatitis and most patients with chronic pancreatitis do not have elevated levels of either serum amylase or serum lipase. The lack of elevation in many cases can be explained by the extensive pancreatic destruction that has occurred in the course of the disease. Because of continued increased renal amylase clearance, urine amylase levels may be increased in chronic pancreatitis, especially with serial measurements. Exocrine pancreatic insufficiency occurs in one third of patients with chronic pancreatitis. In these patients the secretin test and other tests of exocrine pancreatic function are usually abnormal. These patients may also have hyperglycemia, reflecting progressive dropout of pancreatic islets. The finding of low levels of serum immunoreactive trypsin has been correlated with loss of pancreatic parenchyma.

Carcinoma of the Pancreas
Tests of pancreatic function, unfortunately, are rarely helpful in the diagnosis of pancreatic carcinoma. Only 10% of patients have abnormal serum amylase or lipase levels, and steatorrhea occurs only in 10%. Laboratory evidence of biliary tract obstruction is much more common with carcinoma of the head of the pancreas than with carcinoma of the body or tail. Tumor markers of value for case-finding or monitoring treatment include carcinoembryonic antigen and CA19-9 in those neoplasms that express them.

Macroamylasemia

In some instances of malabsorption or alcoholism, patients have one of two forms of serum amylase: (1) the normal molecule and (2) polymers of amylase molecules bound to IgG and IgA molecules. These polymers (macroamylase) are too large to be filtered by the glomeruli, hence these patients have persistently elevated serum amylase. The presence of macroamylasemia is inferred by the finding of a decreased urinary amylase clearance.

Cystic Fibrosis

Cystic fibrosis is the most common lethal hereditary disease in whites. Eight-five percent of patients with cystic fibrosis eventually develop exocrine pancreatic insufficiency. The single best laboratory test to establish the diagnosis of cystic fibrosis remains, by definition, the measurement of the concentration of chloride in exocrine sweat. The elevation of values is so characteristic that more than 99% of children with cystic fibrosis have concentrations of sweat chloride greater than 60 mmol/L (60 mEq/L). Furthermore, there is no disease comparable clinically with cystic fibrosis that also consistently gives elevated sweat chloride values. However, sweat chloride concentrations may not be as dramatically increased in adolescent or adult patients as they are in infants and young children, and many laboratories perform this test poorly. Properly done, pilocarpine is iontophoresed (introduced into the skin by electrical current) onto the forearm. The resulting sweat is absorbed, then analyzed for chloride content. Under precisely controlled conditions, the method is both safe to the patient and reliable.

Elevated serum immunoreactive trypsin levels in neonates have been suggested as a screening mechanism for cystic fibrosis. Heterozygote carriers of the autosomal-recessive gene cannot be separated from the noncarriers on the basis of these tests. Genetic testing now reveals a multiplicity of gene defects and should have clinical benefits soon.

References

Clavien PA, Robert J, Meyer P, et al. Acute pancreatitis normoamylasemia. *Ann Surg.* 1989;210:614-620.

McMahon MJ, Playforth MJ, Rashid SA, et al. The amylase-to-creatinine clearance ratio—a non-specific response to acute illness? *Br J Surg.* 1982;69:29-32.

Speicher CE. *The Right Test: A Physician's Guide to Laboratory Medicine.* Philadelphia, Pa: WB Saunders Co; 1989:94-97.

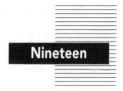
Diabetes Mellitus and Hypoglycemia: Laboratory Tests

Key Points

1. Diabetes mellitus (DM) does not equate to hyperglycemia.
2. Documentation of hyperglycemia is the key to the diagnosis of DM. Appropriate control of testing conditions is mandatory.
3. Urine glucose testing has little if any place in diagnosis or monitoring of diabetes, and has been superceded by fingerstick glucose measurement.
4. Glucose tolerance testing is infrequently required, and is used primarily for gestational diabetes.
5. The glucose tolerance test should not be used to assess symptoms of alleged hypoglycemia.
6. Hypoglycemia is a term that can be used only if the glucose is truly measured and truly low.

Background

The plasma glucose concentration is normally maintained within rather narrow limits during feeding and fasting. Disorders of glucose homeostasis that cause hyperglycemia are common. The incidence of true hypoglycemia is low.

Diabetes Mellitus

In DM the key biochemical manifestation is impaired glucose tolerance. In practice, this hyperglycemia is difficult to document reliably. Because of the medical, legal, and social (insurability) implications associated with DM, the diagnosis should be made with certainty and only under standardized conditions.

Diagnosing DM in patients with classic signs and symptoms of DM, such as polyuria, polydipsia, ketonuria, and rapid weight loss, together with gross and

Table 19.1 Criteria for Diagnosis of DM in Nonpregnant Adults.*

A. Presence of the classic symptoms of diabetes, such as polyuria, polydipsia, ketonuria, and rapid weight loss, together with gross and unequivocal elevation of plasma glucose

B. Fasting plasma glucose concentration ≥7.8 mmol/L (140 mg/dL) more than once

C. Oral glucose tolerance test showing both of the following:
    1. Two-hour plasma glucose concentration ≥11.1 mmol/L (200 mg/dL)
    2. At least one plasma glucose value between zero time and 2 hours ≥11.1 mmol/L (200 mg/dL)

* Any one of the criteria must be met.

unequivocal elevation of plasma glucose, presents no diagnostic difficulty. Biochemical testing is required in asymptomatic patients. All but 2.5% of apparently healthy persons maintain overnight fasting glucose concentrations between 3.9 and 6.1 mmol/L (70 and 110 mg/dL). When the fasting plasma glucose concentration is greater than 7.8 mmol/L (140 mg/dL) on more than one occasion, a diagnosis of DM is made.

The oral glucose tolerance test is utilized when a patient who is clinically suspected of having DM has a persistently normal fasting glucose level (<7.8 mmol/L [140 mg/dL]). The currently accepted criteria for the interpretation of the oral glucose tolerance test have been outlined by the National Diabetes Data Group of the National Institutes of Health (summarized in Tables 19.1-19.4). DM in nonpregnant adults is diagnosed if the 2-hour plasma glucose concentration is greater than 11.1 mmol/L (200 mg/dL) and at least one plasma glucose value between zero time and 2 hours is greater than 11.1 mmol/L (200 mg/dL). A diagnosis of impaired glucose tolerance is rendered if the 2-hour plasma glucose concentration is between 7.8 and 11.1 mmol/L (140 and 200 mg/dL) and at least one value between zero time and 2 hours is greater than 11.1 mmol/L (200 mg/dL). Follow-up studies of patients in this category reveal that a small proportion will revert to normal glucose tolerance, and the majority will remain in the impaired glucose tolerance class. Normal glucose tolerance is defined as a 2-hour plasma glucose concentration less than 7.8 mmol/L (140 mg/dL).

The major impetus for precise control of insulin therapy is prevention of the vascular complications of DM. Optimal control can be achieved but requires self-monitoring of glucose levels and multiple doses of insulin. If properly instructed

Table 19.2 Criteria for Diagnosis of Impaired Glucose Tolerance in Nonpregnant Adults.*

A. Fasting plasma glucose <7.8 mmol/L (140 mg/dL)

B. Oral glucose tolerance test showing both of the following:
    1. Two-hour plasma glucose concentration ≥7.8 mmol/L (140 mg/dL) and <11.1 mmol/L (200 mg/dL)
    2. At least one plasma glucose value between zero time and 2 hours ≥11.1 mmol/L (200 mg/dL)

* Both criteria must be met.

Table 19.3 Criteria for Gestational Diabetes.*

Measurement Time	Glucose Level, mmol/L (mg/dL)
Fasting	5.8 (105)
`1 h	10.5 (190)
2 h	9.2 (165)
3 h	8.0 (145)

* Two or more of the plasma glucose values must be met or exceeded after a 100-g oral glucose load.

and motivated, most patients with DM will make conscientious efforts to maintain good insulin control.

Physicians seeing diabetic patients periodically are faced with the problem of monitoring their degree of control. In the past, the patient's weight, dietary and insulin history, and any home glucose and ketone measurements have constituted the major information about disease control. Testing for glycosylated proteins is now established as the key measurement of ongoing control. Levels correlate with average glucose values obtained by patients in home monitoring programs.

Gestational Diabetes Mellitus

Gestational DM is a separate category, composed of women who first manifest impaired glucose tolerance during pregnancy. Identification of this group is indicated because of an associated increased risk of perinatal morbidity (including malformations) and mortality. Certain clinical features, such as glycosuria, family history of DM, history of stillborn or spontaneous abortion, previous fetal malformation, previous large-for-date newborn, high maternal age, and parity of five or more, are indications for the performance of an oral glucose tolerance test in a pregnant woman. The diagnosis of gestational DM is made when two or more of the following plasma glucose concentrations are met or exceeded after a 100-g oral glucose load: 5.8 mmol/L (105 mg/dL) fasting, 10.5 mmol/L (190 mg/dL) at 1 hour, 9.2 mmol/L (165 mg/dL) at 2 hours, and 8.0 mmol/L (145 mg/dL) at 3 hours. Patients with gestational diabetes are at an increased risk of developing DM 5 to 10 years after parturition. DM in pregnancy is a problem that requires close obstetrical attention. The incidence of complications is related to glucose control as measured by glycosylated hemoglobin. Normalization of glucose restores the probability of favorable outcome.

Table 19.4 Criteria for Normal Glucose Tolerance.*

A.	Fasting plasma glucose concentration <7.8 mmol/L (140 mg/dL)
B.	Oral glucose tolerance test with 2-hour plasma glucose concentration <7.8 mmol/L (140 mg/dL)

* Both criteria must be met.

Hypoglycemia

Hypoglycemia does not always connote pathological hypoglycemia. It has become a fad diagnosis encompassing a variety of constitutional symptoms. Simply remember that plasma (or serum) glucose levels below 3.9 mmol/L (70 mg/dL) occur often in asymptomatic normal people; thus, a "low" glucose level does not always diagnose pathological hypoglycemia. True symptomatic hypoglycemia does need to be diagnosed. Traditionally, hypoglycemia has been categorized two ways. Reactive hypoglycemia is the occurrence of symptoms related to postprandial hypoglycemia within 5 hours of food ingestion. Reactive hypoglycemia usually does not suggest the possibility of serious underlying disease. True organic (fasting) hypoglycemia occurs after the patient passes from the fed to the fasted state. Fasting hypoglycemia usually occurs 6 hours or longer after eating. Patients with fasting hypoglycemia often have a serious underlying disease.

Patients with symptomatic hypoglycemia have autonomic complaints: sweating, palpitations, weakness, and anxiety. Vague constitutional symptoms, such as chronic fatigue or mental dullness, do not represent symptomatic hypoglycemia by themselves. True, or fasting, hypoglycemia is a difficult condition to document. Whipple's triad (symptoms, low plasma glucose levels, and alleviation of symptoms after glucose administration) defines the disorder. Alimentary hypoglycemia is the type most common in patients following gastric surgery.

Fasting hypoglycemia must be measured because it often suggests a serious underlying disorder. Most patients with fasting hypoglycemia are diabetic patients receiving insulin therapy. Ethanol ingestion causes fasting hypoglycemia, especially in children who accidently ingest ethanol and in adults with limited food intake. When generalized liver disease destroys more than 80% of the liver, fasting hypoglycemia can develop. Patients with pituitary or adrenocortical insufficiency can have fasting hypoglycemia due to lack of the counter-regulatory hormone, cortisol. Neonatal fasting hypoglycemia occurs with a variety of disorders and often presents with nonspecific signs and symptoms. Certain large nonpancreatic tumors (eg, retroperitoneal sarcomas) can cause fasting hypoglycemia. A rare but detectable cause of fasting hypoglycemia is an insulinoma. The biochemical hallmark of this tumor is relative hyperinsulinism—inappropriately high serum insulin levels in the presence of hypoglycemia. Surreptitious insulin injection can cause fasting hypoglycemia. Measurements of C peptide levels (a peptide formed during the proteolytic conversion of proinsulin to insulin by the pancreatic islet beta cells) in serum may aid in the recognition of or exclusion of factitious hypoglycemia.

Laboratory Tests of Impaired Glucose Metabolism

Plasma (or Serum) Glucose Concentration

Most clinical laboratories use enzymatic techniques for measuring glucose. These methods are more precise and specific than previously used colorimetric techniques. Nevertheless, plasma or serum glucose measurements are subject to variation. Delayed separation of the plasma or serum from the cells can cause falsely low glucose values, because in 10 mL of whole blood, erythrocyte and leukocyte glycolysis consumes glucose at a rate of about 7.0 mg/h. Some anticoagulant mixtures used for glucose measurements contain sodium fluoride, a glycolytic inhibitor. A variety of emotional and physical stresses can temporarily elevate the plasma or serum glucose level. Transient hyperglycemia is seen in patients receiving large loads of intravenous glucose.

Because of the seriousness of the disorders involved in symptomatic hypoglycemia, glucose determinations should be as accurate as possible and measured in the main laboratory rather than on self-monitoring devices. Several determinations using enzymatic techniques provide reliable results, but screening tests are not reliable in the low range. Age of the patient can greatly influence plasma (or serum) glucose levels. Infants normally have a lower limit for these levels than older children. Adult men have higher limits than women for hypoglycemia. If fasting hypoglycemia is suspected, measurements of plasma (or serum) glucose levels after overnight, 24-, 36-, and 48-hour fasting are required. Serum insulin levels are also useful. The glucose tolerance test should not be part of the workup for symptomatic hypoglycemia.

Urine Glucose Level
Urine glucose values are archaic and should be abandoned.

Ketone Bodies
Recall that acetoacetate is the primary ketone body detected and that others are not detected at all by routine methods. Measurement of acetoacetate in the serum or urine is useful in monitoring patients receiving insulin therapy and in diagnosing ketoacidosis. Beta-hydroxybutyrate may cause ketoacidosis for hours after the routine "ketones" are negative.

Oral Glucose Tolerance Test
The oral glucose tolerance test measures plasma (or serum) glucose concentrations following an oral glucose load of 75 g (in pregnant patients use 100 g). The best results are obtained from ambulatory patients who fast overnight after a period of several days of high carbohydrate intake (150-300 g/d). Hospitalized patients stressed by surgery or serious illness, or patients otherwise subject to major stress, should not be tested because transient glucose intolerance may be exhibited. Age is also an important factor. After 50 years of age, oral glucose tolerance deteriorates rapidly, resulting in increase in plasma or serum glucose measurements of 0.4 to 0.7 mmol/L (8-13 mg/dL) per decade. In contrast, fasting plasma (or serum) glucose increases by only about 0.1 mmol/L (2 mg/dL) per decade of life after age 50 years. Limitations, even in patients optimally tested, result from an unacceptably high level of false-positive and false-negative test outcomes. An abnormal glucose tolerance test does not necessarily mean that symptomatic diabetes is inevitable.

Glycosylated Hemoglobins
The nonenzymatic glycosylation of proteins, including hemoglobin, occurs in hyperglycemic persons. The glycosylation of hemoglobin is thought to be a slow and irreversible process that occurs throughout the life span of the erythrocyte.

Hence, patients with clinically overt DM have an increased percentage of glycosylated hemoglobins (eg, hemoglobin A_{1c}), which reflects hyperglycemia during the preceding few months. Analysis of this protein provides insight into long-term glucose control, and should be routinely monitored.

Serum Insulin Levels

Insulin was the first polypeptide hormone to be measured using the radioimmunoassay technique. Today, however, serum insulin measurements play no role in the routine diagnosis and management of patients with DM. Low levels may be beneath the assay's limit of sensitivity, and insulin-treated patients often develop insulin antibodies, which invalidates the test. Levels are useful in suspected hyperinsulinism.

Microalbuminuria

The American Diabetes Association now recommends annual urine measurement of albumin in diabetics to detect low levels. This predicts progression to nephropathy and vascular complications.

References

Selby JV, FitzSimmons SC, Newman JM, et al. The natural history and epidemiology of diabetic nephropathy. *JAMA.* 1990;263:1954-1960.

Watts NB, Keffer JH. *Practical Endocrinology.* 4th ed. Philadephia, Pa: Lea & Febiger; 1989.

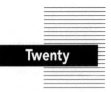
Acid-Base Balance: Laboratory Tests

Key Points

1. Arterial blood gases are required to establish pulmonary function—either hypoxia or ventilatory failure.
2. The pH quantitates the end result of the acid-base process, reflecting either an acute process or chronic compensation.
3. Think of $PaCO_2$ (arterial CO_2 tension) as a measure of respiratory ventilation. pH is inversely related to $PaCO_2$. Think of HCO_3^- (bicarbonate) as a measure of kidney handling of H^+. It is linearly related to pH.
4. Venous blood gases are satisfactory for repetitive evaluation of metabolic state in the absence of concern with oxygen tension. Venous pH is typically 0.03 units lower than arterial pH, and venous pCO_2 is typically 6 to 8 mm Hg higher than arterial pCO_2.

Background

Acute medical problems frequently involve acid-base study, focusing on pH, blood gases, and electrolytes. Common problems include ventilatory insufficiency acutely due to cardiac arrest, pneumonia, or pulmonary infarction; chronic states such as pulmonary emphysema with chronic obstructive lung disease; or a combination of acute and chronic disease, as seen in chronic lung disease patients with superimposed asthma. Metabolic diseases, typically associated with renal compensation, also necessitate acid-base analysis. Review acid-base physiology as needed, and remember the Henderson-Hasselbalch equation:

$$pH = pK + \log [(HCO_3^-)/(H_2CO_3)]$$

Since H_2CO_3 is in equilibrium with dissolved carbon dioxide, and dissolved CO_2 is in equilibrium with pCO_2, the equation can be simplified to $pH\alpha\, HCO_3^-/pCO_2$.

The kidney controls H^+ ion balance by retaining or excreting HCO_3^-; this is affected by the lungs, which increase or decrease CO_2 excretion by altering minute ventilation. Therefore, the pH is proportional to how the kidney handles HCO_3^- and inversely proportional to how the lung handles CO_2. Metabolic acidosis/alkalosis results from primary disturbance of HCO_3^-, and respiratory acidosis/alkalosis results from primary disturbance of pCO_2.

Acid-Base Abnormalities

$PaCO_2$ and HCO_3^-

Use the acid-base abnormalities table (Table 20.1) to resolve acid-base problems, keeping in mind that $PaCO_2$ can be affected rapidly (within minutes) by changes in ventilation, but HCO_3^- is excreted or retained by the kidney only over many hours.

Look first at $PaCO_2$; if this is high there is hypoventilation. Look next at pH; if it is slightly low the hypoventilation is chronic with compensation. The lower the pH the less the compensation and the more acute the hypoventilation (respiratory acidosis). Reverse the logic for hyperventilation (respiratory alkalosis).

If the $PaCO_2$ is low but so is the pH, there is metabolic acidosis. Reverse the logic for metabolic alkalosis.

From the laboratory data alone it can be difficult to distinguish respiratory acidosis from compensated metabolic alkalosis, or a compensated respiratory alkalosis from compensated metabolic acidosis. Here, knowledge of the clinical situation is essential. For instance, if the patient has severe lung disease, hypoventilation is probably causing the high $PaCO_2$.

Compensatory changes are always incomplete. Thus the pH does not return to "normal" and an acidosis or alkalosis exists in the untreated state. After administration of bicarbonate or ventilatory/oxygen therapy the results of blood gas analysis are probably induced by treatment.

Readily available and reliable measurements of blood pH and blood gases as stat tests are now routine. Monitoring arterial blood gases is essential when looking at either oxygen status or ventilation. CO_2 diffuses extremely rapidly through water because of its high solubility and therefore, even in the presence of pulmonary edema, it will continue to be exchanged adequately. The oxygen concentration of the arterial blood will drop promptly, because oxygen diffuses slowly across the alveolar and capillary distances if these are expanded by edema. In cases where one wishes to follow only the pH, venous specimens are satisfactory (in the absence of peripheral vascular collapse such as might be seen during acute cardiac resuscitation). The venous pH is extremely useful to follow metabolic acidosis and alkalosis.

Respiratory Acidosis

Respiratory acidosis results from acute or chronic failure of ventilation. If there is an increased production or retention of CO_2, then the respiratory system increases the rate and depth of respiration by blowing off CO_2. If further com-

Table 20.1 Examples of Acid-Base Abnormalities.*

	PaCO$_2$, mm Hg	HCO$_3^-$, mmol/L	pH
Reference ranges	35-45	23-26	7.36-7.45
Respiratory situations			
Acute hypoventilation; acute respiratory acidosis	60	26	7.25
Acute hyperventilation; acute respiratory alkalosis	25	22	7.58
Chronic hypoventilation; compensated respiratory acidosis	60	33	7.35
Chronic hyperventilation; compensated respiratory alkalosis	25	17	7.45
Metabolic situations			
Acute metabolic acidosis; no respiratory compensation	40	12	7.10
Acute metabolic acidosis; respiratory compensation	22	12	7.36
Acute metabolic acidosis; partial respiratory compensation	18	6	7.12
Acute metabolic alkalosis; no respiratory compensation	36	35	7.60
Acute metabolic alkalosis; respiratory compensation	51	35	7.46
Acute metabolic alkalosis; partial respiratory compensation	64	48	7.50

* Reprinted, with permission, from. A. G. Gornall, *Applied Biochemistry of Clinical Disorders.* 2nd ed. Philadelphia, Pa: JB Lippincott Co; 1986:133.

pensation is needed, renal reabsorption of bicarbonate is increased. The renal response is chronic and does not adjust rapidly in an acute situation.

Respiratory Alkalosis
Respiratory alkalosis is suggested by a low HCO$_3^-$ and raised pH levels. The PaCO$_2$ level drops precipitously when hyperventilation exists, either as an anxiety response or, more likely, as a result of mechanically assisted ventilation at an excessive rate. Occasionally, high-dose salicylates and fever may induce respiratory alkalosis. Compensation is achieved when an increase in renal excretion results in a decrease in the HCO$_3^-$ level. Such compensation is a slow and long process.

Metabolic Alkalosis
Metabolic alkalosis results from prolonged vomiting, provided the individual has normal gastric acid production, or from excessive ingestion of bicarbonate. Compensation results from increased bicarbonate wasting through the kidneys. Respiratory compensation includes decreased ventilation caused by decreased rate and depth of respiration, with CO$_2$ retention.

Metabolic Acidosis
Metabolic acidosis is seen in association with diabetes mellitus as a result of excessive production of ketoacids, with chronic renal failure with impaired clearance of acid products of metabolism, with lactic acidosis occurring in association with generalized or regional ischemia and associated hypoxia, with diarrhea as a result of loss of bicarbonate from intestinal secretions, and with excessive vomiting in an individual who has achlorhydria. In each of these cases there is increased absorption of bicarbonate by the kidney and removal of hydrogen ion through the potassium exchange mechanism. Respiratory compensation occurs in

metabolic acidosis as a result of increased rate and depth of respiration in response to lowered pH. One must consider the necessity of frequent sampling to evaluate the compensatory changes.

Anion Gap

The concept of anion gap is simple: balanced equivalents of positive and negative ions are maintained in plasma. The anion gap, practically speaking, is the difference between the sodium (Na^+) concentration and the sum of chloride (Cl^-) and HCO_3^- concentrations. If there is an increase in the anion gap, it is usually because organic acids have accumulated, often representing a metabolic acidosis. For example, the increased anion gap seen in diabetic ketoacidosis is a result of butyrate and acetoacetate accumulation; in renal failure it results from accumulation of sulfate, phosphate, and organic acids; in shock or hypoxic states it results from lactic acid production; and in myeloma it results from an increase in proteins functioning as anions. On the other hand, a decreased anion gap is almost always the result of hypoproteinemia or, less likely, a laboratory error in electrolyte measurement. In practice, the anion gap is overrated as a case-finding tool because total protein and albumin are measured in most seriously ill patients anyway, and renal failure or ketoacidosis are not likely to be discovered as a result of an abnormal anion gap. Detecting laboratory error by using a decrease in the anion gap is an unusual event, because strict quality control makes such an error unlikely. The decrease in anion gap may be more useful to suggest ketoacidosis.

Serum Lactate

Serum lactate is one of the most underutilized tests easily available from the laboratory. With regional hypoxia/ischemia, there is an outpouring of lactic acid from damaged tissues that is not readily metabolized. Therefore, even if there is no systemic acidosis, there may be a marked regional change. It is possible to measure regional venous, eg, femoral, lactate to assess regional ischemia. Elevated systemic lactate production is more common than generally recognized. It results from low cardiac output and a concomitant fall in PaO_2 concentration, which results in generalized tissue hypoxia.

Summary

Acid-base assessment should not be a guessing game. We have the ability to rapidly, precisely, and, if necessary, repetitively measure pH, blood gases, and electrolytes to provide the numerator and denominator of the acid-base equation. By utilizing patient data and appropriately interpreting laboratory findings, these conditions can be effectively diagnosed and managed.

References

Adrogue HJ, Rashad MN, Gorin AB, et al. Assessing acid base status in circulatory failure, differences in arterial and central venous blood. *N Engl J Med*. 1989;320:1312-1316.

Bleich HL. The clinical implications of venous carbon dioxide tension. *N Engl J Med.* 1989;320:1345-1346.

Gornall AG. *Applied Biochemistry of Clinical Disorders.* 2nd ed. Philadelphia, Pa: JB Lippincott Co; 1986.

Lehmann HP, Majonos JS, Scheer WD. *Review Course in Clinical Chemistry.* Chicago, Ill: ASCP Press; 1987.

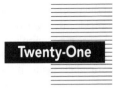

Twenty-One

Urinalysis

Key Point

A properly collected and promptly analyzed specimen is paramount for accurate data.

Background

Urinalysis is performed for two reasons: (1) to detect and assess renal disease and (2) to investigate diseases involving other organ systems that may be reflected in the urine. Most adults excrete 1000 to 1500 mL of urine every 24 hours. Young children excrete less total urine volume than adults but more urine volume per body weight. Adults over 70 years of age may excrete as little as 250 mL/d. In general, there is an inverse relationship between the volume of urine excreted and the specific gravity of the urine. Normal adults void five to nine times each day in amounts of 100 to 300 mL.

Polyuria is the excretion of an increased volume of urine. Polyuria may result from diabetes mellitus (DM) (diuresis caused by increased solute load), diabetes insipidus (lack of antidiuretic hormone [ADH]), drugs (especially caffeine, diuretics, and ethanol), chronic renal failure, renal tubular damage, primary aldosteronism, adrenocortical insufficiency, hyperparathyroidism, increased salt and/or protein intake, and certain psychiatric disorders (eg, psychogenic polydipsia).

Oliguria is a decreased urine volume, to between 100 and 500 mL/d, which is insufficient to excrete the necessary amount of solute. Oliguria can result from a variety of renal diseases as well as from intravascular fluid volume contraction. Anuria is the virtual absence of renal function, with urine production of less than 100 mL/d. Anuria implies severe renal disease, such as complete and/or long-standing urinary tract obstruction or bilateral renal cortical necrosis.

Proper specimen collection is mandatory. All specimens must be collected in clean, dry, and detergent-free containers. The first urine voided in the morning is the preferred specimen for assessing the concentrating capacity of the kidney. It provides the best preserved and most concentrated urinary sediment. However, the most commonly obtained sample is a random urine voided at any time. This specimen may not reveal abnormalities in urine solute content, protein content, or formed elements. If these abnormalities are suspected but not found, a first voided specimen should be examined. Glucosuria is best detected in a postprandial specimen; urobilinogen is most likely to be elevated in urine collected in the afternoon.

A midstream clean-catch specimen is the sample of choice in cases of suspected urinary tract infection because it is necessary to obtain urine that is least contaminated by the epithelium and bacterial flora of the external genitalia. The external genitalia must be thoroughly cleaned with an antiseptic soap and rinsed with sterile water. After micturition is begun, the first few milliliters of urine are discarded, and a midstream sample is collected into a sterile container.

Bladder catherization (in and out) may be safely used to obtain a sterile urine specimen, especially in pediatric patients. Under certain circumstances a sterile urine specimen may be obtained by transcutaneous suprapubic aspiration of the urinary bladder with syringe and needle.

A timed urine collection is used to quantitate excretion of a particular analyte during a fixed period (eg, 2 hours, 12 hours, 24 hours). Timed specimens must be completely collected for the desired period and the volume accurately measured. The specimen must be preserved to prevent bacterial overgrowth and to limit the deterioration of solutes. Refrigeration of the specimen during collection is a satisfactory method of preservation for most routine testing; however, the urine specimen must come to room temperature before testing specific gravity. For certain chemical determinations, preservatives (eg, formaldehyde, thymol, toluene) may have to be added to the container during collection. Most clinical laboratories provide appropriately prepared containers.

Routine Urinalysis

Once the urine specimen is collected, examination should begin promptly. Changes result when urine is left standing at room temperature, providing the principal cause for inaccurate results. After 1 hour at room temperature one must anticipate the following changes in the urine specimen: pH elevation; destruction of erythrocytes and leukocytes; decrease in ketones and glucose, bilirubin, and urobilinogen levels; dissolution of casts; formation or dissolution of crystals (depending on pH); bacterial growth; and development of turbidity, darker color, and pungent odor. If delay is anticipated between collection and examination, the urine should be refrigerated. However, refrigeration may induce precipitates that can obscure the urinary sediment.

As currently performed, routine urinalysis consists of the following tests, explained below: (1) physical properties—color, clarity, odor, pH, specific gravity, and osmolality; (2) chemical characteristics—protein, glucose, blood, bile pigments, ketones, and nitrite/esterase; and (3) sediment constituents—cells, casts, lipids, crystals, microorganisms, tumor cells, and contaminants.

Physical Properties

Color

The normal pale yellow to dark amber color of urine is due primarily to the pigment urochrome and to a lesser extent to the pigments uroerythrin and urobilin. The intensity of color in normal urine is proportional to the quantity of solutes present. The most common cause of abnormal urine color is medication. Red or red-brown urine results from blood, hemoglobin, myoglobin, methemoglobin, or porphyrins, or may follow ingestion of beets or drugs such as phenazopyridine hydrochloride (Pyridium) or phenolphthalein. Intact erythrocytes in urine (hematuria) cause a smoky or cloudy red-brown appearance; free hemoglobin (hemoglobinuria) or myoglobin (myoglobinuria) causes a clear red urine. A red or red-brown urine in females is most often the result of contamination with menstrual blood. Yellow-brown or green-brown urine is caused by bile pigments. Since a highly concentrated normal urine may also be yellow-brown, it is important to chemically confirm the presence of bile pigments. Orange urine results from bile pigments or analgesic substances like phenazopyridine hydrochloride. Bright orange-yellow urine following ingestion of multivitamins is due to excretion of riboflavin or its metabolites. Brown urine may be caused by the formation of methemoglobin from hemoglobin in an acid urine, by melanin (produced by metastatic melanoma), by homogentisic acid (associated with alkaptonuria), or following ingestion of rhubarb, cascara, or senna. Green urine results from acriflavine ingestion, and blue-green urine from ingestion of methylene blue or azure B dye.

Clarity

Normal urine is clear. Cloudy urine most often comes from normal individuals and is due to solute precipitation—phosphates in alkaline urines and urates in acid urines. Pathological conditions causing cloudy urine include excretion of leukocytes (pyuria), erythrocytes (hematuria), bacteria (bacteriuria), and lymph (chyluria). All cloudy or turbid urines must be examined microscopically.

Odor

Urine contaminated with bacteria may smell like ammonia (especially with urease-positive organisms) or putrefaction (if heavily contaminated). Phenylketonuria patients produce urine with a musty odor. Advanced cirrhosis results in a pungent, aromatic odor (fetor hepaticus). Infants with maple syrup urine disease, a disorder of amino acid metabolism, produce maple syrup–smelling urine. An odor of sweaty feet occurs in glutaric acidemia and isovaleric acidemia. Ketonuric patients produce urine that smells like acetone.

Urinary pH

The kidneys share responsibility with the lungs for maintaining chemical homeostasis of plasma. Whereas the lungs are primarily involved in the excretion of carbon dioxide, the kidneys have a dual role in acid-base homeostasis. The renal tubules reabsorb nearly all of the filtered bicarbonate, principally in the proximal nephron. In addition, tubules excrete the daily plasma load of nonvolatile organic acids as titratable acid and ammonium. Renal acid-base control exerts more long-standing effects than the short-term pulmonary mechanism. In a steady state, the net acid excretion (titratable acid + ammonium - bicarbonate) must equal the amount of acid added to the extracellular fluid from diet, metabolism, and fecal alkali losses. At physiological pH levels, very few free hydrogen ions are present. Hence, urinary pH determinations do not measure total acid excretion. The urinary pH does reflect the urine acid excretion in a qualitative manner.

Normal urine is usually slightly acid (pH, ~6; range, 4.5-8.0). A specimen with pH less than 4.5 was probably collected in an acid-contaminated container. A urine pH greater than 8.0 reflects bacterial contamination producing alkalization after collection. A diet high in protein produces an acid urine; a predominantly vegetable diet results in a urine pH greater than 6. The urine excreted shortly after a meal will be slightly more alkaline than normal, corresponding to a postprandial metabolic alkalosis that results from the production of gastric acid (the "alkaline tide"). At night, respiratory acidosis that occurs during sleep results in the production of a more acid urine.

In some cases the urinary pH reflects a pathological process. Most patients with systemic acid-base abnormalities have urinary pH changes that reflect renal compensation. Table 21.1 illustrates expected findings. Some patients with prolonged and severe hypokalemia may have persistent aciduria despite metabolic alkalosis. There are two forms of renal tubular acidosis that are caused by defective tubular function. Both show systemic acidosis accompanied by persistently alkaline urine (the pH cannot be lowered below 6 or 6.5). The proximal form is caused by a defect in reabsorption of bicarbonate, the distal form by a failure to maximally acidify the urine. Persistently alkaline urine may also be excreted by patients with pyelonephritis or renal tubular necrosis.

Urinary pH must be measured on fresh urine because the pH tends to rise in standing urine due to loss of carbon dioxide to the atmosphere and production of ammonia by urease-positive bacteria.

Specific Gravity

Each day approximately 170 L of glomerular filtrate are formed but only 1 to 1.5 L of urine are excreted. Water and solute ingestion, renal tubular function, and the effects of ADH affect urine solute content. Reduced or absent ADH secretion or impaired renal tubular responsiveness to ADH can result in excretion of a persistently dilute urine. Conversely, the excretion of a persistently concentrated urine could result from sustained or inappropriate ADH secretion, an exaggeration of proximal tubular fluid reabsorption, or impaired solute resorption in the loop of Henle and distal nephron. In general, a clinical assessment of the concentrating capacity of the kidneys may be obtained by measuring the urine volume and the urinary solute content.

Quantitatively, the most important urine solutes are urea, sodium, chloride, sulfate, and phosphate. Measurements of urine specific gravity and osmolality assess urinary solute content. More specialized tests include measurement of free water and osmole clearances and provocative tests of renal concentrating and diluting capacities.

The specific gravity of a solution is the ratio of the mass per unit volume of the solution to the mass per unit volume of distilled water. Hence, the specific

Table 21.1 Urinary pH in Systemic Acid-Base Disorders.

Disorder	Urinary pH	Change in Urine Composition
Metabolic acidosis	Acid	Increased titratable acidity and ammonium
Metabolic alkalosis	Alkaline	Decreased ammonium
Respiratory acidosis	Acid	Increased ammonium
Respiratory alkalosis	Alkaline	Increased bicarbonate

gravity is a relative measure by weight of the amount of dissolved urinary solutes. Although normally the major solutes of urine are inorganic compounds of comparable molecular weight, a specimen may contain other compounds of much higher molecular weight. Of particular importance are proteins, glucose, dyes, and radiographic contrast material. These compounds raise the specific gravity out of proportion to their concentration. Under these circumstances a measurement of the number of solute molecules present in the urine, the urine osmolality, would be more useful.

Normally, an adult should be able to concentrate urine to a specific gravity of 1.016 to 1.022. A first morning urine with a specific gravity of 1.023 or greater after overnight fluid deprivation indicates normal concentrating capacity. Although this test is quite sensitive for impaired renal concentrating capacity, an abnormal test result is nonspecific and cannot distinguish possible causes. Provocative tests of renal diluting capacity are of little practical value. Extremely high specific gravities (eg, 1.060) indicate the presence of a high-molecular-weight substance (eg, radiographic contrast material). Hyposthenuria means a persistently low urine specific gravity (less than 1.007). Isosthenuria means a fixed urine specific gravity, usually 1.010.

DM is associated with increased urinary volume and elevated specific gravity due to urinary glucose, which increases the solute content. Diabetes insipidus results in a large urinary volume with low specific gravity, as loss of ADH adversely affects the renal concentrating mechanism. Renal tubular disease is often manifested early by a loss of the concentrating capacity of the kidneys; the patient is no longer able to produce urine with a specific gravity greater than 1.018. Later in the course of disease the capacity to dilute urine is lost and the patient can only produce an isosthenuric urine. Variations in urine solute content do not always produce noticeable changes in urine volume.

Osmolality

Osmolality and osmolarity are measures of the number of solute molecules within a solution. The molecular weight of the individual solute molecules does not affect these measures; hence, they are a more accurate measurement of solute concentration than is specific gravity. Osmolality is the ratio of the number of solute molecules to the weight of the solution; osmolarity is the ratio of the number of solute molecules to the volume of the solution. In practice urine osmolarities and osmolalities are considered equivalent, although theoretically they are not.

The osmolality of urine is variable and greatly affected by diet. For a normal adult on the usual American diet, a normal fluid intake will result in a urine osmolality of 500 to 800 mmol/kg (mOsm/kg) of water. Of the 800 mmol (mOsm), approximately 330 mmol (mOsm) come from urea molecules and the remaining 470 mmol (mOsm) from sodium, potassium, chloride, and phosphate ions. Under conditions of dehydration, the kidneys concentrate urine to 800 to 1400 mmol (mOsm). During water diuresis a normal patient should produce a dilute urine of 40 to 80 mmol (mOsm). A high protein diet will increase the urine osmolality; a salt-free diet will decrease it. Normally the ratio of urine to serum osmolality is between 1.0 and 3.0. In cases of oliguria due to acute tubular damage, the ratio is usually less than 1.2. When the glomerular filtration rate is impaired and there is oliguria, the ratio is usually greater than 1.2. In cases of polyuria, osmotic diuresis causes a ratio greater than 1.0, whereas water diuresis and diabetes insipidus cause a ratio less than 1.0.

Chemical Characteristics

Protein

Normal urine contains small amounts of protein. The majority of this protein (50%-70%) comes from plasma and the remainder from tubular and lower urinary tract sources. A random 100-mL urine specimen normally contains 0.002 to 0.008 g of protein. The upper limit of normal for protein excretion in the urine is 0.15 g/d. Daily urine protein excretion in excess of 0.15 g is, by definition, proteinuria. Patients with very high urine volumes can excrete sufficient protein daily to have proteinuria, but each urine specimen might not have a protein concentration high enough to be detected by screening methods.

Urine proteins resemble the normal plasma proteins. Because of the molecular size and electrostatic charge barrier of the glomerulus, very little albumin is filtered. Most of the filtered albumin is reabsorbed and catabolized by the proximal tubular epithelial cells. The majority of proteins excreted in the urine are globulins. Several normal urinary proteins are not found in plasma—primarily the Tamm-Horsfall mucoprotein originating in the distal renal tubules and collecting ducts, and proteins of seminal, prostatic, and urethral origin.

Although proteinuria suggests renal disease, not all proteinuria is caused by renal dysfunction. Transient proteinuria usually does not indicate renal disease. There are two recognized types of transient proteinuria. Postural proteinuria, observed in approximately 3% to 5% of healthy adolescents and young adults, occurs when the person is upright and disappears when the person is recumbent. Functional proteinuria is associated with physiological conditions. It may be caused by fever, unaccustomed physical exercise, exposure to heat or cold, emotional stress, or congestive heart failure. People with transient proteinuria can have associated urinary sediment abnormalities. Both proteinuria and sediment changes disappear when the causative factor is removed. Transient proteinuria is related more to alterations in renal hemodynamics than to changes in glomerular permeability. Persistent proteinuria, on the other hand, usually indicates renal disease. Even without any obvious clinical or laboratory evidence of renal disease, all instances of persistent proteinuria should be considered presumptive evidence of renal disease.

Heavy proteinuria (more than 4 g/d) is usually caused by renal diseases that greatly increase glomerular permeability. It is characteristic of nephrotic syndrome, and associated with acute and chronic glomerulonephritis, lupus nephritis, amyloidosis, and severe renal venous congestion. Moderate proteinuria (0.5-4 g/d) may be seen with any disease just listed. In addition, it is seen in nephrosclerosis, pyelonephritis with hypertension, preeclampsia, diabetic nephropathy, multiple myeloma, and toxic renal damage. Minimal proteinuria (<0.5 g/d) may be associated with chronic pyelonephritis, renal tubular disorders, polycystic renal disease, and the inactive phases of glomerular diseases. All cases of postural and functional proteinuria produce minimal proteinuria. Proteinuria may be absent in acute pyelonephritis, chronic pyelonephritis, obstructive uropathy, renal calculi, renal tumors, and congenital malformations.

Most renal disease causing proteinuria is associated with albumin excretion. This pattern is seen in glomerular diseases, due to loss of the selective filtering ability of the glomeruli. Excretion of low molecular weight proteins caused by their impaired reabsorption is a pattern typical of diseases of the renal tubular epithelium and interstitium. A third pattern, the loss of one specific protein or protein fragment, is characteristic of monoclonal gammopathies (eg, multiple myeloma, Waldenström's macroglobulinemia). In these disorders there is overproduction and increased filtration of Bence Jones protein, one of the immunoglobulin light chains (kappa or lambda).

In most (but not all) cases the degree of proteinuria correlates with the severity of renal disease, but significant, even advanced renal disease can exist in the face of minimal or absent proteinuria. The simplest screening test for proteinuria is the colorimetric method, using a reagent strip that contains a pH indicator dye. The degree of color is proportional to the degree of proteinuria. This method has the advantages of being simple and not too sensitive (0.15-0.30 g/L is the lowest detectable amount). Concentrated urine with a high specific gravity may show trace levels of protein, even though total daily excretion of protein is normal. Clinical judgment is needed to evaluate the significance of trace amounts. The colorimetric method is fairly specific for protein; drugs and radiographic contrast media will not be falsely detected by this method; however, contamination of the urine with quaternary ammonium compounds (some antiseptics and detergents) or with skin cleansers containing chlorhexidine may produce false-positive results. The indicator dye reacts very well in the presence of albumin; however, the dye is much less sensitive to other proteins (hemoglobin, Bence Jones protein, globulins) and may not detect these.

Precipitation methods are used as confirmatory tests for protein. These include the precipitation of proteins by heat and acetic acid, sulfosalicylic acid, or trichloroacetic acid, and allow the semiquantitation of protein according to the degree of turbidity produced. In general, precipitation methods are more sensitive than the colorimetric method. Neither method detects the amount of protein found in normal urine. Unlike the colorimetric method, precipitation methods may produce urinary turbidity in the presence of certain drugs (eg, tolbutamide) or radiographic contrast material.

Three methods are used to detect Bence Jones proteinuria. A screening test is based on precipitation of these proteins with toluene sulfonic acid. Gradually heating urine allows one to detect Bence Jones proteinuria because the protein precipitates at 40°C to 60°C but redissolves near 100°C. The best method is protein electrophoresis.

Recent attention has been given to more sensitive assays of urine albumin that measure low levels of albuminuria not detected by routine screening methods. Normal urine contains little albumin (<0.03 g/L), fivefold less than the amount detected by the urine reagent strip (dipstick). Excretion of albumin in excess of this amount, but in quantities not detected by the dipstick, has been referred to as "microalbuminuria." It may identify early injury to the glomerular capillary basement membrane in patients with DM, for which therapeutic intervention may be important. Assay of a timed overnight collection provides more accurate information than testing a random urine specimen.

Glucose and Other Sugars

Glucose is freely filtered by the glomeruli and then reabsorbed by the renal tubules. The tubules have a maximum reabsorption capacity for glucose such that with normal renal blood flow a blood glucose concentration in excess of 8.3 to 10.0 mmol/L (150-180 mg/dL) (hyperglycemia) results in the presence of glucose in the urine (glucosuria). This blood glucose concentration is termed the "renal threshold" for glucose. The glucosuria of DM is caused by this mechanism. A large amount of glucose in the urine induces an osmotic diuresis which results in the polyuria and polydipsia typical of DM and a relatively high urine specific gravity. Glucosuria does not by itself mean DM; exaggerated and prolonged postprandial hyperglycemia is required for diagnosis. However, glucosuria is a hallmark of the disease and every patient with glucosuria should be evaluated for DM.

Glucosuria due to hyperglycemia can result from diseases other than DM, including Cushing's syndrome, pancreatic islet-cell tumors, hyperthyroidism, pheochromocytoma, destructive pancreatic disease (eg, carcinoma, pancreatitis), central nervous system disorders (eg, brain tumors, hypothalamic disease, asphyxia), disturbances of metabolism (eg, glycogen storage disease, feeding after starvation, liver disease, uremia, obesity), trauma (eg, thermal burns, bone fractures), infections, and certain drugs, such as steroids.

Glucosuria in the absence of hyperglycemia is termed renal glucosuria, a defect of the renal tubular glucose reabsorptive mechanism, resulting in glucosuria at normal or slightly elevated blood glucose concentrations. Hyperglycemia and abnormal glucose tolerance are not features of renal glucosuria. Renal glucosuria can occur as a primary renal disorder or secondary to toxic renal injury. It can be an isolated defect or a component of multiple tubular defects (Fanconi's syndrome). Glucosuria without hyperglycemia also may occur during pregnancy; the mechanism is a reduced maximum reabsorption capacity for glucose.

There are two methods for detecting glucosuria: copper reduction tests and enzymatic tests. Copper reduction tests are not specific for glucose and rely on the reducing properties of glucose and other sugars. These tests are available commercially as Benedict's test or Clinitest® tablets (Miles Laboratories Inc, Elkhart, Ind). Sugars other than glucose (fructose, galactose, pentose, lactose, maltose), as well as nonsugar reducing agents (eg, ascorbic acid, uric acid, creatinine, and certain drug metabolites), will give positive results. In infants and young children, the copper reduction test is a good screening test for galactosemia. The threshold for glucosuria detection by the Clinitest® method is 8.3 to 13.9 mmol/L (150-250 mg/dL).

Enzymatic tests for glucosuria utilize the enzyme glucose oxidase, which is specific for glucose. All multiple reagent test strips use the enzymatic method. In addition to increased specificity, the enzymatic tests are also more sensitive (2.8-5.6 mmol/L [50-100 mg/dL]) than copper reduction tests. The only substance causing a false-positive enzymatic test reaction is hypochlorite bleach (eg, Clorox), used to clean urine specimen containers. Hence, enzymatic tests are the preferred method for detecting glucosuria. Ascorbic acid (vitamin C) in concentrations of 2840 μmol/L (50 mg/dL) or greater may inhibit the reaction, causing a false-negative test in specimens containing small amounts of glucose (≤5.6 mmol/L [100 mg/dL]).

Identification of urinary sugars other than glucose is occasionally necessary. Urine sugars usually tested are galactose, lactose, fructose, and pentose. Of these, galactose is the most important. Galactosemia is a treatable metabolic disorder causing galactosuria, liver damage, mental retardation, and cataracts in infants. This disorder often is diagnosed by finding a urine that reacts positively with a copper reduction test but negatively with an enzymatic test. Positive identification of galactose or any other nonglucose sugar in the urine requires chromatography.

Blood Hemoglobin and Related Pigments

Blood in the urine occurs in two forms: intact erythrocytes (hematuria) or hemoglobin pigment (hemoglobinuria). Normal urine contains 0 to 2 erythrocytes per high-power field (HPF). Approximately 2000 red blood cells (RBCs) per milliliter of urine must be present to be identified microscopically. The dipstick is less sensitive and detects between 10,000 and 50,000 intact erythrocytes per milliliter (5-20 RBCs/HPF) or 0.15 to 0.62 g/L of free hemoglobin in the urine. A negative dipstick test for hemoglobin or RBCs does not exclude occult blood in the urine; a microscopic examination for hematuria should be performed when clinically indicated. Erythrocytes may hemolyze in urine so that hemoglobinuria and hematuria both may be present.

Hematuria can result from renal disease or lower urinary tract disease. Hemoglobinuria can result from urinary tract bleeding with hemolysis of cells within the urine, or from intravascular hemolysis. Hemoglobin in the plasma is bound to the protein haptoglobin. If plasma hemoglobin exceeds 1.3 to 1.5 g/L (130-150 mg/dL), the binding sites are saturated and hemoglobin circulates free in the plasma. The glomerulus is permeable to free hemoglobin but not to the haptoglobin-hemoglobin complex. Once haptoglobin is saturated, hemoglobinuria appears. The finding of hemoglobinuria without hematuria in a fresh urine sample indicates clinically significant hemoglobinemia. The combination of a positive test for hemoglobin and a normal urinary sediment in the absence of intravascular hemolysis suggests that the urine specimen was not fresh when examined, resulting in cell lysis. Proteinuria usually accompanies hemoglobinuria. However, the chemical test for hemoglobin is much more sensitive than is the chemical test for protein. Three interfering situations are worthy of note: (1) Large amounts of urinary ascorbic acid will inhibit the test for hemoglobin. (2) Urine specimens with significant bacterial contamination may contain sufficient peroxidase activity to produce a false-positive test for hemoglobin. (3) Urine specimen containers contaminated with hypochlorite bleach may cause a false-positive reaction.

Myoglobin is not present in normal urine. Myoglobinuria may result from severe traumatic injury to muscle (crush syndrome), thermal burns, toxic muscle injury (eg, snake venom), primary muscle disease, and severe and unaccustomed exercise ("march" myoglobinuria), and in spontaneous paroxysmal myoglobinuria. Myoglobin is a much smaller molecule than hemoglobin (17,000 vs 64,000 molecular weight). Like hemoglobin, myoglobin contains peroxidase activity so that myoglobinuria will produce a positive dipstick test for hemoglobin. If the hemoglobin test is positive but the physician suspects myoglobinuria, the urine sediment can be examined microscopically for hematuria, or the urine can be chemically tested for myoglobin by salt precipitation or spectrophotometry.

Bile Pigments

Two bile pigments may be detected in urine: bilirubin and urobilinogen (Table 21.2). Conjugated (water-soluble) serum bilirubin in excess of 18 to 34 µmol/L (1-2 mg/dL) is excreted into the urine. Both hepatocellular diseases and obstructive biliary tract diseases may produce bilirubinuria before jaundice becomes apparent. Urinary bilirubin excretion is enhanced by alkalosis. The reagent strip can detect urine levels of 13.7 µmol/L (0.8 mg/dL), whereas the Icto® test tablet (Miles Laboratories Inc) can detect levels as low as 0.9 to 1.7 µmol/L (0.05-0.1 mg/dL). False-positive reactions occur when chlorpromazine metabolites are present. False-negative results may occur with high levels of ascorbic acid or in urine that has been exposed to light for several hours.

Urobilinogen is produced by bacterial action on bilirubin within the intestinal lumen. Urobilinogen is partially absorbed into the portal circulation and a small amount is excreted into the urine. The majority is excreted by the liver. Urinary and fecal urobilinogen levels may be increased in hemolytic anemia. Urinary urobilinogen levels are increased with hepatocellular disease because injured hepatocytes fail to excrete absorbed urobilinogen (enterohepatic circulation). Decreased or absent urine urobilinogen may accompany complete biliary tract obstruction.

Fresh urine must be examined when assaying urobilinogen. Urine levels up to 1.0 Ehrlich unit are normal; a negative result is not always reliable. False-negative results occur when phenazopyridine hydrochloride or azo dyes are present in the urine. The test is not specific for urobilinogen; other compounds give false-positive results.

Ketones

The three major ketone bodies (or ketones) produced as the result of hepatic fatty acid metabolism are acetone (2% of urinary ketones), acetoacetic acid or diacetic acid (20%), and beta-hydroxybutyric acid (78%). Ketones are products of the incomplete metabolism of fat, and their presence is indicative of ketoacidosis. The ketones are readily excreted into urine, where they produce ketonuria. Ketonuria is commonly seen in patients with poorly controlled DM. It is important in any patient with DM to test the urine for ketonuria as well as glucosuria.

Ketonuria is detected by testing the urine for acetoacetic acid using alkaline nitroprusside. The test does not react with beta-hydroxybutyric acid or acetone.

Table 21.2 Bile Pigments in Urine.

	Normal Urine	Hemolytic States	Hepatocellular Disease	Biliary Obstruction
Urobilinogen	Normal	Increased	Increased	Negative/Decreased
Bilirubin	Negative	Negative	Positive/Negative	Positive

Because of this, there may be occasions when a patient with significant ketoacidosis and ketonuria has a negative test for urine ketones. Diabetic patients who are hypoxic have impaired conversion of beta-hydroxybutyric acid to acetoacetic acid. Patients with lactic acidosis and diabetic patients with hyperosmolar coma do not have ketoacidosis or ketonuria. False-positive results (usually reflected as trace amounts) may occur in highly pigmented urines or in those containing large quantities of levadopa metabolites.

Several conditions and diseases other than DM produce ketoacidosis and ketonuria. These include exposure to cold, violent exercise, starvation or cachexia, eclampsia, uncontrollable emesis during pregnancy, anesthesia, von Gierke's disease (type I glycogen storage disease), inborn errors of fatty acid oxidation, high-fat and low-carbohydrate (ketogenic) weight-reduction diets, and acute febrile illnesses and toxic states accompanied by vomiting and diarrhea. The common denominator of all these conditions, including DM, is the use of fatty acids, rather than carbohydrates, for energy.

Nitrite and Leukocyte Esterase

The nitrite and leukocyte esterase tests have become available as part of the dipstick portion of the urinalysis and should be used in tandem. They offer some indication of bacteriuria or pyuria without the need for microscopic examination of the urinary sediment. They have allowed the dipstick alone to be used as a screening test in asymptomatic patients without evidence of urinary tract disease, thus eliminating the need for unnecessary microscopic examinations. These tests should not supplant microscopic examination in symptomatic patients or in patients with a likelihood of urinary tract disease.

The nitrite test to detect bacteriuria depends on the reduction of urine nitrate to nitrite by bacteria within the bladder. The test should be performed on a first morning specimen, or on a urine sample collected at least 4 hours or more following the previous voiding. This allows organisms that might be present in the bladder sufficient time to metabolize urinary nitrate. Positive reactions on stale urine may be due to bacterial proliferation within the specimen after voiding.

The nitrite test is specific for gram-negative organisms. Negative results occur with pathogens such as enterococci, streptococci, or staphylococci, which do not form nitrite. The sensitivity is only 60% when compared with micobiological procedures, but a positive reaction suggests significant bacteriuria ($>10^5$ organisms per milliliter). Large amounts of ascorbic acid decrease the sensitivity of the test. False-positive reactions are produced by medication that turns urine red or that turns red in acid medium (such as phenazopyridine).

The leukocyte esterase test is used to detect pyuria. Microscopic detection and quantification of leukocytes in urine can be unreliable because of cell lysis or variability in the performance of the microscopic examination. The leukocyte esterase test detects both lysed and intact leukocytes. The test is capable of detecting the equivalent of 5 to 15 leukocytes per HPF and is at least as sensitive as light microscopy for the detection of pyuria. Elevated glucose concentrations (>166 mmol/L [3 g/dL]), high specific gravity, the presence of cephalexin, cephalothin, or high concentrations of oxalic acid may interfere. Tetracycline may reduce the reactivity of the assay and high concentrations of the drug may cause false-negative reactions. Nitrofurantoin colors the urine brown and may mask the color reaction. Neutropenic patients may have false-negative results. Contamination from vaginal neutrophils will give false-positive results. The negative predictive value of a combined negative nitrite/esterase test is greater than 95%.

Sediment Constituents

First voided urine is the best specimen to examine because the urine is most concentrated and cellular elements are best preserved. After the urine has been examined and tested for appropriate physical properties and chemical constituents, it should be promptly centrifuged and the sediment examined as soon as possible. The protocol for microscopic examination follows:

1. If any delay (>30-60 min) is anticipated, preserve the urine with a few drops of 10% formalin. Refrigeration can also be used but dense precipitation of crystals initiated by refrigeration may obscure the sediment.
2. Mix the urine well. Place a 10- to 15-mL aliquot into a centrifuge tube and centrifuge for 5 minutes at 2000 rpm.
3. Decant the supernatant and resuspend the sediment in 1 mL of supernatant. Mix well. Save the supernatant for possible confirmation tests.
4. Place one drop of the resuspended sediment on a glass slide. A coverslip without mounting medium is used to protect the microscope's objective lenses.
5. Adjust the light source by closing the diaphragm and lowering the condensor to obtain maximum contrast.
6. Scan the specimen under low-power (100x) magnification. Omission of this step may cause the observer to overlook some large casts. Pay close attention to the edges of the cover slip.
7. Identify the various casts, cells, and crystals under high-power (400x) magnification.
8. Record the number of cells per HPF (400x) and the number of casts per low-power field (100x).

Cells

Erythrocytes. Erythrocytes in urine (hematuria) are usually round or spherical rather than biconcave. They are easily hemolyzed in alkaline or dilute urine, and crenated in concentrated urine. The finding of RBC casts localizes the cause of hematuria to the kidney. Associated proteinuria also suggests renal origin. Hematuria may be the only abnormality of the urinary sediment in cases of urinary calculi or neoplasms of the urinary tract. Whereas microscopic hematuria can occur with a variety of disorders, gross hematuria is characteristic of only a few, which include viral cystitis, urinary calculi, neoplasms of the urinary tract, IgA nephropathy, hypercalciuria, polycystic kidney disease, and poststreptococcal glomerulonephritis.

Leukocytes. Leukocytes identified in the urinary sediment are usually polymorphonuclear leukocytes. The multilobed nucleus can usually be seen. More than 50 leukocytes per HPF and/or clumps of leukocytes in the sediment suggest acute infection, eg, acute pyelonephritis or acute urethrocystitis. However, pyuria (>5 polymorphonuclear leukocytes per HPF) may be the earliest sign of acute glomerulonephritis. Leukocyte casts locate the disease within the kidney. Urinary calculi often are accompanied by pyuria. Repeated episodes of pyuria despite negative urine cultures suggests either renal tuberculosis or lupus nephritis. Eosinophils in the urinary sediment suggest an allergic interstitial nephritis. Lymphocytes suggest tuberculosis. All leukocytes are rapidly lysed in alkaline or hypotonic urine. A glitter cell is a leukocyte that contains separated, refractile granules exhibiting brownian movement. Formerly, they were thought to be pathognomonic of acute pyelonephritis, but it is recognized that they may appear in normal hypotonic urines.

Epithelial Cells. Epithelial cells are commonly found in urinary sediment, and some may be difficult to distinguish from leukocytes. Renal tubular epithelial cells are the smallest epithelial cells and can be found in normal urine. They are round, slightly larger than a leukocyte, with a round nucleus and moderately abundant, clear cytoplasm. They originate in the renal tubules and increased numbers are seen in conditions associated with acute tubular damage (eg, acute tubular necrosis, acute pyelonephritis, necrotizing papillitis, acute renal allograft rejection). Oval fat bodies are renal tubular epithelial cells and/or macrophages containing ingested lipid, which may be refractile or exhibit a Maltese cross-formation under polarized light. Transitional epithelial cells originate from the renal pelvis, ureter, or bladder epithelium. These cells have more cytoplasm than renal tubular cells, and are cuboid or caudate (if from the renal pelvis), with a large nucleus. They may be seen in inflammatory states. Malignant transitional epithelial cells, especially in large clumps, may be recognized. Squamous epithelial cells are very large, polygonal cells with angulated edges. These cells originate in the urethra and are of no diagnostic importance.

Casts

Casts are cylindrical, agglutinated masses formed in the lumens of the distal nephron and passed to the urine. The width of a cast is determined by the diameter of the nephron segment in which it formed. Most casts are narrow, the width of three to four leukocytes. They are believed to originate in the distal convoluted tubules or the first part of the collecting ducts. Broad casts are formed by stasis in the distal portion of the collecting ducts or in the ducts of Bellini. They have been termed renal failure casts because of their association with advanced renal disease. The cells within casts soon disintegrate, and their cytoplasmic and nuclear material appears as granular fragments (granular cast). Eventually, the cellular debris within casts becomes a refractile, homogeneous mass (waxy cast).

A "telescoped urinary sediment" is a sediment containing a mixture of all types of casts and inflammatory cells.

Hyaline Casts. Hyaline casts are composed of precipitated, gelled protein (especially Tamm-Horsfall protein). They are transparent, homogeneous, and colorless. Their optical density is only slightly greater than the background; hence, they are often missed. Furthermore, hyaline casts are soluble in hypotonic urine. Those with tapered ends are referred to as cylindroids. During their formation, they may entrap other elements within the hyaline matrix. This is the origin of hyaline cellular casts, hyaline granular casts, and hyaline fatty casts. Increased excretion of hyaline casts occurs after exercise, with dehydration, and with proteinuria. Hyaline casts are the only casts that may be found in small numbers in normal individuals.

Erythrocyte Casts. Erythrocyte casts in fresh urine specimens are yellow-brown to red-brown. Sometimes the individual erythrocytes may be seen; often, only cellular ghosts remain. Degenerated erythrocyte casts that retain the hemoglobin pigment are termed pigmented, or hemoglobin, casts. The finding of pigmented, coarsely granular casts should raise the suspicion of hemoglobin casts. It is important to remember that hemoglobin pigment fades rapidly in standing urine. Erythrocyte casts suggest glomerular disease; hemoglobin casts suggest glomerular disease or intravascular hemolysis. Erythrocyte casts also may be found in patients with malignant nephrosclerosis or acute tubular necrosis. The importance of thoroughly searching the urine for erythrocyte casts in cases of hematuria cannot be overemphasized, as their presence localizes the source of bleeding to the kidney.

Leukocyte Casts. Leukocyte casts are tight aggregates of leukocytes within a pale protein matrix. The leukocytes are often degenerating and/or admixed with other cell types. They may be mistaken for epithelial cell casts or clumps of leukocytes, but they are more tightly packed with cells and have a definite cylindrical shape. Leukocyte casts suggest renal tubular and/or interstitial disease, especially acute inflammation. These casts are typical of acute and chronic pyelonephritis and interstitial nephritis, but they may also be seen in acute glomerulonephritis.

Epithelial Cell Casts. Epithelial cell casts are composed of renal tubular epithelial cells, sometimes grouped into distinct rows. It is often difficult to distinguish pure epithelial cell casts from leukocyte casts. In general, epithelial cell casts in the urinary sediment have the same significance as abnormal numbers of single renal tubular epithelial cells—severe tubular damage.

Granular Casts. Granular casts result either from degeneration of cellular casts or by direct aggregation of plasma proteins into the Tamm-Horsfall matrix. They are colorless, have sharp outlines, and may be dense. Both coarse and fine granular casts occur. Granular casts may be observed in any form of acute or chronic renal disease or congestive heart failure. They are commonly found in association with proteinuria.

Waxy Casts. Waxy casts are believed to represent end-stage degeneration of epithelial cell casts. They are composed of yellow, highly refractile, homogeneous material with sharp outlines, irregular ends, and prominent cracks or fissures. Waxy casts imply localized nephron obstruction and oliguria. They are seen in advanced renal disease. Broad waxy casts are the most ominous of all casts to be found in the urinary sediment.

Fatty Casts. Fatty casts are coarse granular casts composed mainly of lipid material. The lipid material is refractile and anisotropic under polarized light. Fatty casts are often found in the company of oval fat bodies.

Lipiduria

Lipiduria, the presence of fat in the urine, is of clinical importance. It may occur in three forms: free fat droplets, oval fat bodies, or fatty casts. Lipiduria, when associated with heavy proteinuria, suggests the nephrotic syndrome. The nephrotic syndrome is characterized by severe proteinuria, hypoalbuminemia, edema, hyperlipidemia, and lipiduria. Lipiduria, primarily as free fat droplets, can also be seen in nonrenal conditions that release lipid into the blood stream, eg, fractures of long bones or atheromatous emboli. Lipiduria can be detected by routine microscopy, microscopy with polarization, or lipid stains (eg, oil red O).

Crystals

Crystals within the urinary sediment are not usually indicators of renal disease. They are morphologically varied and interesting, but their presence rarely gives the physician useful information. A convenient grouping of common urinary crystals is shown in Table 21.3.

Microorganisms

Bacteria. A clean-catch specimen and quantitative urine culture is the most reliable way to document significant bacteriuria (>10^5 bacteria per milliliter). Alternatively, bacteria in a Gram's-stained smear of an uncentrifuged urine specimen indicates significant bacteriuria. Bacilli are most commonly seen. Specificity may be increased by quantitating the number of organisms per oil immersion field. This simple procedure is an excellent method for rapid screening of urine. However, a negative screen does not exclude infection, especially in females, who may have urethrocystitis with low bacterial counts. Acid-fast stains of urine should not be used for the detection of mycobacterial infections, because smegma contains nonpathogenic acid-fast organisms. Urine culture is the preferred method.

Fungi. The most common fungus found in urine is *Candida*, especially in patients with DM. Although budding yeast cells are characteristic, occasional pseudohyphal forms occur. Yeast from vaginal infection may contaminate the urine.

Parasites. *Trichomonas* is the most common parasite observed in urine; its presence indicates a vaginal infection. Urine samples with fecal contamination may contain ova characteristically found in the stool, eg, pinworm eggs. In endemic areas, ova of *Schistosoma haematobium* may enter the urine from the bladder.

Table 21.3 Crystals Found in Normal and Abnormal Urines.

Normal Urines

Alkaline urines
  Ammonium biurate: yellow-brown spheres, often with spines ("thornapple" crystals)
  Ammonium magnesium phosphate (triple phosphate): colorless, three- to six-sided prisms ("coffin lid" crystals)
  Calcium phosphate: stellate prisms or wedge shapes
  Calcium carbonate: tiny, colorless spheres or "dumbbells"
  Amorphous phosphates: fine yellow-brown precipitate of crystalline material of varying size and shape
Acid urines
  Amorphous urates: tiny yellow-brown granules of varying shape but generally uniform size
  Uric acid: most polymorphic of the crystals; usually yellow or red-brown prisms or rhomboids
  Calcium oxalate: refractile, often tiny, octahedrons ("envelopes")

Abnormal Urines

Sulfonamides: needle-like sheaves or round forms with radial striations; rarely seen with the currently used sulfa drugs
Cystine: hexagonal plates
Leucine: yellow, refractile spheres with radial and concentric striations
Tyrosine: fine, dark yellow needles arranged in sheaves or clumps
Ampicillin: masses of long, thin, colorless crystals; seen in acid urine
Radiographic contrast material: flat, four-sided plates or long, thin rectangles; seen in urines with very high specific gravity; may mimic cholesterol crystals
Cholesterol: notched, rectangular plates; may be mimicked by x-ray dye

Viral Inclusions. Epithelial cells with viral inclusions, for instance the nuclear and cytoplasmic inclusions of cytomegalovirus, may be recognized in the urine. Usually Papanicolaou-type stains are necessary to observe the characteristic inclusions.

Tumor Cells

Urine sediment may reveal malignant epithelial cells exfoliated from the renal pelvis, bladder wall, or urethra. Renal cell carcinoma is rarely diagnosed in this manner.

Contaminants

Contaminants can be numerous and are important to recognize so they are not confused with pathological entities. Common contaminants are spermatozoa, mucus strands, fabric, pollen, hair, talc, and starch granules.

References

Graff L. *Handbook of Routine Urinalysis*. Philadelphia, Pa: JB Lippincott Co; 1983.

Haber M, ed. *Urinary Sediment: A Textbook Atlas*. Chicago, Ill: ASCP Press; 1981.

Wilson JD, Braunwald E, Isselbacher KJ, et al, eds. *Harrison's Principles of Internal Medicine*. 12th ed. New York, NY: McGraw-Hill Inc; 1991.

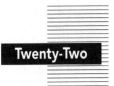
Renal Function Tests

Key Points

1. For estimating glomerular filtration rate (GFR), measurement of creatinine clearance on a 24-hour urine sample is the most convenient method and closest to the "gold standard" inulin-clearance test.
2. The 24-hour urine sample for creatinine clearance must be carefully and fully collected.
3. Serum creatinine concentration has a reciprocal relationship to the GFR and can be used to estimate it.
4. In severe renal disease, the urea clearance, averaged with creatinine clearance, compensates for the vagaries of both.

Background

Renal glomerular filtration provides the focus for workup of suspected renal impairment. Laboratory evaluation of glomerular filtration is one of the most useful and widely used renal function tests. In most renal diseases the GFR is an accurate index of the degree of damage to the kidney. Tubular function tests are less straightforward but provide useful data.

Tests of Glomerular Filtration

The methods used in the laboratory evaluation of GFR are all based on the concept of renal clearance. This concept is, in turn, based on the axiom that the rate of removal from the plasma of any solute must equal the simultaneous rate of excretion of that solute into the urine. Renal clearance of any substance is expressed as the volume of plasma freed of that substance by renal activity per unit of time. Mathematically, the renal clearance formula is written:

$$C_x = [(U_x)(V)]/P_x$$

where C_x indicates renal clearance of substance x per unit of time, U_x indicates urine concentration of substance x, V indicates urine volume flowing per unit of time, and P_x indicates plasma concentration of substance x.

If it is known that a particular substance is handled almost exclusively by the glomeruli, the clearance rate of that substance will accurately estimate the blood flow to the glomeruli. An ideal substance would be one that is freely filtered from the plasma by the glomeruli and would be inert without renal absorption, secretion, or metabolism. Inulin is such a compound, and the clearance of inulin is the standard against which other methods are compared. Because it is expensive, time-consuming, requires intravenous injection, and necessitates multiple inulin assays (not commonly available) in plasma and urine, it is not frequently done. However, all estimates of GFR by other methodologies are compared with the inulin clearance.

Endogenous Creatinine Clearance

Endogenous creatinine clearance in a 24-hour urine sample provides a widely used method to determine GFR. Creatinine is an end product of creatine metabolism in muscle. Its production and release from muscle is rather constant and only minimally dependent on physical activity, protein intake, and protein catabolism. After release, creatinine gains access to the plasma and is excreted exclusively by the kidney. The excretion of creatinine is dependent almost entirely on the process of glomerular filtration, although tubular secretion contributes slightly. Because of this tubular secretion, the clearance of endogenous creatinine would be higher than the normal GFR as measured by inulin clearance. However, because of the methodology commonly utilized in the creatinine assay, the tubular secretion component is fortuitously compensated and the end result is close to the inulin clearance. As a result, the endogenous creatinine clearance can be used as a reasonable approximation of the GFR. However, as the GFR is reduced, there is proportionally more urine creatinine from tubular secretion, so that creatinine clearance overestimates the true GFR. While inulin and radioisotope clearances more accurately evaluate true GFR, neither shares the advantages of universal availability, reliability, simplicity, safety, and low cost of creatinine clearance. Furthermore the creatinine clearance answers the questions most important to physician and patient: (1) Is the GFR normal or abnormal? and (2) If abnormal, is the GFR stable or changing (a means of assessing the course or rate of progression of the renal disease)?

One very real disadvantage of the endogenous creatinine clearance measurement on urine must be remembered. Despite very accurate clinical measurements of serum and urine creatinine concentrations, inaccurate or incomplete urine collection produces an erroneous value. For this reason, special attention must be given to assuring that the urine specimen is completely collected.

Normal values for the GFR by endogenous creatinine clearance are variable with age and sex. At birth, the GFR is very low, in the range of 20 mL/min per 1.73 m^2 of body surface area. This increases to about 50 mL/min per 1.73 m^2 of body surface area by 4 weeks of age. By 1 year of age, the value is comparable with that of a young adult (100 mL/min per 1.73 m^2 of body surface area). Past 40 years of age, creatinine clearance decreases by 1 mL/min per year. There is also a sex difference, since males have 20% higher values than females (120 mL/min vs 100 mL/min).

Serum Creatinine Concentration

Serum creatinine concentration normally varies with muscle mass and ranges from 54 to 90 μmol/L (0.6-1.0 mg/dL) in women and 70 to 117 μmol/L (0.8-1.3 mg/dL) in men (varying slightly depending on the individual laboratory). It varies little throughout the day and from one day to the next. Values in infants less than 1 year of age are less than 90 μmol/L (1 mg/dL).

Glomerular function can be estimated by measurement of the serum creatinine concentration alone. There is a reciprocal relationship between serum creatinine levels and GFR, so serum creatinine levels can give an estimate of glomerular filtration. Any reduction in glomerular filtration imposes a limitation on creatinine excretion; this impedance to excretion, in the face of a continued constant release of creatinine from muscle, leads to an accumulation of creatinine throughout total body water and thus to a rise in serum concentration. Accumulation continues until a new steady state is achieved in which the daily quantity of filtered (and therefore excreted) creatinine matches the amount released into the circulation by metabolism each day. Thus, the serum creatinine concentration should be interpreted as an index of glomerular function only in the patient who is in a steady state.

The serum creatinine concentration doubles for every 50% reduction in GFR. For example, a patient with a normal serum creatinine concentration of 90 μmol/L (1 mg/dL) has approximately 50% of normal glomerular function remaining when the serum creatinine concentration is 180 μmol/L (2 mg/dL), and 25% of normal function remaining when the serum level is 360 μmol/L (4 mg/dL). Therefore, a small increase in creatinine concentration above the normal level implies a much larger percent change in glomerular function than the same absolute increase in serum creatinine when renal function is already moderately impaired. In a child, who is likely to have a normal serum creatinine of 40 μmol/L (0.5 mg/dL), a change in serum creatinine level from 45 to 90 μmol/L (0.5-1.0 mg/dL) represents a loss of 50% of GFR. Unfortunately, chemical measurements of serum creatinine are less accurate in this low range than at higher levels.

There are certain instances where the plasma creatinine levels can increase but there is no change in the GFR: excess production of creatinine (eg, massive rhabdomyolysis); the presence of drugs that decrease creatinine secretion by the proximal tubule (eg, cimetidine); and compounds that are measured with true creatinine if the alkaline picrate assay is used (eg, acetoacetic acid in ketoacidosis). Hence, in practice one must (1) be sure of the accuracy of serum creatinine measurements, (2) know the clinical situation of the patient, and (3) know the medications the patient is taking before making clinical judgments based solely on laboratory determinations of serum creatinine. Furthermore, as previously noted, the fraction of creatinine excreted by tubular secretion increases as the GFR falls. Moreover, for various reasons, the creatinine excretion is less in patients with chronic renal failure. Therefore, the actual GFR in patients with chronic renal failure is much lower than that predicted by any given serum creatinine concentration.

Blood Urea Nitrogen

Blood urea nitrogen (BUN), though widely used to assess glomerular filtration, is a less satisfactory measurement than the serum creatinine concentration for two reasons: (1) urea clearance varies with the rate of urine flow, and (2) the plasma concentration of urea is dependent on nitrogen metabolism as well as renal function. Urea is not only filtered by the glomeruli but is also partially reabsorbed (20%-50%) by the tubules. In a well-hydrated normal person ingesting a diet of average composition, the BUN is approximately 3.6 to 5.4 mmol/L (10-15 mg/dL). A low BUN, less than 2.9 to 3.6 mmol/L (8-10 mg/dL) in adults, is frequently associated with overhydration. A BUN of 3.6 to 5.4 mmol/L (10-15 mg/dL) almost always indicates normal glomerular function in the euvolemic patient with normal liver function. A BUN in the range of 18.0 to 53.5 mmol/L (50-150 mg/dL) is beyond the level anticipated from variations in urine flow or nitrogen balance alone and thus implies impairment of renal function, which may have prerenal, renal, or postrenal cause. Finally, a markedly elevated BUN (eg, 53.5-89.0 mmol/L [150-250 mg/dL]) is virtually conclusive evidence of severe impairment of renal function.

The BUN level is not as reliable as the serum creatinine level in evaluating renal function, because there are factors that can enhance urea production as well as conditions where there is increased reabsorption. There are similar objections to use of urea clearance as a measure of GFR, because under the best of circumstances the urea clearance as measured by the BUN is only one half to three quarters that of an inulin clearance. However, there is one circumstance where the urea clearance test can be of some value. In patients with severe renal disease, the creatinine clearance grossly overestimates the GFR while the urea clearance continues to underestimate the true GFR. As a result, a better estimate of the true GFR can be obtained if a creatinine clearance and a urea clearance are averaged together.

Radioisotopic methods have been developed for evaluating the GFR by using the radioisotopes ^{51}Cr-ethylenediaminetetraacetic acid, ^{125}I-iothalamate, ^{125}I-diatrizoate, vitamin B_{12}, and ^{99m}Tc-diethylenetriamine pentacetic acid. The filtration rate measured by these techniques appears to approximate inulin clearance. These isotopic techniques are not universally available, however, and they require specialized equipment not needed for measurement of creatinine or BUN.

Tests of Tubular Function

Compared with the use of inulin clearance as a measure of glomerular function, no single test of renal tubular function can be as specific because the renal tubules carry out many different functions. Studies of the maximal capacity of the tubules to reabsorb glucose or to secrete p-aminohippurate are approximate indices of functional tubular mass, but such studies are too complex for clinical purposes. As a substitute, tests of concentration and dilution have been used to detect early renal tubular damage and to follow the functional progression of pathological processes.

Renal Concentrating Capacity

This is a test of renal function. To maintain plasma water within the narrow limits of 280 to 290 mmol/kg (mOsm/kg) water, urine excretion and water intake must be balanced. Urine production (normally about 1 L/d) is balanced between total fluid intake and loss from other sites such as lung, skin, and stool. An important part of this homeostasis is the mechanism of dilution or concentration of urine by the kidney. The urine has a tremendous range of diluting and concentrating ability, with the tonicity of the urine varying between 40-1200 mmol/kg (mOsm/kg) water. If urine has a concentration less than that of plasma (280-290 mmol/kg [mOsm/kg] water) it is considered dilute or hypotonic. If the concentration of the urine is greater than plasma, the urine is considered concentrated or hypertonic. Most normal individuals excrete a total of 450 to 600 mmol (mOsm) of solute per day. How concentrated the urine becomes determines the volume of urine that must be excreted for the body to lose this solute load. Assuming the maximum concentrating ability of the kidney is intact, the minimum normal volume of urine that must be excreted before the patient is considered oliguric is in the range of 500 mL/d (0.5 L [daily urine output] x 1200 mmol/L [mOsm/L] [maximum concentrating capacity of kidney] = 600 mmol [mOsm] [required daily solute loss]). Clearly, if some of the concentrating ability of the kidney has been lost, then a greater volume of urine excretion is necessary for the patient to avoid becoming azotemic. Thus, the ability of the kidney to concentrate urine forms the basis of another test of renal function.

The essential ingredients of renal concentrating capacity studies are: (1) a stimulus for renal water conservation (usually a suitable period of fluid restriction) and (2) a method for assessing urine tonicity (eg, osmolality or specific gravity). Instead of directly measuring the osmolality of urine by comparing the freezing point with that of distilled water, it has been found that the specific gravity very closely approximates osmolality. Specific gravity is easily measured with a hydrometer or with a dipstick. Another method commonly used for measuring urine tonicity utilizes a refractometer; the refractive index correlates well with the specific gravity. High levels of protein, glucose, or radiopaque contrast medium markedly elevate hydrometer readings but affect refractometer results less. Alkaline urine and large amounts of protein affect dipstick results.

Plasma specific gravity is 1.010, so urine with a specific gravity below this figure is dilute and above, concentrated. Very dilute urine containing 50 mmol/kg (mOsm/kg) water has a specific gravity of about 1.001. A moderately concentrated urine specimen with an osmolality of 800 mmol/kg (mOsm/kg) water has a specific gravity of 1.020. If a random urine sample has a specific gravity of 1.022 or greater (without glucose, protein, or radiopaque contrast medium being present), then the kidney concentrating ability is considered normal and no further testing is necessary.

If the patient persistently presents with dilute urine, then a test of concentrating ability may be necessary. Generally, an overnight period of water deprivation is sufficient. Water deprivation in a persistently polyuric patient with markedly increased urine flow should be of shorter duration (4-6 hours), and the patient must be carefully monitored so that marked dehydration does not occur (frequent checks of body weight) or to make sure the patient is not drinking water.

If a patient shows an inability to concentrate urine, a number of factors can be responsible. (1) If endogenous antidiuretic hormone (ADH) secretion is reduced or absent, then the patient has neurogenic diabetes insipidus. This can occur idiopathically or following head trauma in which there is damage to the posterior pituitary or hypothalamus. (2) If ADH is being secreted but the tubular epithelium of the collecting duct is unresponsive and remains impermeable to water, the condition is called nephrogenic diabetes insipidus. This is seen in a variety of clinical settings, including marked renal insufficiency, drugs (such as demethylchlortetracycline and lithium carbonate), and hypercalcemia. In rare instances it is an inherited disorder. (3) If the tonicity of the medulla is impaired, the kidney is incapable of concentrating urine, which can occur if there is deficient sodium resorption in the ascending limb of Henle's loop. Drugs such as furosemide (a diuretic), for instance, inhibit active sodium transport in Henle's loop. Medullary tonicity can also be impaired by washing out the solute gradient with compulsive water-drinking. A protein-restricted diet can also limit the ability of the kidney to concentrate urine. Medullary ischemia (eg, in sickle cell renal disease) also impairs renal urine concentration.

As part of the urine concentrating test, a small dose of ADH is often used either to alleviate the need for prolonged dehydration or, in the polyuric patient, after the patient is dehydrated. The response to ADH in the polyuric patient helps separate the different forms of diabetes insipidus from compulsive water-drinking. In compulsive water-drinking, the concentrating ability approaches normal, whereas in diabetes insipidus (either neurogenic or nephrogenic) the urine concentrating ability of the kidney is low.

As can be seen, lack of concentrating ability by the kidney is nonspecific and is present in a variety of conditions. The kidney in almost any glomerular or interstitial renal disease eventually shows impaired concentrating ability. However, those diseases that primarily affect the papillary and medullary portions of the kidney (eg, obstructive uropathy or polycystic disease) show the greatest defects in urine-concentrating capacity.

Tests of Renal Diluting Capacity

Although diluting capacity is impaired in renal disease, a test of this function has limited diagnostic usefulness. There is also a small but definite risk of water intoxication in the patient with renal disease. These factors make a water-loading test of little practical value in the assessment of renal function.

References

Danovitch GM. Evaluation of renal function. In: Massry SG, Glassock RJ, eds. *Textbook of Nephrology*. Baltimore, Md: Williams & Wilkins; 1983:11.28-11.34.

Kassirer JP, Harrington JT. Laboratory evaluation of renal function. In: Schrier RW, Gottschalk CW, eds. *Diseases of the Kidney*. 4th ed. Boston, Mass: Little, Brown & Co Inc; 1988:393-441.

Rose BD. Clinical assessment of renal function. In: *Pathophysiology of Renal Disease*. New York, NY: McGraw-Hill Inc; 1987:1-39.

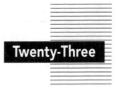

Twenty-Three

Calcium and Phosphorus Metabolism

Key Points

1. Measurements of ionized calcium most accurately assess pathological calcium states.
2. Ionized calcium can be reliably measured in all acute care laboratories using anaerobic technique (due to the acute impact of pH, and thus pCO_2, on the ionized fraction).
3. Serum parathyroid hormone (PTH) is now sensitively and specifically measured using the newer two-site immunoradiometric analysis method for intact (whole-molecule) PTH.
4. Hyperparathyroidism is common but may be asymptomatic; it is often discovered by an elevated screening serum calcium and confirmatory elevated PTH and ionized calcium levels.
5. Hypercalcemia associated with malignancy consistently is coupled with a low PTH level except in the rare neoplasm that produces the whole PTH molecule.
6. Measurement of PTH and ionized calcium levels permits accurate diagnosis of hypoparathyroidism.

Background

Of the many tests developed to assess parathyroid function and the status of calcium and phosphorus metabolism, only a few have proven to be both informative and practical to implement. These include serum and urine calcium concentrations and serum inorganic phosphate concentration in conjunction with measurements of serum PTH (Figure 23.1).

Calcium

Calcium, a common element in the human body, is tightly controlled by complex biological mechanisms. Ninety-nine percent of the calcium an adult possesses is

Figure 23.1 Major Hormonal Regulators of Calcium Homeostasis.*

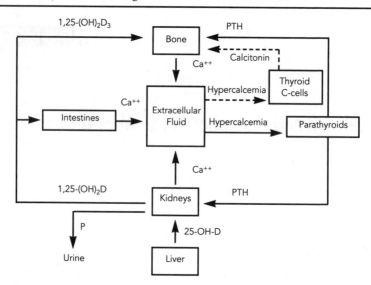

* Reprinted, with permission, from J. Woo and D. C. Cannon. In: J. B. Henry, ed. *Clinical Diagnosis and Management by Laboratory Methods.* Philadelphia, Pa: WB Saunders Co; 1991. Chapter 8.

skeletal, where it is incorporated in the extracellular crystalline hydroxyapatite matrix for bone strength. The remainder exists in extracellular fluid, in blood plasma, or in cell cytosol in an exchangeable calcium pool available for incorporation into bone or for cell functions.

Calcium participates in vitally important physiological functions, acting as an enzyme cofactor through reversible combination with calmodulin, a small protein found in all nucleated cells. Such important cell functions as cell motility, adhesion, ciliary action, and mitosis are influenced by this complex. Some clotting factors utilize calcium, and, in addition, calcium activates contraction of the myosin fibril in striated muscle.

Membrane calcium regulates membrane permeability and neurotransmitter release, and diminishes neuromuscular excitability. On the cell surface, extracellular ionized calcium controls the secretions of cells in endocrine organs, such as parathyroid, thyroid (C cells), and pancreas.

Calcium is excreted in feces, urine, and sweat, and must be replenished by dietary intake. Only about 25% of dietary calcium is absorbed, and the average US diet can easily be calcium-deficient, especially if dairy products are not consumed. Relatively more calcium is required during growth, pregnancy, lactation, and the postmenopausal years.

Phosphate

Phosphate is the form phosphorus assumes in the human adult body. It is distributed evenly between extracellular and intracellular locations, in contrast to the mainly extracellular location of calcium. Intracellular phosphate is present mainly in organic macromolecules such as phospholipids, phosphoproteins, and phosphonucleotides, which are termed "organic phosphates." A lesser amount exists intracellularly as "inorganic phosphate," which is vital to high-energy transfer reactions within the cell.

Most of the extracellular inorganic phosphate is incorporated into hydroxyapatite and so participates in the dynamic process of bone mineralization and mineral release. Chronic hypophosphatemia contributes to rickets and osteomalacia, since phosphate is a major player in forming appropriately mineralized bone.

Phosphate is utilized in myriad cellular activities. As phospholipid it serves as a structural unit for all cell membranes. When present as phosphoprotein, it drives cellular energy metabolism and even gene replication. Because phosphate is a substrate for oxidative phosphorylation, it plays a role in generation of cellular energy. Additionally, glycogen breakdown requires phosphate to produce glucose. Dietary phosphate intake is generally adequate in the average US diet.

Three hormones are the main regulators of calcium and inorganic phosphate homeostasis: PTH, calcitonin, and 1,25-dihydroxyvitamin D (1,25-$(OH)_2$D), the active form of vitamin D.

Tests for Calcium and Phosphorus Homeostasis

Calcium

Calcium is present in plasma in three forms: ionized, protein-bound, and complexed (mainly to phosphate, bicarbonate, and citrate). Since the ionized fraction is the physiologically active form, the protein-bound and complexed forms act as a pool to help maintain the ionized fraction in tight equilibrium. Under normal conditions, the concentration of total serum or plasma calcium is 2.5 mmol/L (10 mg/dL), and that of the ionized fraction is 1.125 mmol/L (2.5 mEq/L). Because even small variations in calcium concentration can signify disease states, methods for measurement need to be highly precise and accurate. Blood should be drawn on a fasting patient in usual phlebotomy posture with minimal prephlebotomy venostasis by the tourniquet. Prolonged (more than 3 minutes) veno-occlusion will falsely increase the total calcium value. Using ethylenediaminetetraacetic acid (EDTA) or oxalate anticoagulants in the blood tube invalidates the calcium analysis.

Almost half of the serum calcium is reversibly bound to protein (albumin and globulins), so any fluctuation in the protein available for binding will affect the measurable total calcium. Hyperproteinemia causes an increase in total serum calcium concentration because the protein-bound fraction increases. For practical purposes an elevated protein-bound calcium level in the presence of normal ionized calcium concentration occurs only in dehydration with hemoconcentration or in paraproteinemias such as myeloma. The total serum calcium elevation is mild and proportional to the relative hyperproteinemia. Rehydration restores normocalcemia. Significant hypoproteinemia decreases the total serum calcium, so an increase in the ionized calcium fraction is hidden by a normal total serum calcium level in that condition. Low plasma protein level is the most common cause of hypocalcemia in a hospital population.

True hypocalcemia may be caused by hypoparathyroidism or vitamin D deficiency (rare in the United States due to enriched food). Hypoparathyroidism is most often secondary to thyroid or parathyroid surgery.

Hypocalcemia, if severe, will cause tetany; however, clinical tetany is not specific for hypocalcemia. Tetany can also occur in patients with systemic alkalosis or magnesium depletion.

A simple rule states that a reduction or increase in the serum albumin concentration of 10 g/L will result in a corresponding 0.2 mmol/L (0.8 mg/dL) reduction or increase in the total serum calcium concentration.

Formulas for "corrected" total calcium exist that take into account the patient's total serum protein or albumin values.

$$Corrected\ Ca = Total\ Ca/(0.6 + Total\ Protein/194)$$
$$Corrected\ Ca = Total\ Ca + 0.1(40 - Albumin)/6$$

Obviously, these correction formulas are misleading if the proteins are qualitatively abnormal. Plasma acid-base balance can also affect the ionized fraction. Since alkalosis causes a reduction in the circulating ionic calcium fraction, tetany may occur in the presence of normal total serum calcium. Conversely, since an acid pH increases ionization of calcium, and therefore of the ionized calcium fraction, a normal total serum calcium level in states of chronic acidosis may falsely obscure the presence of an elevated ionized calcium concentration.

In summary, appropriate levels of ionized calcium in extracellular fluid are needed for essential bodily processes. The ionized calcium level in blood regulates the secretion of parathyroid hormone. Low ionized calcium levels stimulate parathyroid hormone secretion and high ionized calcium levels suppress parathyroid hormone secretion.

Hypercalcemia can be life-threatening, although mild forms are common and cause few symptoms. Malignant disease and primary or tertiary hyperparathyroidism are the two main causes of pathological hypercalcemia. Malignant tumors cause hypercalcemia by two mechanisms: direct bone involvement by the tumor (primary or metastatic), or indirect bone involvement via secretion of hormonally active compounds produced by the tumor that affect calcium homeostasis (eg, "PTH-like substance").

Primary hyperparathyroidism (PTH is secreted in excess of levels required for calcium homeostasis) is caused by gland hyperplasia or adenoma. Tertiary hyperparathyroidism is the development of autonomous elevated PTH secretion after longstanding stimulation. These conditions both result in hypercalcemia. Secondary hyperparathyroidism is the longstanding hypertrophy (stimulation) due to chronic hypocalcemia.

Renal stones, peptic ulcer, muscle weakness, hypertension, osteopenia, or bone cyst can all signal primary hyperparathyroidism. All of these can present subtly. Always correlate the PTH results with the serum calcium, keeping renal status in mind. Other, rarer causes of hypercalcemia include thyrotoxicosis, immobilization of patients due to bed rest, accelerated bone turnover (eg, Paget's disease of bone), vitamin A or D intoxication, the milk alkali syndrome, sarcoidosis, and adrenocortical insufficiency.

Quantitation of urine calcium is most useful with a 24-hour collection of urine and when the dietary intake of calcium is known. Quantitative urine calcium measurement is the preferred test for evaluating hypercalciuria. A calcium clearance related to creatinine can be a good screening test for hypercalciuria, a common correlate with renal stones. The absence of calcium in the urine suggests a low serum calcium concentration.

Serum Inorganic Phosphorus Concentration

Serum inorganic phosphorus concentration and all other phosphorus measurements require a serum specimen free of hemolysis to preclude an artefactual contribution to serum inorganic phosphate from the large organic phosphorus fraction in erythrocytes. A fasting morning specimen eliminates the effects of circadian rhythm and carbohydrate metabolism that can cause variation in serum phosphorus concentration.

Serum phosphorus levels are higher in growing children and young adults, because growth hormone causes elevation of serum inorganic phosphorus levels. When the serum phosphorus concentration exceeds the renal threshold, phosphorus is excreted in the urine in direct proportion to the serum concentration. The action of PTH on the renal tubular cells blocks renal tubular reabsorption of phosphate. Cyclic adenosine monophosphate (cAMP), the intracellular "second messenger," mediates this inhibition of reabsorption, which leads to decreased serum phosphorus concentration. Hyperphosphatemia is seen with an absence of PTH, in end-organ refractoriness to PTH (eg, renal tubular cAMP is defective or absent), and with a decreased glomerular filtration rate (eg, renal failure). Decreased serum phosphorus to levels of 0.30 to 0.80 mmol/L (1.0-2.5 mg/dL) is seen (but not consistently) in patients with primary hyperparathyroidism, after glucose administration, in vitamin D deficiency, and with gram-negative bacteremia. Severe hypophosphatemia (levels <0.30 mmol/L [1.0 mg/dL]) occurs with alcohol withdrawal, nutritional recovery after starvation, hyperalimentation, administration of certain antacids, and severe burns.

Parathyroid Hormone

PTH is synthesized by the four small parathyroid glands, each as part of a paired set situated close to or on the posterior inferior and posterior superior surface of the thyroid gland.

PTH is a single-chain polypeptide of 84 amino acids that in circulation is cleaved into fragments. Intact (active) PTH attaches to hormone-specific receptors on the plasma membranes of its target cells and is excreted by the kidney. The N-terminal fragment is biologically active as well. The inactive midmolecule and C-terminal fragments are removed exclusively by renal excretion, and if renal function is impaired, immunoassays directed to these fragments will give increased values. These differences in excretion of active and inactive fragments pose assay problems. Biologically active hormone levels are very low normally (about 10 pmol/L, or 0.1 ng/mL when determined by immunoassay). Since it appears that intact PTH is the dominant biologically active plasma form, its measurement by immunoradiometric analysis (IRMA) technique is preferred.

The main role of PTH is the regulation of the extracellular fluid calcium concentration, so its targets are the renal tubule and bone-modeling unit. Osteoclasts, osteocytes, and the calcium resorbing cells of the renal (mainly distal) tubules are stimulated by PTH. PTH also stimulates the production of active vitamin D. The concentration of ionized calcium in the blood regulates, via a feedback loop, the synthesis and secretion of PTH. Decreasing levels of ionized serum calcium stimulate PTH synthesis and secretion within minutes; increasing levels of ionized calcium suppress secretion. PTH affects the level of plasma phosphorus, but the plasma phosphorus level does not in turn directly control PTH secretion. Increased blood phosphate does, however, stimulate PTH secretion indirectly, thereby moving calcium and phosphate into bone, decreasing resorption of mineral from bone, and increasing calcium phosphate complexes in plasma. This leads to a decrease of plasma ionized calcium, thereby stimulating PTH secretion. Since phosphate retention occurs with chronic renal failure, elevation of the plasma PTH level is a feature of this condition.

In summary, PTH affects serum calcium homeostasis by increasing renal tubular calcium and decreasing renal tubular inorganic phosphate reabsorption, stimulating osteoclast bone resorption (along with $1,25\text{-}(OH)_2D_3$) and stimulating the hydroxylation of inactive vitamin D.

Calcitonin

Calcitonin is produced by the C cells of the thyroid gland. Its main function is inhibition of bone calcium and phosphate resorption when PTH and vitamin D levels are high, thereby lowering serum calcium. It has little apparent role in calcium homeostasis because when calcitonin is absent after thyroidectomy hypercalcemia does not occur. Calcitonin-secreting tumors, in turn, do not induce hypocalcemia. Low plasma concentration is the rule in healthy adults.

Vitamin D and Metabolites

Vitamin D and metabolites come from two main sources. Vitamin D_3 (cholecalciferol) is produced in the skin by the action of sunlight and is also present in animal food sources. Vitamin D_2 (ergocalciferol) is a semisynthetic source produced from plants that is used as a food additive. Only a few minutes of skin exposure to sunlight a day provides a very efficient means of acquiring vitamin D. Fish oils, liver, eggs, and butter are the only natural foods that contain significant amounts of the vitamin. Due to the addition of the semisynthetic vitamin to enrich foods, mainly milk, the US diet meets the daily requirements of vitamin D. Usually, only breastfed infants and strict vegetarians that do not eat eggs or milk become deficient.

Before vitamins D_2 and D_3 become active, each undergoes two hydroxylations, catalyzed by specific enzymes. These important metabolites, produced in the kidney, are 1,25-dihydroxyvitamin D_3 ($1,25\text{-}(OH)_2D_3$) and 24,25-dihydroxyvitamin D_3 ($24,25\text{-}(OH)_2D_3$).

$1,25\text{-}(OH)_2D_3$ is the most potent of the metabolites. It stimulates cell membrane transport of calcium. When calcium mobilization is required, as with hypocalcemia, vitamin D deficiency, hyperparathyroidism, or hypophosphatemia, hydroxylation activity is stimulated and synthesis of $1,25\text{-}(OH)_2D_3$ takes place. When calcium mobilization is either not needed (when calcium levels are normal) or would be detrimental (in hypercalcemia), hydroxylation ceases and $1,25\text{-}(OH)_2D_3$ is converted to $24,25\text{-}(OH)_2D_3$, which has no bone calcium mobilization action. In the healthy individual on a diet containing adequate calcium, the plasma contains a small but detectable amount of $1,25\text{-}(OH)_2D_3$ and large amounts of $24,25\text{-}(OH)_2D_3$.

$1,25\text{-}(OH)_2D_3$ exhibits three main actions: it stimulates calcium reabsorption from bone (acting along with PTH); it stimulates calcium absorption from the small bowel; and it increases calcium reabsorption in the distal renal tubules.

References

Bowers GN Jr, Brassard C, Sena SF. Measurement of ionized calcium in serum with ion-selective electrodes: a mature technology that can meet the daily service needs. *Clin Chem.* 1986;32:1437-1447.

Fraser D, Jones G, Kooh SW, Radde IC. Calcium and phosphate metabolism. In: Tietz NW, ed. *Textbook of Clinical Chemistry.* 3rd ed. Philadelphia, Pa: WB Saunders Co; 1986.

Hackeng WH, Lips P, Netelenbos JC, Lips JM. Clinical implications of estimation of intact parathyroid hormone (PTH) versus total immunoreactive PTH in normal subjects and hyperparathyroid patients. *J Clin Endocrinol Metab.* 1986;63:447-453.

Mangin M, Webb AC, Dreyer BE, et al. Identification of a cDNA encoding a parathyroid hormone–like peptide from a human tumor associated with humoral hypercalcemia of malignancy. *Proc Natl Acad Sci USA.* 1988;85:597-601.

Nussbaum SR, Zahradnik RJ, Lavigne JR, et al. Highly sensitive two-site immunoradiometric assay of parathyrin, and its clinical utility in evaluating patients with hypercalcemia. *Clin Chem.* 1987;33:1364-1367.

Pollard A, Pritzker KP, Grynpas MD. Disorders of calcium magnesium and bone metabolism. In: Gornall AG, ed. *Applied Biochemistry of Clinical Disorders.* 2nd ed. Philadelphia, Pa: JB Lippincott Co; 1986.

Woo J, Cannon DC. In: Henry JB. *Clinical Diagnosis and Management by Laboratory Methods.* 18th ed. Philadelphia, Pa: WB Saunders Co; 1991. Chapter 8.

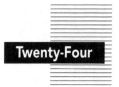
Thyroid Function Tests

Key Points

1. The test of choice for screening or initiating thyroid dysfunction workup is the highly sensitive thyroid-stimulating hormone (TSH) test. If this is abnormal, order free thyroxine (T_4) in the ambulatory patient.
2. Free T_4 assays are diagnostically unreliable in acutely ill patients, especially those taking multiple drugs.
3. Total T_4 assay frequently can be misleading due to the variable concentrations of thyroid-binding globulin. Greater than 99% of T_4 is protein-bound.
4. Thyrotropin-releasing hormone (TRH) stimulation test should be ordered in equivocal cases because response to TRH (or rise in TSH) excludes primary hyperthyroidism.
5. Thyroid replacement is optimized by measurement of TSH. On replacement therapy, TSH should be measurable and not increased. On T_4 suppression/cancer therapy, TSH should be undetectable.

Background

Thyroid hormones are necessary for normal growth and development. They have a stimulating effect on many cell metabolic processes.

Thyroliberin (TRH) from the hypothalamus controls the anterior pituitary release of thyrotropin (TSH). In turn, TSH stimulates the thyroid gland to produce both T_4 and triiodothyronine (T_3). This production creates negative feedback for the pituitary, normalizing output of TSH. If T_3 and T_4 are produced in excess, the feedback will block further release of TSH. In peripheral tissues, T_4 is converted to T_3, the physiologically active product, and to a lesser extent reverse T_3. Thyroid hormone is bound to protein—T_4 is 99.97% bound (0.03% free),

Table 24.1 Factors That Increase and Decrease TBG.

Increase
  Estrogens (pregnancy, exogenous hormones)
  Being a newborn
  Porphyria
  Acute hepatocellular disease
  Having hereditary TBG increase
  Phenothiazines
  Chronic liver disease

Decrease
  Androgens
  Anabolic steroids
  Diphenylhydantoin
  Phenylbutazone
  Salicylates
  Major illness
  Hereditary TBG deficiency
  Surgical stress
  Nephrotic syndrome
  Acromegaly
  Chronic liver disease
  Hypoproteinemia

and T_3 is 99.7% bound (0.3% free). Only the free unbound fraction is metabolically active, while the bound fractions constitute a storage form. Circulating free T_4 approximates 10 to 31 pmol/L (0.8-2.4 ng/dL) and free T_3, 7 pmol/L (480 pg/dL). Therefore the amount available to assay is small, which limits its precision and accuracy. Thyroxine-binding globulin (TBG), thyroxine-binding prealbumin, and albumin all bind thyroxins (Table 24.1).

When working up possible thyroid disease it is critical to recognize that each person has his/her own narrow range of "normal" for thyroxine, a more narrow range than is encountered in the wider population's "normal range." This narrower range of biological activity for each person means that the pituitary response to small fluctuations of free T_4 or free T_3 results in a prompt response in the TSH level. A small increase of free T_4 may suppress TSH in the absence of clinical signs and symptoms. These apparently small laboratory value shifts can be significant to the patient.

Hyperthyroidism and Its Diagnosis

Overt hyperthyroidism occurs in 0.5% to 1.0% of people but subclinical disease is much more frequent. The symptoms and signs of hyperthyroidism include weight loss, muscular weakness, hair loss, skin changes, nervousness, tachycardia, palpitations, and tremor. In reality there are many patients with significant disease who have nonspecific presentation. Clinical diagnosis often requires biochemical testing because findings can be nonspecific and associated with other diseases, especially in the elderly patient.

The commonest cause of hyperthyroidism is Grave's disease (Table 24.2). A diffusely enlarged nontender smooth thyroid, and infiltrative ophthalmopathy

Table 24.2 Causes of Hyperthyroidism.

Grave's disease

Subacute thyroiditis

Toxic adenoma

Toxic nodular goiter

Exogenous thyroid hormones

Struma ovarii

and dermopathy (pretibial myxedema) constitute the disease elements, not all of which are evident at diagnosis.

Grave's disease is an autoimmune disorder with thyroid-stimulating antibodies committed to TSH receptor binding. This causes thyroid hyperactivity with consequent suppression of TSH.

Thyroid-Stimulating Hormone

TSH is now the test of choice for routine "screening" or, in combination with free T_4, for initial assessment of suspected thyroid abnormality. The American Thyroid Association recommendations should be read in detail. Unaffected by varying levels of binding proteins, TSH levels in the ambulatory population clearly separate the hyperthyroid patient from the euthyroid person. Assays are widely available with a sensitivity to 0.1 mU/L, sufficient for the outpatient environment. In this setting TSH is measurable in euthyroidism and absent in hyperthyroidism, and the level predicts the TRH response.

Rarely, a TSH assay with sensitivity to even lower levels is indicated. In the profoundly ill patient, eg, one with septic shock, TSH falls in the absence of hyperthyroidism. In such cases the most sensitive assay is informative because some TSH will be detected. It is apparent that there is no completely trouble-free approach to thyroid assessment; however, the highly sensitive TSH is the least disturbed by interfering processes. Obviously, a severely ill patient, especially one taking interfering medication, may be difficult to evaluate. Remember the following when utilizing the highly sensitive TSH test:

1. TSH may remain suppressed for a lengthy period following correction of hyperthyroidism. Thus, monitor free T_4 or T_3 levels in such cases.

2. In patients with severe nonthyroidal illness, TSH may be transiently low when the patient is ill or high when recovering.

3. Dopamine and glucocorticoids suppress TSH.

4. TSH is not a reliable indicator of thyroid function in patients with pituitary or hypothalamic disease.

5. TSH may be inappropriately normal or high in the syndrome of peripheral resistance to thyroid hormone.

Thyroxine

T_4 serum levels are reliably assayed. Free T_4 is the preferred test of T_4 because it assays active hormone, and direct methods are now routinely available.

If one is uncertain of the diagnosis after measuring TSH and subsequently quantitating the degree of abnormality with a free T_4, then the TRH stimulation test should be performed. After obtaining a baseline TSH, 500 mg (1 ampule) of TRH is injected and repeated samples are obtained at 20, 30, and 60 minutes. A normal TSH response excludes primarily hyperthyroidism. No response suggests pituitary disease. This provides the "gold standard" to diagnose conventional hyperthyroidism in equivocal cases.

During treatment for Grave's disease, monitoring serum free T_4 is superior to the measurement of TSH because TSH remains suppressed for weeks after the restoration of the eumetabolic state.

Factitious hyperthyroidism is commonly seen in health care workers who have access to T_4 therapy in the absence of clinical need.

Several tests of thyroid function are no longer considered as helpful as those discussed herein. Early attempts to measure approximations of thyroid hormone level included protein-bound iodine followed by total T_4 tests; now the free T_4 test is preferred.

T_3 assay is of interest in one condition: T_3 toxicosis. In this condition, hyperthyroidism is recognized by suppressed TSH but the free T_4 level is normal, which suggests excess production of T_3. Therefore, measurement of T_3 is appropriate in this situation.

"T_3 uptake," now known as the thyroid hormone–binding ratio, has always been confusing to clinicians because its name has no relevance to the T_3 level. In fact, it is not a measure of thyroid function but rather gives an estimation of amount of TGB and was useful in evaluating total T_4 abnormalities due to TBG abnormalities. Since total T_4 is not now the preferred test, T_3 uptake is no longer needed.

Free thyroxine estimates (FT$_4$ index, or FTI, or T_7) provided a rough approximation of free T_4; with direct free T_4 assays, it is no longer ordered.

Hypothyroidism and Its Diagnosis

Overt hypothyroidism has an incidence of 1% to 2% in the general population—2% to 4% if subclinical disease is included. Signs and symptoms include fatigue, personality change, decreased mental and physical output, hoarseness, constipation, muscle cramps, dry skin, and peripheral edema. Nearly all hypothyroidism is caused by thyroid gland failure. This gland burnout can be the final pathway after thyroiditis or goiter. Pituitary or hypothalamic failure is uncommon.

The underlying thyroiditis can be asymptomatic or associated with symptoms of inflammatory disease.

Thyroid autoantibodies (antithyroglobulin and antimicrosomal antibody) can be helpful in defining etiology. The underlying etiology, while appropriate to document, does not affect treatment, which consists of daily oral L-thyroxine replacement to bring the TSH into the low normal range. An elevated TSH and low T_4 define the disease. The severity of the primary hypothyroidism can be deduced from the free T_4 level. In the recently hospitalized patient acutely ill with nonthyroidal disease, there may be a transient TSH elevation to levels of 20 to 30 mU/L while recovery is ongoing. In these patients a definitive diagnosis and the initiation of treatment for hypothyroidism should be delayed.

References

Cle GG, Hayid A. Sensitive thyrotropin assays: analytic and clinical performance criteria. *Mayo Clin Proc.* 1988;63:1123-1132.

Morris JC, Hay ID, Nelson RE, et al. Clinical utility of thyrotropin receptor antibody assays: comparison of radioreceptor and bioassay methods. *Mayo Clin Proc.* 1988;63:707-717.

Surks MI, Chopra IJ, Mariash CN, et al. American Thyroid Association guidelines for use of laboratory tests in thyroid disorders. *JAMA.* 1990;263:1529-1532.

Watts NB. Use of a sensitive thyrotropin assay for monitoring treatment with levothyroxine. *Arch Intern Med.* 1989;149:309-312.

Watts NB, Keffer JH. *Practical Endocrinology.* 4th ed. Philadelphia, Pa: Lea & Febiger; 1989.

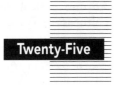

Twenty-Five

Adrenocortical Function Tests

Key Points

1. Adrenocortical hormone insufficiency or excess is uncommon, but must be considered frequently in differential diagnosis.
2. Cortisol is the main product of the adrenal cortex and should be assayed directly.
3. Adrenocortical insufficiency equates with insufficient hydroxycorticoids and is diagnosable by a cosyntropin challenge test. This test may be falsely negative during the several weeks following acute loss of pituitary function.
4. Cushing's syndrome is typically manifest by hypercortisolism, which is quantified by measurement of 24-hour urinary free cortisol.
5. Dexamethasone suppression with a low (1-mg) dose readily screens out most people who do not have Cushing's syndrome.
6. Hyperaldosteronism is rare and must be worked up in a controlled setting, with a patient's volume and salt normalized adequately.

Background

The human adrenal cortex has three steroid-secreting layers from outer to inner: the zona glomerulosa produces aldosterone, a mineralocorticoid that regulates extracellular fluid volume (as part of the renin-angiotensin system) and potassium metabolism; and the zona fasciculata and inner zona reticularis, which together synthesize and secrete glucocorticoids (such as cortisol) and the sex steroids (such as testosterone and estrogen precursors).

The glucocorticoids and sex hormones are under hypothalmic-anterior pituitary corticotropin (ACTH) control. Excess or insufficient production of the cortical hormones produces diseases that may be life-threatening. Accurate diagnosis is important.

Adrenocortical Hypofunction: Diseases and Associated Laboratory Tests

Patients with adrenocortical hypofunction have either primary (Addison's disease) or secondary (pituitary) adrenal insufficiency and a low level of serum cortisol. Addison's disease is commonly due to autoimmune destruction of the adrenal cortex. Infection, hemorrhage into the gland, metastatic tumor, acquired immunodeficiency disease (AIDS), and surgical removal of the adrenal glands also cause adrenal insufficiency.

Addison's Disease
Patients with Addison's disease typically have deficiencies of glucocorticoids and mineralocorticoids, abnormal skin pigmentation, and depletional hyponatremia. Deficiency of other hormone systems can result in hypothyroidism, hypoparathyroidism, hypogonadism, and diabetes mellitus, as well as pernicious anemia through related autoimmune mechanisms. The possibility of multiple endocrine system deficiencies should be considered when evaluating Addison's disease, but patients with secondary adrenocortical hypofunction have only glucocorticoid deficiency. These patients typically lack the skin pigmentation abnormalities found in Addison's disease, but they may have dilutional hyponatremia and characteristically have evidence of other pituitary hormonal deficits. Secondary adrenal insufficiency often occurs in patients who have just completed corticosteroid therapy. Cessation of either short-term or long-term therapy can produce acute clinically significant adrenocortical insufficiency if the patients are stressed by events such as surgery or infections.

Cortisol Assay
In the initial workup of a patient with suspected adrenocortical hypofunction, one should immediately utilize the corticotropin stimulation test. Plasma cortisol level is measured at baseline, then a low dose (250 mg) of synthetic corticotropin (cosyntropin) is given intramuscularly or intravenously. Plasma cortisol is again measured at 30 and 60 minutes after injection. Patients in addisonian crisis can have the screening corticotropin test performed simultaneously with the initiation of dexamethasone therapy. A normal response (elevation of the plasma cortisol level by at least 280 nmol/L [10 µg/dL]) excludes the diagnosis of adrenocortical hypofunction. Subnormal responses to this test must be further evaluated with more elaborate tests. Mineralocorticoid deficiency in Addison's disease is usually reflected by intravascular volume contraction, hyponatremia, and hyperkalemia. Aldosterone levels are not routinely measured in patients evaluated for Addison's disease because this function is lost only if the entire cortex is destroyed.

Highly specific measurements of plasma cortisol levels are now routinely available by immunoassay, with no cross-reaction with dexamethasone. Elevations of plasma cortisol levels can be caused by elevation of circulating transcortin levels (as in pregnancy or estrogen therapy), increased corticotropin secretion from stress, and a variety of drugs. Urinary excretion of cortisol and its metabolites was formerly assayed by measurement of 24-hour 17-hydroxycorticosteroids (17-OHCS). Immunoassay is now available for measuring the free cortisol excreted unchanged in the urine and is the preferred method. This measurement directly reflects the level of free cortisol in the plasma and therefore is the test of choice for cortisol excretion. Circadian rhythms greatly influence plasma cortisol levels, and hence the sample timing must be planned. Levels are normally highest in the early morning.

Two complicated laboratory tests can help distinguish primary from secondary adrenocortical hypofunction. The prolonged corticotropin stimulation test is a test of adrenal cortical responsiveness. Synthetic corticotropin is administered intravenously at a dosage of 5 U/h for 8 hours. Plasma cortisol levels are measured before and after corticotropin infusion. No response after prolonged stimulation to overcome atrophy of disuse (less than a twofold rise in cortisol levels) implies primary adrenocortical hypofunction (Addison's disease). A normal response implies pituitary dysfunction and proves adrenal cortical responsiveness (secondary hypofunction); these patients must be further evaluated for other pituitary deficits.

The metyrapone test estimates corticotropin reserve and is useful only after proving adrenal cortical responsiveness to be normal. Metyrapone is a compound that competitively blocks the enzymatic conversion of 11-deoxycortisol to cortisol in the adrenal cortex. Reduced plasma levels of cortisol, produced after metyrapone administration, cause a stimulation of corticotropin secretion by the pituitary. This increase in corticotropin causes increased production of 11-deoxycortisol (and other cortisol precursors) but not cortisol. Response to metyrapone can be monitored by measuring either plasma 11-deoxycortisol levels (a cortisol precursor) by radioimmunoassay or, more recently, corticotropin itself. The effectiveness of the 11-hydroxylation blockade should be assessed by measuring the plasma cortisol level, which drops dramatically after administration of metyrapone to trigger corticotropin response.

The major value of the metyrapone test is to confirm secondary adrenocortical hypofunction in patients in whom this diagnosis is suspected but not established. Patients with secondary hypofunction will have no response to metyrapone, and thus metyrapone administration can potentially precipitate an addisonian crisis. Addisonian crisis is a medical emergency. Serum electrolytes and glucose, blood urea nitrogen, and plasma cortisol levels should be obtained in these patients. Corticotropin (cosyntropin) can be administered while therapy with dexamethasone is initiated.

Measurement of plasma corticotropin levels is available, with an assay that is sensitive, specific, and stable. The corticotropin level is substantially elevated in primary adrenal insufficiency and low or "normal" in secondary adrenal insufficiency. Corticotropin shows diurnal variation and pulsatile secretion, and has a short half-life. It should be collected and transported on ice and frozen if not assayed at once.

Adrenocortical Hyperfunction: Diseases and Associated Laboratory Tests

Three clinical syndromes result from adrenocortical hyperfunction: Cushing's syndrome (excess cortisol), Conn's syndrome (aldosteronism, ie, excess aldosterone), and adrenogenital syndrome (excess steroids). Combined syndromes occur.

Cushing's Syndrome

Three laboratory tests are useful in the initial evaluation of a patient with suspected Cushing's syndrome. One of the earliest, but inconstant, biochemical alterations is the loss of the normal nocturnal decline in plasma cortisol levels. Patients with Cushing's syndrome often have no decline in evening plasma cortisol levels, even though random morning plasma cortisol values may not be elevated. Plasma cortisol levels in fully expressed Cushing's syndrome do not fall below 220 to 280 nmol/L (8-10 μg/dL), and evening plasma cortisol levels range from 410 to 830 nmol/L (15-30 μg/dL) (normal values for evening are 80-280 nmol/L [3-10 μg/dL]).

The overnight dexamethasone suppression test is the preferred screening test. One milligram of dexamethasone is given orally at 11:30 PM, and the plasma cortisol level is measured at 8 AM the following morning. Timing of the dexamethasone administration is important, and the drug must be given orally to prevent inadequate suppression. If Cushing's syndrome is present, the 8 AM plasma cortisol level will be typically above 280 nmol/L (10 μg/dL); normally, this value would fall to well below 140 nmol/L (5 μg/dL).

Patients suspected of having Cushing's disease who show equivocal suppression should be further evaluated by measuring their 24-hour urinary free cortisol levels. In usual practice, the screening dexamethasone suppression test is 97% sensitive. False-positive results occur in patients who are acutely ill, are under severe stress (eg, postoperatively), have thyrotoxicosis, and are taking drugs (eg, barbiturates) that accelerate the hepatic metabolism of cortisol and dexamethasone. The urinary free cortisol level is almost invariably elevated in a 24-hour collection from patients with Cushing's syndrome. Although this measurement approaches 100% sensitivity in patients with Cushing's disease, it is subject to errors because of the requirement of a 24-hour urine collection. Persistently normal 24-hour urinary free cortisol levels exclude the diagnosis of endogenous Cushing's syndrome; low levels are usually seen in patients with exogenous Cushing's syndrome due to suppression by synthetic steroids.

In present clinical practice, the most common cause of Cushing's syndrome is exogenous (synthetic) glucocorticosteroid therapy (iatrogenic) for a nonendocrine disorder. Three pathological conditions may also produce Cushing's syndrome: (1) autonomous function of an adrenocortical lesion, benign or malignant (25%-30% of cases); (2) excessive stimulation of the adrenal cortex by pituitary secretion of corticotropin (pituitary Cushing's disease) (60%-70%); and (3) excessive stimulation of the adrenal cortex by ectopic production of corticotropin (usually from a nonendocrine tumor) (5%-10%). A variety of laboratory tests are available to distinguish between these causes. The high-dose (or formal) dexamethasone suppression test is often used to identify adrenal neoplasms, which show no suppression with both the low-dose (screening) and the high-dose (formal) test. Some patients with ectopic corticotropin hypersecretion show similar results. Patients with (pituitary) Cushing's disease typically show suppression during the high-dose test but no suppression with the low-dose test. Other laboratory tests used for differentiating among the causes of Cushing's syndrome include the metyrapone test, the corticotropin stimulation test, and plasma corticotropin levels. Currently, the corticotropin-releasing hormone test appears to further simplify the differential diagnosis.

Adrenocortical carcinomas are notoriously inefficient at steroid hormone synthesis; therefore, most patients with these tumors do not develop clinical or biochemical changes until the tumors are quite large. Patients with the ectopic ACTH syndrome often manifest signs and symptoms of the primary tumor and/or its metastases, most often a bronchogenic carcinoma of the lung.

Conn's Syndrome

Conn's syndrome, or primary (low-renin) aldosteronism, is a rare condition characterized by hypertension, hypokalemia, renal potassium wasting, increased levels of plasma aldosterone (measured by radioimmunoassay), and decreased levels of plasma renin activity (measured in the basal state and after stimulation). Although primary aldosteronism is an uncommon cause of hypertension, it is potentially a surgically correctable form of hypertension and should be looked for in appropriate patients. The biochemical calling card of primary aldosteronism is unprovoked hypokalemia in hypertensive patients. Other causes for hypokalemia (especially chronic thiazide diuretic therapy) must be excluded.

Once the diagnosis of primary aldosteronism is considered, further evaluation should be conducted to identify patients with resectable adrenocortical adenomas. Several provocative tests are used to verify the diagnosis of primary aldosteronism. After 4 hours of upright posture and intravenous saline infusion for volume expansion or low-salt diet, patients with primary aldosteronism due to an adrenocortical adenoma will have no change in their plasma aldosterone levels or plasma renin activities. Many patients will require biochemical analysis of adrenal vein blood levels of aldosterone and renin and/or complicated imaging studies before laparotomy.

Adrenogenital Syndrome

The gonads secrete the major sex steroids (testosterone in men and estradiol in women). The adrenal cortex is an important source of the minor sex steroids (estradiol in men and testosterone in women). Some adrenocortical steroids such as dehydroepiandrosterone and delta-4-androstanedione are peripherally converted into sex steroids, primarily testosterone. Radioimmunoassays are available for testosterone, estradiol (E2), and estrone (E1). Measurements of the latter two compounds have replaced measurements of total urinary estrogens.

Adrenogenital syndromes encompass multiple genetic disorders of deficient adrenocortical hormone synthesis or function, accompanied by adrenal hyperplasia. These disorders include partial, discrete enzymatic defects in cortisol biosynthesis and target all malfunction. Complete enzyme deficiencies would result in fatal absence of cortisol production. The decreased cortisol production that characterizes these disorders causes an increase in corticotropin secretion leading to bilateral adrenocortical hyperplasia (congenital adrenal hyperplasia). To compensate for the decreased cortisol production, therefore, the adrenal cortices of these patients greatly overproduce steroid hormone precursor compounds proximal to the particular enzymatic blocks. Many of these compounds exhibit androgenic and/or mineralocorticoid activity, thus giving rise to distinctive clinical features.

The majority of cases have a deficiency of either the 21-hydroxylase or the 11-hydroxylase enzyme. These patients develop the virilizing adrenogenital syndrome (classical congenital adrenal hyperplasia). Most patients are identified in infancy or childhood, and there is a broad spectrum of clinical expression. Females typically have ambiguous genitalia while the male neonate may appear normal. Biochemically, these patients have increased serum testosterone levels and increased urinary 17-ketosteroid levels. In addition, patients with the 21-hydroxylase deficiency have normal or low urinary free cortisol levels (and 17-OHCS levels) and markedly elevated plasma 17-hydroxyprogesterone levels (a good marker for this deficiency). Patients with the 11-hydroxylase deficiency have elevated urinary 17-OHCS levels (primarily due to increased amounts of 11-deoxycortisol metabolites), low urinary free cortisol levels, elevated plasma and urine 11-deoxycortisol levels, and increased levels of the mineralocorticoid 11-deoxycorticosterone (a good marker for this deficiency). Patients with a 21-hydroxylase deficiency may or may not have urinary sodium loss (depending on whether aldosterone production is diminished), whereas patients with an 11-hydroxylase deficiency typically have urinary sodium retention and hypertension. Other enzyme deficiencies are rare, or the infants do not survive in utero.

Rarely, congenital hyperplasia is recognized in adult life. Syndromes of androgen overproduction are rarely detected in postpubertal men, but even subtle syndromes may be identified in postpubertal women. Androgen excess in women can cause hirsutism or virilization. Virilized women may be evaluated for either ovarian or adrenocortical lesions. Most hirsute women have no identifiable cause.

References

Biemond P, de Jong FH, Lamberts SWJ. Continuous dexamethasone infusion for seven hours in patients with the Cushing syndrome. *Ann Intern Med.* 1990;112:738-742.

CRH Test in the 1990's. *Lancet.* 1990;2:1416. Editorial.

Raff H, Findling JW. A new immunoradiometric assay for corticotropin evaluated in normal subjects and patients with Cushing's syndrome. *Clin Chem.* 1989;35:596-600.

Watts NB, Keffer JH. *Practical Endocrinology.* 4th ed. Philadelphia, Pa: Lea & Febiger; 1989.

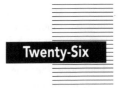
Pituitary Function Tests

Key Points

1. The pituitary gland is functionally multifaceted; there is no single test for pituitary function as a whole.
2. Measurement of both the tropic hormone and the target gland hormone is necessary in view of the feedback relationship, eg, corticotropin (ACTH)/cortisol, thyroid-stimulating hormone/free thyroxine (TSH/FT$_4$).
3. The study of one tropic hormone and its target organ does not nececessarily relate to the integrity of the remaining hormones; each must be studied.
4. Measure prolactin when pituitary disease is suspected because prolactinomas are the most common hypersecreting adenomas.

Background

Anterior pituitary evaluation requires recognition of the basic principles of endocrine physiology, especially feedback loops. Output of pituitary (tropic) hormones is modulated by both hypothalamic inhibiting or releasing hormones and the hormones produced by the pituitary's peripheral target glands. Therefore, measurement of a single hormone level, whether it be of hypothalamic, pituitary, or target gland origin, usually provides inadequate data.

A feedback mechanism implies that each substance produced in response to its initiating hormone provides appropriate feedback for the next step in the chain. For instance, when the peripheral glands (thyroid, adrenal, or gonads) produce adequate levels of hormone in response to the pituitary tropic hormones, the peripheral hormones feed back to the pituitary, thereby modulating the pituitary tropic hormone response. This is called "closed loop feedback." The pituitary gland, however, is not the "master gland," for it is modulated by the hypothalamus. A variety of factors acting on the central nervous system, including stress, anxiety, response to cold, and various central nervous system biochemical mediators, influence hypothalamic production of releasing hormone (designated with the suffix -liberin) and inhibiting factors (designated with the suffix -statin). Therefore, the negative feedback from the peripheral gland hormone is one of many modulating factors acting on the pituitary.

There are several cardinal principles to remember to understand pituitary gland function and feedback: (1) The physiology is complex; however, it is fundamentally ordered. (2) We can measure the peripheral gland hormones and the tropic hormones with ease and accuracy. (3) By knowing the hormone interactions and feedback, one can define intact physiology or its pathological counterpart (Table 26.1).

The human 24-hour diurnal cycles affect hormone levels. Corticotropin has a maximal effect or level between 2 AM and 4 AM and falls to its lowest level in the evening. This results in concomitant changes in the level of cortisol. TSH peaks between 8 PM and midnight and may have significant variation, but it is not commonly addressed clinically. Growth hormone and prolactin both reach their highest levels shortly after the onset of sleep. Throughout the day there are other (ultraradian) cycles that are superimposed on the circadian 24-hour rhythm. Consequently, hormone levels are frequently less informative when only a single serum sample is analyzed. This is also true of luteinizing hormone (LH), follicle-stimulating hormone (FSH), and testosterone. To integrate the peaks and valleys, one should pool aliquots of serum from three samples taken at intervals of 15 to 30 minutes.

Anterior Pituitary Disorders

Isolated deficiency and excess states exist for each of the hormones, and they frequently exist in combination. Therefore, no one test can "screen" for pituitary deficiency or excess. Based on the patient's clinical findings, both tropic and target gland hormones need to be assayed. Commonly, either stimulation or suppression tests to determine the integrity of the normal physiological response to appropriate agents also needs to be included.

Pituitary adenomas are the most common pituitary neoplasm and are more common than realized (from 1%-25% of patients in autopsy series). They may be associated with either hypofunction or hyperfunction. Workup includes anatomic assessment of sella turcica ("Turkish saddle") by the use of imaging techniques; assessment of visual field defects and movement abnormalities of the eyes as a result of involvement of nearby cranial nerves III, IV, and VI; hypothalamic functional assessment, including central temperature regulation, appetite, emotions, and sleep pattern; increased intracranial pressure; cerebrospinal fluid rhinorrhea; seizures; and change in mental status, as well as assessment of the posterior pituitary. Thyroid and adrenal disorders are discussed elsewhere (Chapters 24 and 25, respectively).

Growth Hormone Excess

Growth hormone excess is typically due to a pituitary adenoma. Occurrence prior to the closure of the epiphyses results in gigantism; following closure of the epi-

Table 26.1 Endocrine System Interactions.

Hypothalamus	Anterior Pituitary	Target Organ/Gland
Somatoliberin (SRH) aka growth hormone-releasing hormone (GRH)	Releases somatotropin (STH) aka growth hormone (GH)	Bones, cartilage, soft tissues
Somatostatin (SIF) aka growth hormone-inhibiting hormone	Inhibits somatotropin (STH) aka growth hormone (GH)	Bones, cartilage, soft tissues
Thyroliberin (TRH) aka thyrotropin-releasing hormone	Releases thyrotropin (TSH) aka thyroid-stimulating hormone	Thyroid (thyroxin)
Corticoliberin (CRH) aka corticotropin-releasing hormone	Releases corticotropin (ACTH) aka adrenocorticotropic hormone	Adrenal (cortisol)
Gonadoliberin (LHRH) aka gonadotropin-releasing hormone	Releases follitropin (FSH) aka follicle-stimulating hormone	Gonads (estrogen, progesterone, testosterone spermatogenesis)
Dopamine (DA) aka prolactin-inhibiting factor (PIF)	Releases lutropin aka luteinizing hormone (LH); inhibits prolactin (PRL)	Breast milk-producing units

physes, the result is acromegaly. Failure of growth hormone suppression during glucose administration (glucose tolerance test) diagnoses the autonomous output of growth hormone. Serum samples should be obtained for growth hormone and somatomedin-C, because the latter is the induced product of growth hormone stimulation. In the postnatal period somatomedin-C, also known as "sulfation factor" because it induces cartilaginous chondroitin sulfate, is the most prominent of the "insulin-like growth factors."

Growth Hormone Deficiency
Growth hormone deficiency is commonly worked up using a variety of tests measuring the growth hormone level in response to sleep, L-dopa administration, insulin-induced hypoglycemia, arginine infusion, vasopressin, or glucagon. Growth hormone deficiency is a complex problem and should be assessed by experts.

Prolactin
Prolactin induces the mammary gland to produce milk. Prolactin is also secreted by the most common hormone-secreting pituitary tumor, the prolactinoma. Many women with this tumor are asymptomatic, but galactorrhea, amenorrhea, and infertility may occur. It is estimated to occur in 1 in 1000 women. Prolactin can also be elevated as a result of drug therapy, including phenothiazines, tricyclic antidepressants, antihypertensives (including reserpine and methyldopa), and procainamide derivatives. To document hyperprolactinemia, a baseline prolactin level should be obtained, avoiding friction on the skin of the nipples or chest even from clothing, since this may raise the physiological basal level. Extreme elevation is often associated with pituitary tumors, while lower levels are seen in non-neoplastic conditions. Exclusion of hypothyroidism is essential because prolactin is increased by the thyrotropin-releasing hormone (TRH) mechanism in primary hypothyroidism. Evaluation by an endocrinologist is appropriate. Surgery or medical therapy with bromocriptine has been highly successful.

Gonadal Hormone Deficiency

Workup in the female can be exceedingly complex. Gonadal function testing, especially when the patient presents with infertility, can be a challenge, and many cases require referral to a gynecologic endocrinologist for definitive evaluation and treatment. Appropriate initial study includes documentation of hormonal cycling by measuring basal body temperature and by assaying appropriate serum hormone levels. In an amenorrheic patient, after excluding pregnancy with a highly sensitive measure of human chorionic gonadotropin, serum levels of prolactin, LH, FSH, estradiol, and progesterone should be obtained. If there are marked elevations of FSH and LH, it is apparent that there is no gonadal feedback to the pituitary, promptly-focusing the problem on the gonads. On the other hand, if there is appropriate cycling with a normal physiological retention of the rise in LH at midcycle followed by progesterone elevation, one has gone a long way toward clarifying the picture.

Gonadal effects on vaginal mucosal and endometrial cells make the Pap smear and endometrial biopsy, respectively, cost-effective ways of evaluating hormone influence.

If the menstrual cycle is abnormal, measurement of prolactin can point to pituitary tumor.

In the male, it is simpler to study the deficiency state. Serum levels of testosterone, LH, and FSH plus a sperm count should be included in the initial workup. The examination of sperm in a semen sample for motility and morphology is crucial in the investigation of infertility. These initial data should be available when a patient is referred by a primary care physician to a specialist.

Gonadal Hormone Excess

Gonadal hormone excess is generating interest, with the realization that gonadotropin-secreting pituitary adenomas are far more common than previously recognized. Usually, hypersecretion has little clinical effect, but these adenomas are often recognized because their expanding volume in the limited space of the sella results in headaches, visual disturbances, or hypopituitarism. The most reliable single test is the measurement of the gonadotropin free alpha subunit. These tumors have been found to respond to TRH and, when challenged, show an elevation of FSH and LH in response to TRH stimulation. This is an unexplained but useful diagnostic tool.

In summary, in all cases of pituitary and related endocrine disturbance, one must consider the basic physiology, measure the hormone levels at appropriate times, and integrate the results with physiological expectations. This permits confident exclusion or recognition of disease.

Posterior Pituitary Disorders

There are two posterior pituitary hormones, oxytocin and vasopressin (also known as antidiuretic hormone [ADH]). Oxytocin causes breast milk release and promotes contraction of estrogen-sensitized uterine smooth muscle at delivery. Synthetic injectable preparations can be utilized at this time. No hypofunction or hyperfunction states are relevant to testing.

ADH acts on the collecting duct system of the kidney as an antidiuretic, increasing water reabsorption and concentrating the urine. Its deficiency results in diabetes insipidus, the exertion of a large volume of very dilute urine. This diagnosis is established by measurement of the serum ADH level as well as urine and serum osmolality. Compulsive water-drinking (psychogenic polydipsia), often without conscious awareness on the part of the disturbed individual, needs to be excluded by controlled observation by preventing ingestion of water, thus allowing the kidney to concentrate the urine. Typically in this condition, a dilute serum osmolality in addition to a dilute urine osmolality reveals an appropriate response to pathologically excess water intake.

Nephrogenic diabetes insipidus also needs to be excluded. It results from inability of a chronically diseased kidney to respond to endogenous ADH. A hemoconcentrated serum osmolality plus persistently dilute urine exists. If one does not have an assay for ADH readily available to confirm appropriate secretion of ADH, one can administer ADH to determine if the diuresis can be reversed. If the cause is amyloidosis or myeloma kidney, then administration of ADH fails to reverse the persisting renal water loss.

True diabetes insipidus results from failure of the posterior pituitary to produce ADH and is typically seen following surgery or as a result of a destructive pituitary process. In this setting, one promptly reverses the inappropriate urine diuresis by the administration of ADH, the deficient hormone.

Remember to monitor both serum and urine osmolality, simultaneously collected, to most meaningfully follow up as well as diagnose this condition.

Excess ADH seen with "syndrome of inappropriate ADH secretion" may follow cranial trauma, may be associated with tumors (especially of the lung), or may occur as a result of medication. In syndrome of inappropriate ADH secretion, there is "drowning" of the internal milieu with persistent concentration of urine in spite of hypotonic serum, resulting from an inability to excrete an excess water load. Treatment to correct this condition must proceed slowly to avoid "central pontine myelinolysis." It may be treated with water restriction. If seizures occur resulting from hyponatremia, an antagonist such as demeclocycline may be administered, along with furosemide (Lasix) and a mildly concentrated (intravenous) form of saline. This causes greater water than sodium loss. This complex and critical condition should be approached carefully. If it is suspected emergently, measure the serum and urine osmolality and put serum into an appropriate container to freeze for subsequent measurement of ADH.

References

Gornall AG. *Applied Biochemistry of Clinical Disorders.* 2nd ed. Philadelphia, Pa: JB Lippincott Co; 1986.

Molitch ME. Gonadotroph-cell pituitary adenomas. *N Engl J Med.* 1989;324:626-627.

Watts NB, Keffer J H. *Practical Endocrine Diagnosis.* 4th ed. Philadelphia, Pa: Lea & Febiger; 1989.

Watts NB, Tindall GT. Rapid assessment of corticotropin reserve after pituitary surgery. *JAMA.* 1988;259:708-711.

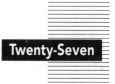

Twenty-Seven

Erythrocyte Disorders

Key Points

1. Hemoglobin and hematocrit levels define the degree of anemia. The red blood cell (RBC) indices and blood smear examination provide a morphological classification that, together with the reticulocyte count, allows correlation with physiological causes of anemia. These initial "routine" studies provide a basis for focusing the confirmatory laboratory tests.

2. The three major categories of anemia are blood loss, impaired RBC production, and accelerated RBC destruction (hemolysis), and each category has numerous causes.

3. The major manifestation of acute blood loss is hypovolemia. With chronic blood loss, iron deficiency anemia may develop.

4. Anemias resulting from impaired RBC production include nutritional deficiencies, bone marrow suppression in chronic illnesses, primary bone marrow failure, and a variety of bone marrow infiltrative processes.

5. Iron deficiency is the most common microcytic hypochromic anemia. It is distinguished from anemia of chronic disease by iron studies and from ß-thalassemia trait by hemoglobin A_2 levels.

6. Megaloblastic anemias nearly always result from vitamin B_{12} or folate deficiency. These deficiency states are distinguished by serum B_{12}, serum folate, and RBC folate levels. The Schilling test can identify the mechanism of vitamin B_{12} deficiency.

7. Aplastic anemia and anemias due to marrow replacement processes are normocytic-normochromic and usually manifest a decreased reticulocyte count, thrombocytopenia, and/or leukopenia.

8. Hemolytic anemias are due to primary abnormalities of the RBC (inherited) or abnormalities in the RBC environment (acquired). They are identified by demonstrating increased RBC destruction (bilirubin, haptoglobin, lactate dehydrogenase [LD] levels) and a compensatory increased rate of erythropoiesis (reticulocyte count).

9. Blood smear examination is particularly useful in assessment of hemolytic anemias; identification of specific poikilocytes may lead to a diagnosis.

10. Plasma hemoglobin, urine hemoglobin, and urine hemosiderin are found in cases of intravascular hemolysis and serve to distinguish intravascular from extravascular (macrophagic) destruction of RBCs.

Background

Anemia is a reduction in the RBC mass and hemoglobin (HGB) concentration of the blood. The usual criteria for defining the degree of anemia are the blood concentration of hemoglobin, expressed in grams per liter (grams per decaliter), and the packed RBC volume (hematocrit [HCT]), expressed as a fraction (percent) of total volume. Other studies useful in the initial assessment of anemia are total RBC count, RBC indices, blood smear examination, and reticulocyte count. RBC indices include the following:

1. Mean cell volume (MCV): the average volume of an RBC, expressed in femtoliters (cubic micrometers)—[HCT/RBC] = MCV
2. Mean cell hemoglobin (MCH): the average content (mass) of hemoglobin per RBC, expressed in picograms—[HGB/RBC] = MCH
3. Mean cell hemoglobin concentration (MCHC): the average concentration of hemoglobin in a given volume of packed RBCs, expressed in grams per liter (grams per decaliter)—[HGB/HCT] = MCHC
4. RBC distribution width (RDW): the coefficient of variation of RBC volume.

RBC indices may be calculated as shown above, but in most laboratories instruments directly measure or automatically calculate them. Adult reference ranges are shown in Table 27.1.

Anemias may be classified using MCV, MCHC, and RDW, which correspond to the size, color, and degree of anisocytosis (size variably) of RBCs on a blood smear. These morphological classes, based on RBC indices, correlate with physiological causes of anemia.

An MCV between 76 and 100 fL (μm^3) means that the average RBC size is normal, or normocytic. An MCV of 75 fL (μm^3) or less defines microcytosis, most often associated with an abnormality of hemoglobin synthesis. An MCV of more than 100 fL (μm^3) defines macrocytosis, which in the absence of increased reticulocytes usually indicates an abnormality of nuclear maturation. RBCs are normochromic when the MCHC is normal (330-370 g/L [33-37 g/dL]). A low MCHC is associated with disorders of hemoglobin synthesis, so that the RBCs become hypochromic. An MCHC above the normal reference range is rarely encountered. Using the MCV and MCHC, anemias may be categorized into one of the following groups: (1) normocytic-normochromic, (2) microcytic-normochromic, (3) microcytic-hypochromic, and (4) macrocytic-normochromic.

The RDW is a measure of RBC anisocytosis (variation in cell size); the higher the RDW the greater the degree of anisocytosis. The RDW is most useful in the differential diagnosis of microcytic anemia. Patients may have a decreased MCV and normal RDW (microcytic homogenous anemia), which are the usual findings

Table 27.1 Adult Reference Ranges for Hematology.*

	Système International (SI)			Conventional		
	Units	Men	Women	Units	Men	Women
Hemoglobin (HGB)	g/L	136-172	120-150	g/dL	13.6-17.2	12.0-15.0
Hematocrit (HCT)	1	0.39-0.49	0.33-0.43	%	39-49	33-43
Erythrocyte count (RBCs)	$\times 10^{12}$/L	4.3-5.9	3.5-5.0	$\times 10^6$/mm^3	4.3-5.9	3.5-5.0
Reticulocyte count	%	0.5-1.5		%	0.5-1.5	
Absolute number	$\times 10^9$/L	10-75		/mm^3	10,000-75,000	
Mean cell volume (MCV)	fL	76-100		μm^3	76-100	
Mean cell hemoglobin (MCH)	pg	27-33		pg	27-33	
Mean cell hemoglobin concentration (MCHC)	g/L	330-370		g/dL	33-37	
RBC distribution width (RDW)	—	11.5-14.5		—	11.5-14.5	

* Reference ranges vary among laboratories. The reference ranges for the laboratory providing a result should always be used when interpreting a laboratory test.

in anemia of chronic disease and thalassemia minor, or a decreased MCV and increased RDW, as would be expected in iron deficiency.

The studies discussed above are components of the complete blood count (CBC). Appropriate interpretation of the information provided by the CBC, together with careful evaluation of a blood smear, focuses the laboratory assessment of anemia on a specific group of confirmatory tests. Time and expense is reduced when these initial studies are used correctly.

Normal RBC Production and Destruction

RBC Production
As RBC precursors (normoblasts) mature in the bone marrow they become smaller, the nuclear chromatin becomes condensed, hemoglobin content increases, and ribonucleic acid (RNA) decreases. When maturation is nearly complete the small pyknotic nucleus is extruded from the cell. RBCs ordinarily remain in the marrow for 48 to 72 hours after loss of their nucleus as the cytoplasm continues to mature. The RBC then enters the circulation as a reticulocyte.

In a normal individual, RBCs circulate for approximately 120 days. In the steady state the marrow produces and replaces about 1% of the circulating RBCs each day. Young RBCs circulate as reticulocytes for approximately 24 hours. On routinely stained blood smears they appear slightly blue or polychromatophilic and are larger than the other RBCs. A reticulocytic count is performed using a

Table 27.2 Reticulocyte Counts in Anemia.

Anemias with increased reticulocyte counts
  Hemolytic anemias (sustained reticulocytosis)
  Acute blood loss (transient reticulocytosis)
  Response to treatment of deficiency states
  Marrow recovery from exogenous suppression

Anemias with decreased reticulocyte counts
  Deficiency states (iron, vitamin B_{12})
  Anemia of chronic illness
  Hypoplastic (aplastic) anemia
  Bone marrow replacement processes (leukemia, fibrosis, metastasis)
  Dyserythropoietic states (congenital and acquired)
  Iatrogenic bone marrow suppression

---

stain that is more specific for reticulocytes and stains the residual RNA in a "reticulum"-like pattern. An increased reticulocyte count is evidence of bone marrow response to anemia. A decreased or inadequately elevated reticulocyte count in an anemic patient is indicative of bone marrow failure or lack of normal response.

As the hematocrit level and RBC count drop, the percentage of reticulocytes will increase even if the absolute number of reticulocytes remains unchanged. It is important, therefore, to report the reticulocyte count in absolute numbers or to correct the percent reticulocyte count based on an expected normal hematocrit of 0.45 (45%). The correction is made as follows:

Reticulocyte count reference range = 0.005 to 0.015 (0.5%-1.5%) or
10 to 75×10^9/L (10,000-75,000/mm^3) (absolute)
Corrected reticulocyte count = (uncorrected count) x
(patient's hematocrit/45)

This corrected reticulocyte percentage is accepted as reflective of the actual bone marrow response.

Reticulocyte counts are increased in anemias caused by RBC loss or premature destruction. They are usually diminished in anemias caused by a deficiency state or bone marrow failure (Table 27.2).

RBC Catabolism

Normal RBC destruction and catabolism occurs extravascularly in reticuloendothelial cells (Figure 27.1). Under normal conditions, only a small number of RBCs undergo intravascular destruction. This mechanism becomes more important in cases of intravascular hemolytic anemia.

Evaluation for Specific Types of Anemia

Anemias may be separated into three major categories: blood loss, impaired RBC production, and accelerated RBC destruction (hemolyis), each of which has numerous etiologies.

Figure 27.1 Catabolic Pathway of Red Blood Cells.*

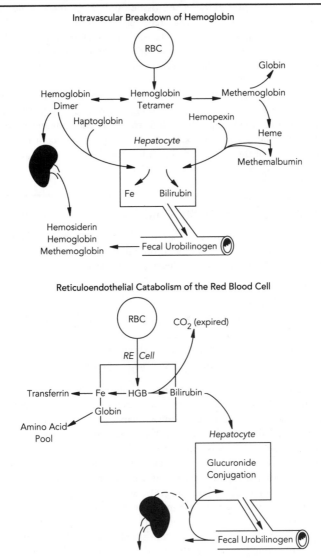

Intravascular Breakdown of Hemoglobin

Reticuloendothelial Catabolism of the Red Blood Cell

* Reprinted, with permission, from R. S. Hillman and C. A. Finch, *Red Cell Manual.* 5th ed. Philadelphia, Pa: FA Davis Co; 1985:19-20.

Anemia Due to Blood Loss

Anemia may result from acute traumatic blood loss, surgery, or abnormal hemostasis. Chronic blood loss may occur with occult bleeding from the gastrointestinal tract or other sites, or from chronic heavy menstruation or multiple pregnancies. In acute blood loss the initial clinical findings may relate to hypo-volemia. Anemia is demonstrable when tissue fluid enters the vascular space to compensate for the volume loss, thus reducing the concentration of RBCs by dilution. The diagnosis is made by the history and physical findings. The RBCs are normocytic and normochromic. The reticulocyte count is elevated within 2 or 3 days and peaks at 7 to 10 days following acute bleeding.

Changes associated with chronic blood loss are usually insidious. Initially, the bone marrow compensates with a mild reticulocyte response and the hemoglobin and hematocrit levels remain normal. In time, iron stores may become depleted due to loss of iron-containing RBCs, and iron deficiency anemia evolves. The RBC indices are microcytic-normochromic or microcytic-hypochromic, depending on the severity of the iron deficiency. The reticulocyte count may be normal, decreased, or mildly but inadequately increased.

Anemias Due to Impaired RBC Production

Anemias due to impaired RBC production are seen with nutritional deficiencies, bone marrow suppression effects of a chronic illness, primary bone marrow failure, and a variety of bone marrow infiltrative or replacement processes.

Nutritional Deficiencies

Nutritional deficiencies result when dietary substances essential for normal erythropoiesis are either lacking in the diet, lost from the body, or abnormally absorbed or incorporated. Cytoplasmic maturation defects and nuclear maturation defects may result from deficiency states, causing anemia.

Iron Deficiency Anemia. Iron is an essential component of the heme portion of the hemoglobin molecule. Iron deficiency anemia (microcytic-hypochromic) results from inadequate amounts of iron available to maintain a normal rate of hemoglobin synthesis. Iron deficiency is the most common cause of microcytic-hypochromic anemia. Patients initially have microcytic-normochromic RBCs, which progress to ones that are microcytic and hypochromic. As the process evolves there is increased anisocytosis and poikilocytosis (abnormally shaped cells). Mild to moderate thrombocytosis is present in many patients.

The recognition of a microcytic-hypochromic anemia should instigate evaluation of iron status. Measurement of the total serum iron (TSI), total iron-binding capacity (TIBC), and transferrin saturation should be obtained. Transferrin is an iron transport protein, and the TIBC is a direct measure of the amount of iron that can be added to unsaturated transferrin binding sites and an indirect measurement of serum transferrin concentration. The transferrin saturation is the ratio of TSI to TIBC expressed as a percentage. A saturation less than 15% indicates iron deficiency. In iron deficiency, the TSI level is decreased, the TIBC increased, and the transferrin saturation decreased.

The serum ferritin and free erythrocyte protoporphyrin (FEP) levels are useful supplementary tests in the differential diagnosis of microcytic anemias. Measurement of serum ferritin has largely eliminated the need for bone marrow examination to determine iron stores. Serum ferritin roughly parallels tissue fer-

Table 27.3 Relationship of Cytoplasmic Maturation Defect Anemias and Red Blood Cell Indices: Morphological Classification.

Physiological Basis of Anemia	Morphological (Indices) Classification		
	MCV-MCHC	MCHC-RDW	Poikilocytosis
Cytoplasmic maturation defect anemia (abnormalities in hemoglobin synthesis)			
Iron deficiency			
Early	Microcytic-normochromic	Microcytic-heterogeneous	+
Late	Microcytic-hypochromic	Microcytic-heterogeneous	+
Iron reutilization defect (anemia of chronic disease)	Normocytic-normochromic or Microcytic-normochromic	Normocytic-homogeneous	−
β-Thalassemia minor	Microcytic-normochromic or Microcytic-hypochromic	Microcytic-homogeneous or Microcytic-heterogeneous (less heterogeneous than iron deficiency)	+ +

ritin levels and therefore is a good estimation of tissue iron stores. Levels are decreased in iron deficiency anemia. Serum ferritin results must be interpreted with caution in patients with underlying hepatocellular disease, malignant neoplasms, and inflammatory diseases, because in these conditions ferritin may be disproportionately high relative to the actual storage iron. FEP accumulates when heme synthesis is impaired. In disorders of heme synthesis (eg, iron deficiency, anemia of chronic disease, lead poisoning, porphyria) RBC FEP is increased.

The two most important cytoplasmic maturation defect anemias that must be distinguished from iron deficiency are iron reutilization defect anemias (anemia of chronic disease), usually associated with a chronic inflammatory illness, and ß-thalassemia trait (Table 27.3). In both of these conditions, the RBCs are microcytic but usually normochromic or only mildly hypochromic. Their distinction from an early iron deficiency anemia is important because of therapeutic considerations.

Patients with anemia of chronic disease have iron reutilization defects secondary to their chronic illness, resulting in reduced TSI levels and decreased TIBC. The percent transferrin saturation may also be reduced but generally not to the level of that in iron deficiency anemia. Serum ferritin and bone marrow iron stores are normal or increased in iron reutilization defects and serve to distinguish anemia of chronic disease from iron deficiency.

ß-Thalassemia minor (trait) is the heterozygous state of an inherited abnormality of synthesis of the beta globin chains of hemoglobin. A microcytic slightly hypochromic anemia of mild degree usually occurs. Patients with ß-thalassemia trait generally have normal iron studies and a normal FEP. Hemoglobin A_2 is elevated and is the definitive test for ß-thalassemia trait. In contrast, the hemoglobin A_2 level is normal or decreased in iron deficiency and normal in iron

Table 27.4 Laboratory Findings in Microcytic-Hypochromic Anemias.

Test	Reference Range	Iron Deficiency	Iron Reutilization Defect	Thalassemia
Total serum iron (TSI), μmol/L (μg/dL)	(M) 10-25 (55-140) (F) 5-22 (30-125)	D	N or D	N or I
Total iron binding capacity (TIBC) μmol/L (μg/dL)	(M) 45-74 (253-415) (F) 45-73 (249-409)	I	N or D	N or D
Transferrin saturation (TSI/TIBC)	(M) 20%-55% (F) 20%-55%	< 15%	15%-30%	N or I
Serum ferritin, μg/L	(M) 30-200 (F) 20-150	< 12	> 12	N or I
Free erythrocyte protoporphyrin, μmol/L (μg/dL)	0.18-1.60 (10-90)	I	I	N
Hemoglobin A_2	2%-3.5% of total hemoglobin	N or D	N	I (3.5% -7.5%)

D = decreased; N = normal; I = increased

reutilization defects. Laboratory findings in microcytic-hypochromic anemias are shown in Table 27.4.

Vitamin B_{12} and Folate Deficiency Anemia (Megaloblastic Anemia). Megaloblastic anemias result from abnormal nuclear maturation. Deficiency of either vitamin B_{12} or folate leads to impaired deoxyribonucleic acid (DNA) synthesis and retardation of cell mitosis. RNA synthesis, however, is less impaired and proceeds more normally. This asynchrony results in nuclear cytoplasmic dissociation in the affected cell populations. Hematopoietic cells replicate rapidly and are highly vulnerable to deficiencies of vitamin B_{12} or folate. The term megaloblastic anemia is commonly used, but is too restrictive, because leukopenia and thrombocytopenia are often present in addition to anemia, and a megaloblastic state may exist in the absence of anemia.

Two groups of laboratory tests for the diagnosis of megaloblastic anemias are those used to define the anemia as megaloblastic and those that identify the specific cause.

The tests used to identify megaloblastic anemias include the CBC, blood smear examination, and, occasionally, bone marrow examination. The RBCs are macrocytic-normochromic and the red cell distribution width is increased. The reticulocyte count is reduced. The blood smear shows prominent anisocytosis and oval-shaped macrocytes. Platelets and leukocytes may be reduced. Some of the neutrophils are larger than normal and/or exhibit nuclear hypersegmentation (more than five nuclear segments.) If a bone marrow examination is performed, characteristic morphological changes are observed, including abnormally large RBC precursors with striking nuclear-cytoplasmic asynchrony, delicate nuclear chromatin, and prominent (open) parachromatin in a hypercellular marrow.

Table 27.5 Serum Vitamin B$_{12}$ and Serum and Red Blood Cell Folate Measurement in Megaloblastic Anemia.

	Reference Ranges		Vitamin B$_{12}$ Deficiency	Folate Deficiency	Negative Folate Balance	Combined B$_{12}$ and Folate Deficiency
	Système International (SI)	Conventional				
Serum vitamin B$_{12}$	150-750 pmol/L	200-1000 pg/mL	↓	N	N	↓
Serum folate	4-22 nmol/L	2-10 ng/mL	N or ↑	↓	↓	↓
Red blood cell folate	550-2200 nmol/L	140-960 ng/mL	N or ↓	↓	N	↓

N = normal; ↑ = increased; ↓ = decreased

Most of the abnormal erythroid percursors in advanced megaloblastic states are destroyed in the bone marrow. The combination of anemia, a reduced reticulocyte count, and erythroid hyperplasia in the marrow is referred to as ineffective erythropoiesis.

Serum vitamin B$_{12}$, serum folate, and RBC folate measurements are used to identify the deficiency leading to macrocytic anemia. The changes in these parameters in the various deficiency states are shown in Table 27.5.

Folate deficiency is related to inadequate dietary intake in most cases, although it can, uncommonly, result from intestinal absorption failure. In contrast, vitamin B$_{12}$ deficiency is rarely due to dietary lack and nearly always evolves from failure to absorb B$_{12}$ normally. Absorption failure may be due to gastric intrinsic factor deficiency (pernicious anemia) or failure of the ileum to absorb B$_{12}$-intrinsic factor complex. Rarely, competition with intestinal helminths or microorganisms may lead to B$_{12}$ deficiency.

The mechanism of vitamin B$_{12}$ deficiency can be assessed by the Schilling test, which is a measurement of the capacity to absorb orally administered radiolabeled vitamin B$_{12}$. If failure to adequately absorb B$_{12}$ is observed, the test is repeated with simultaneous oral administration of intrinsic factor. This technique distinguishes between intrinsic factor deficiency and failure of the ileum to absorb B$_{12}$-intrinsic factor complex.

Gastric acidity testing to identify achlorhydria, commonly associated with pernicious anemia, is nonspecific because achlorhydria may occur in individuals without pernicious anemia. Gastric analysis for intrinsic factor is more useful but is not widely available.

Serum intrinsic factor blocking antibodies may be demonstrated by radioassay in 50% to 60% of patients with pernicious anemia. Their presence in a patient with megaloblastic anemia is essentially diagnostic of pernicious anemia.

The deoxyuridine suppression test of bone marrow DNA synthesis is highly sensitive for B$_{12}$ or folate deficiency. Abnormal findings may be demonstrated before hematologic changes occur. When modified and applied on blood lymphocytes, the test may detect deficiency states in patients treated with hematinics prior to adequate evaluation of their anemia. Urinary excretion of methylmalonic acid is increased in most cases of vitamin B$_{12}$ deficiency and not in folate defi-

Table 27.6 Causes of Aplastic Anemia.

Constitutional aplasia
  Fanconi's anemia
  Familial aplastic anemia
Physical and chemical agents
  Radiation exposure
  Toxic substances, eg, benzene, antineoplastic agents
Hypersensitivity to drugs
  Chloramphenicol
  Phenylbutazone
  Tripelennamine
Viral infections
  Hepatitis A
Pregnancy
Thymoma

ciency. These measurements are rarely necessary in the assessment of megaloblastic anemias.

Other causes of macrocytic anemia include alcoholism, liver disease, dyserythropoietic bone marrow disorders, reticulocytosis, hypothyroidism, and heavy metal intoxication, but the MCV rarely reaches levels above 110 to 115 fL (μm^3) in these disorders. When the MCV exceeds this level, megaloblastic anemia should be strongly suspected; the MCV in megaloblastic anemia is often above 120 fL (μm^3) and may be as high as 160 fL (μm^3). Other morphological changes that point to megaloblastic anemia are the presence of oval macrocytes and hypersegmented neutrophils. Target cells and acanthocytes are common in liver disease, and polychromatophilic RBCs are abundant in cases of reticulocytosis.

Primary Bone Marrow Failure

Primary bone marrow failure is also a cause of impaired RBC production. Aplastic or hypoplastic anemia results from an inherited or acquired primary defect in hematopoiesis. The term aplastic anemia is a misnomer because there is usually also a reduction in platelets and leukocytes. Aplastic pancytopenia would be a more descriptive term. Several causes of aplastic anemia have been identified (Table 27.6), but many cases are idiopathic.

RBC indices are normal in aplastic anemia. Reticulocytes, platelets, and leukocytes are decreased. Blood smear examination shows normocytic-normochromic anemia with minimal anisocytosis and poikilocytosis; polychromatophilic erythro-

Table 27.7 Indications for Bone Marrow Examination in the Evaluation of Anemia.

Normocytic-normochromic anemias with a low reticulocyte count and normal iron studies
Anemias associated with other cytopenias
Anemias with circulating normoblasts
Normocytic anemias with circulating abnormal leukocytes or myeloblasts

Table 27.8 Bone Marrow Infiltrative and Replacement (Myelophthisic) Processes.

Hematologic malignancies
  Leukemia
  Lymphoma
  Plasma cell myeloma
Metastatic tumors
Primary myelofibrosis
Metabolic bone diseases
Granulomatous infections
Storage diseases

---

cytes are absent or decreased in number. Other blood cells are usually decreased but are morphologically normal. The diagnosis is confirmed by a bone marrow examination that reveals a markedly hypocellular marrow with reduction in erythroid and, usually, all other hematopoietic cells. Anemia with other cytopenias is generally an indication for a bone marrow examination (Table 27.7).

Pure (isolated) RBC aplasia is less common than generalized aplasia except for the transitory arrest of erythropoiesis that may occur in association with viral infections, eg, parvovirus. RBC aplasia may be congenital (Blackfan-Diamond syndrome) or acquired. Acquired forms are associated with thymoma in about half of the cases.

RBCs are normocytic-normochromic and the reticulocyte count is markedly reduced. The platelet and leukocyte counts are normal in RBC aplasia. The bone marrow shows reduction or absence of erythroid precursors.

Bone marrow infiltrative and replacement processes (myelophthisic anemia) include numerous disorders that invade or encroach on the bone marrow resulting in suppression of hematopoiesis (Table 27.8).

The anemia-associated marrow replacement is usually normocytic and normochromic. The reticulocyte count may be decreased, normal, or increased. There is usually reduction of blood leukocytes and/or platelets. A leukoerythroblastic reaction (nucleated RBCs and immature neutrophils) is characteristically observed in blood smears. A bone marrow examination usually reveals the nature of the marrow infiltrative process.

Anemias Due to Accelerated Hemolytic Destruction of RBCs

Hemolytic anemias result from an accelerated rate of RBC destruction. It may be more appropriate to refer to this group as hemolytic disorders; many patients with moderate chronic hemolysis do not become anemic because they are able to completely compensate for the increased rate of RBC destruction by increased RBC production.

Two basic types of abnormalities result in premature RBC destruction, abnormalities intrinsic to the RBC structure or composition and extrinsic abnormalities in the RBC environment. Hemolytic disorders are classified according to the location of the defect leading to hemolysis (intrinsic or extrinsic) or they are classified

Table 27.9 General Classification of Hemolytic Anemias.

Hereditary hemolytic anemias
  RBC membrane abnormalities
  Hemoglobinopathies
  Enzymopathies

Acquired hemolytic anemias
  Immune
  Nonimmune
  Intravascular pathology (microangiopathic)
  Physical agents
  Chemical agents
  Infectious agents
  Plasma lipid abnormalities
  Hypersplenism
  Intracellular abnormalities
    (paroxysmal nocturnal hemoglobinuria)

---

by the hereditary or acquired nature of the defect (Table 27.9). The two classifications correspond very closely; intrinsic RBC defects are nearly always hereditary, and disorders due to extrinsic causes of hemolysis are nearly always acquired. Hemolysis may also be viewed according to the site of RBC destruction, extravascular or intravascular.

The blood smear is the single most useful laboratory study in the initial evaluation of a patient with hemolytic anemia. There are several morphological changes in blood smears that are indicative of a hemolytic disorder, and some point to a specific etiology. The blood smear findings may narrow the differential diagnosis and provide information that can direct the subsequent anemia workup, often saving considerable time and expense.

Increased polychromatophilic RBCs, corresponding to the increased reticulocyte count, is a hallmark of hemolytic anemias. The polychromatophilic cells in hemolytic anemias are often excessively basophilic, which is indicative of a shift of bone marrow reticulocytes into the blood ("shift reticulocytes"). Normoblastemia may also be present, particularly in children. This results from the greatly increased rate of erythropoiesis and premature release of RBCs from the marrow.

Poikilocytosis of specific types is strongly associated with particular hemolytic disorders. For example, abundant spherocytes suggest either hereditary spherocytosis or an autoimmune hemolytic disorder, while RBC fragments, particularly in association with thrombocytopenia, suggest a microangiopathic hemolytic anemia.

Three categories of laboratory tests useful in the evaluation of hemolytic anemias following the CBC and blood smear evaluation are: tests to identify increased RBC destruction, tests to demonstrate a compensatory increase in the rate of erythropoiesis, and tests to recognize changes found only in particular varieties of hemolytic anemia and useful in the differential diagnosis. The first two categories are aimed at establishing the existence of a hemolytic state and have no causative specificity. Studies in the third category are used to establish the cause of hemolysis. Usually, only a few judiciously selected studies are necessary to identify the cause of a hemolytic disorder.

Tests to Identify Increased RBC Destruction

Increased catabolic products of hemoglobin accompany hemolytic disorders because the heme portion of the hemoglobin molecule is catabolized at a greatly accelerated rate. Excretion of heme catabolites, which can be measured in the clinical laboratory, are increased proportionately.

Hyperbilirubinemia, the increased serum concentration of unconjugated bilirubin present in hemolytic states, is dependent on two factors: the rate at which it is formed and the rate of bilirubin conjugation and excretion by the liver. For these reasons the serum bilirubin level is an unreliable index of the rate of hemolysis; frequently, patients with moderate to mild hemolysis will have no increase in serum bilirubin. Values above 86 µmol/L (5 mg/dL) are uncommon with hemolytic anemia except in infancy.

Fecal urobilinogen excretion is a more sensitive index of hemolysis than is serum bilirubin level and is increased when bilirubin levels are normal. The validity of the test depends on the accuracy of the collected 4-day fecal specimen. Because fecal urobilinogen production depends on intestinal bacteria, low values may be found in patients taking broad-spectrum antibiotics.

Serum haptoglobin is an alpha$_2$ globulin that rapidly binds free plasma hemoglobin. The hemoglobin-haptoglobin complex is quickly removed by the liver. Levels may rapidly decrease or disappear from the plasma because there is no compensatory increase in haptoglobin production in hemolytic states. With significant intravascular hemolysis, haptoglobin rapidly disappears. Even when hemolysis is predominantly extravascular there may be decreased haptoglobin levels.

Decreased RBC survival can be determined by measuring the half-disappearance time of infused chromium-labeled RBC. Patients with the most severe anemia have the shortest half-disappearance time. RBC survival studies should be reserved for particularly difficult diagnostic problems. They are time-consuming, expensive, and rarely necessary. Uptake studies for identifying the site of RBC sequestration should be performed with RBC survival studies. The information obtained from uptake studies may be helpful when splenectomy is a consideration for control of a chronic hemolytic disorder.

Serum LD is elevated in hemolytic disorders. The increase results from liberation of erythrocyte LD into the plasma. Elevated serum LD is not specific for hemolysis but in the appropriate clinical context and in combination with other laboratory studies is a useful test in the diagnosis of hemolytic anemias.

Hemoglobinemia, hemoglobinuria, and hemosiderinuria all accompany intravascular RBC destruction, with release of hemoglobin into the plasma. If plasma hemoglobin exceeds haptoglobin binding capacity, hemoglobinemia results. Hemoglobin dimers are excreted into the urine, causing hemoglobinuria. The hemoglobin dimers are partially reabsorbed by the renal proximal convoluted tubule epithelial cells. The hemoglobin iron is incorporated in the epithelial cells as hemosiderin and ferritin. Iron-containing tubular cells are later sloughed into the urine, resulting in hemosiderinuria.

Table 27.10 summarizes the laboratory indications of RBC destruction.

Laboratory Indications of a Compensatory Increase in Erythropoiesis

Laboratory indications of a compensatory increase in erythropoiesis include all of the following: increased reticulocytes, bone marrow erythroid hyperpla-

Table 27.10 Laboratory Indications of Increased RBC Destruction.

Increased catabolic products of heme
 Hyperbilirubinemia—unconjugated
 Increased fecal urobilinogen
Decreased serum haptoglobin
Decreased RBC survival time as measured by ^{51}Cr-tagged RBCs
Increased serum lactic dehydrogenase activity
Increased plasma hemoglobin, urine hemoglobin, urine hemosiderin

sia, increased plasma iron transport rate, and increased erythrocyte iron turnover rate.

Sustained reticulocytosis in the blood is one of the most reliable signs of increased RBC production. In hemolytic anemia, reticulocytes are persistently increased. This may be reflected in RBC indices as a macrocytic MCV.

The bone marrow is hypercellular with erythroid hyperplasia in hemolytic disorders. The hyperplasia varies according to the degree of anemia and RBC survival time. The ratio of granulocyte to erythroid precursors is decreased.

Ferrokinetic studies, using radiolabeled iron, trace iron as it moves from the plasma to the bone marrow and to the circulating RBCs. Because iron is intimately related to hemoglobin synthesis, ferrokinetic studies make it possible to evaluate rates and sites of erythropoiesis. Plasma iron transport rate is a measure of total erythropoiesis and reflects the degree of erythroid hyperplasia. Erythrocyte iron turnover rate is a measure of effective erythropoiesis and correlates with reticulocyte production. Both of these parameters are increased in hemolytic anemia. These tests are unnecessary in the large majority of patients with hemolytic anemia because other tests, ie, reticulocyte count, are simpler, less expensive, and nearly as accurate.

Tests to Further Classify Hereditary Hemolytic Anemias and Aid in Differential Diagnosis

Hereditary hemolytic anemias are intrinsic to the RBC and include abnormalities of the RBC membrane, the structure and synthesis of the hemoglobin molecule, and the RBC enzyme system. Approximately half of the more than 30 laboratory tests available for the evaluation of anemia pertain specifically to the differential diagnosis of hemolytic disorders. These tests should be requested only when the existence of a hemolytic disorder has been established. Some of these will be discussed in the context of the individual types of hemolytic anemia.

RBC Membrane Abnormalities. Most membrane abnormalities are due to defects in membrane skeletal proteins. The resultant instability of the membrane skeleton leads to loss of cell membrane, spontaneous fragmentation, and permanent deformation. The abnormal-shaped cells are removed from the circulation by macrophages in the spleen and elsewhere in the reticuloendothelial system. The most commonly encountered hereditary RBC membrane disorder that routinely causes significant hemolysis is hereditary spherocytosis; it occurs in about 1 in 5000 individuals. Hereditary spherocytosis is usually of autosomal-dominant inheritance. The family history is of considerable importance in the diagnosis. Physical examination generally identifies splenomegaly. The degree of hemolysis varies considerably between patients; some have a severe hemolytic disease, others may be asymptomatic.

The diagnosis of hereditary spherocytosis is usually established by the following sequence of laboratory studies:

1. Blood smears show increased polychromatophilic RBCs and microspherocytes (small RBCs that lack central pallor).
2. Hemolysis is associated with abnormal laboratory results (reticulocytosis, increased unconjugated bilirubin, decreased haptoglobin, etc).
3. Other causes of spherocytosis are excluded, ie, a negative Coombs' test eliminates immune hemolytic anemia.
4. Osmotic fragility is increased and greatly exaggerated after 24 hours of in vitro RBC incubation.
5. A positive family history is established.

Spherocytes have decreased surface area/volume and are more sensitive to osmotic stress than are normal RBCs. When incubated with hypotonic saline solutions spherocytes lyse at higher concentrations of sodium chloride than do normal cells; osmotic fragility is increased. (RBCs with excess membrane, such as those found in hypochromic anemias, have decreased osmotic fragility.) Increased osmotic fragility is a hallmark of hereditary spherocytosis but may also be observed in other types of anemia, such as autoimmune hemolytic anemia. Osmotic fragility is usually dramatically increased in hereditary spherocytosis compared with other conditions following in vitro incubation of the cells for 24 hours.

Several other hereditary RBC membrane disorders result in variable degrees of hemolysis, including hereditary elliptocytosis, hereditary stomatocytosis, and hereditary pyropoikilocytosis. All of these are rare and are usually suspected by observation of specific types of poikilocytes on blood smears.

Hemoglobinopathies

Structurally Abnormal Hemoglobins. The amino acid sequence of a globin chain is altered in structurally abnormal hemoglobin. This abnormal sequence may be due to single or multiple amino acid substitutions, deletions, or additions. Those most commonly associated with hemolysis are hemoglobin S (sickle cell anemia), hemoglobin C, and unstable hemoglobins. The anemia associated with hemoglobinopathies may result from retarded synthesis of hemoglobin and ineffective erythropoiesis, in addition to hemolysis. The diagnosis of a hemoglobinopathy is often suggested by clinical data and RBC morphology on a peripheral blood smear, eg, sickle cells, target cells, and hemoglobin C crystals. For the most common hemoglobinopathies, including hemoglobins S, C, E, and others, the diagnosis may be confirmed by hemoglobin electrophoresis.

Screening tests are available for the identification of hemoglobin S in sickle cell disease (homozygous) and sickle trait. The solubility test is most commonly used. It is performed on a solution of lysed RBCs. The hemoglobin in the solution is reduced by addition of dithionite. Deoxyhemoglobin S is insoluble in a concentrated phosphate buffer and is easily distinguished from normal hemoglobins. The metabisulfite preparation, or "sickle prep," is a wet mount of whole blood mixed with a 2% solution of sodium metabisulfite, a reducing substance, to enhance deoxygenation. Deoxygenated cells containing hemoglobin S will sickle. The preparation is studied under the microscope. Positive or suspicious test results should always be confirmed by hemoglobin electrophoresis. Both homozygote and heterozygote states will manifest positive results, and false positives can occur with either of these screening tests.

Unstable hemoglobins are rare disorders that may result in chronic hemolysis. The abnormality occurs at the point that heme binds to globin in the hemoglobin molecule. The abnormal hemoglobin is easily denatured, and Heinz bodies (denatured hemoglobin) are formed. As Heinz bodies become numerous they cause the RBC membrane to become rigid. The cells are removed by the spleen. Studies that may be used to identify an unstable hemoglobin include Heinz body stains, heat denaturation test, isopropanol precipitation test, and hemoglobin electrophoresis.

Heinz bodies can be demonstrated by a special stain on a blood smear. The heat denaturation and isopropanol precipitation tests cause rapid precipitation of unstable hemoglobins in hemolysates. Other hemoglobins do not precipitate as rapidly. Most unstable hemoglobins cannot be characterized by routine hemoglobin electrophoresis. Special techniques, including isoelectric focusing, are required.

Thalassemia Syndromes. In thalassemia syndromes there is an imbalance of globin chain production but the chains are structurally normal. The most common of these syndromes are the homozygous and heterozygous states of α- and ß-thalassemia. Anemia in the thalassemia syndromes results from retarded cytoplasmic maturation due to abnormal synthesis of hemoglobin, ineffective erythropoiesis, and hemolysis. The hemolysis is due to precipitation of the excess normal unaffected alpha or beta globin chain on the RBC membrane. The membrane becomes rigid and the cell is removed from the circulation. The diagnosis is usually made by family studies, blood smear examination, and hemoglobin electrophoresis.

RBC Enzymopathies. The most common RBC enzyme deficiency is glucose-6-phosphate dehydrogenase (G6PD). It occurs in 3% to 7% of the population in the United States and is most common in black males and people of Mediterranean extraction. All other RBC enzyme deficiencies associated with hemolytic anemias are rare.

Hemolysis in patients with G6PD deficiency results from the exhaustion of the normal RBC energy system, which leads to denaturation of hemoglobin and formation of Heinz bodies. In the most common form of G6PD deficiency, hemolysis occurs only after exposure to an oxidant substance. Heinz bodies may be pitted out of the RBCs by macrophages. The poikilocytes that result are called "bite" cells or "blister" cells and are observable on blood smears. The tests used to diagnose G6PD deficiency include the Heinz body stain (nonspecific), G6PD screening tests (spot test), and a quantitative assay for G6PD.

The enzyme content of reticulocytes and other young RBCs is often near normal in G6PD deficiency. Quantitative assays performed shortly after a hemolytic episode may not reflect the deficiency state. Therefore, these studies should be performed at a later time.

Table 27.11 Hemolytic Anemias Characterized by Intravascular Hemolysis.

Microangiopathic and other "traumatic" hemolytic anemias

Certain immunohemolytic anemias
    Transfusion reaction due to ABO isoantibodies
    Paroxysmal cold hemoglobinuria
    Some autoimmune hemolytic anemias

Paroxysmal nocturnal hemoglobinuria

Anemias associated with certain infections, ie, clostridium, malaria

Anemias caused by certain chemical agents
    Acute drug reaction associated with G6PD deficiency
    Snake and spider venoms

Tests to Further Classify Acquired Hemolytic Anemia

Acquired hemolytic anemia (Table 27.9) has many possible causes, which are often separated into two major groups, immune and nonimmune.

Acquired Autoimmune Hemolytic Anemia. Acquired autoimmune hemolytic anemia can be divided into either warm or cold types, as well as into primary or secondary forms. Primary refers to an idiopathic process with no apparent underlying disease, while secondary refers to a hemolytic process appearing in association with an underlying disease such as systemic lupus erythematosus or malignant lymphoma. The laboratory evaluation of the immune hemolytic anemias is detailed in the section on blood bank tests (Chapter 30).

Acquired Nonimmune Hemolytic Anemia. Acquired nonimmune hemolytic anemia results from a variety of physical, chemical, and infectious causes. In these hemolytic anemias there is often a significant degree of intravascular hemolysis (Table 27.11). This is in contrast to most of the hereditary hemolytic disorders, in which RBC destruction occurs extravascularly in macrophages. Hemoglobinemia, hemoglobinuria, and hemosiderinuria distinguish intravascular hemolysis from extravascular hemolysis.

Microangiopathic Hemolytic Anemia and Related Disorders. The cause of hemolysis in microangiopathic hemolytic anemia is traumatic injury to the RBCs as they pass through small vessels that are partially obstructed by fibrin strands. Characteristic fragmented RBCs result from tearing of the RBC membrane by the fibrin strands.

The many diseases associated with microangiopathic hemolytic anemia (Table 27.12) have a common underlying microvasculitis and damaged vascular endothelium; disseminated intravascular coagulation may be present.

RBC fragmentation and thrombocytopenia are the characteristic blood smear findings in microangiopathic hemolysis. Leukocytosis and a leukoerythroblastic reaction are often present. Other abnormal laboratory findings may include increased plasma fibrin degradation products and clotting factor abnormalities. Hemoglobinemia, hemoglobinuria, and hemosiderinuria may be demonstrable. Iron

Table 27.12 Disorders Associated With Microangiopathic Hemolytic Anemia.

Thrombotic thrombocytopenic purpura

Hemolytic uremic syndrome

Metastatic carcinoma (particularly mucin-secreting)

Disseminated intravascular coagulation

Severe hypertension

Eclampsia

Collagen vascular diseases

Giant capillary hemangioma (Kasabach-Merritt syndrome)

Cardiac valve disease and prosthetic valves (macroangiopathic)

---

deficiency may complicate chronic RBC fragmentation disorders, due to excessive iron loss in the urine. Hypochromic RBCs and abnormal iron studies may result.

Hemolytic Anemia Due to Drugs and Chemical Agents. The most common are oxidant agents in patients with G6PD deficiency or in individuals with normal RBCs when given very high doses of oxidant drugs. The findings in these hemolytic disorders were covered in the discussion of the RBC enzymopathies earlier in this chapter.

Several other chemicals may induce hemolysis by a variety of pathophysiological mechanisms. They generally result from accidental exposure and include arsine, lead, copper, and insect venoms.

Infectious Diseases. Infectious diseases that cause hemolytic anemia include malaria, babesiosis, and clostridium sepsis. The mechanism of injury varies from direct invasion of RBCs by the microorganism (as in malaria and babesiosis) to disruption of the RBCs by substances produced by the microorganisms (as in severe clostridial infections). Diagnosis is made by identification of the infectious organisms morphologically or by culture.

Plasma Lipid Abnormalities. Plasma lipid abnormalities, primarily those associated with liver disease, may cause mild to moderate hemolytic disorders. These are generally recognized by the observation of target cells and acanthocytes (spiculated RBCs) on a blood smear. Hemolysis presumably occurs because of deposition of lipids on the RBC membrane that alter the optimal ratio of membrane lipid components.

Splenomegaly. Splenomegaly can affect RBCs through hyperfunction (hypersplenism), splenic pooling (sequestration), and dilution. Hemolytic anemia results from hyperfunction of the spleen (hypersplenism). In effect, RBCs are removed from the circulation by splenic red pulp macrophages. Demonstration of splenic enlargement and RBC sequestration is necessary for diagnosis. Other hereditary and acquired hemolytic anemias must be excluded before attributing an anemia to splenic hyperfunction.

Paroxysmal Nocturnal Hemoglobinuria. Paroxysmal nocturnal hemoglobinuria (PNH) is a rare disorder caused by an acquired membrane defect that renders erythrocytes exquisitely sensitive to complement. The best screening test for this disorder is the sucrose hemolysis test. If this test is positive the diagnosis can be confirmed by the acidified-serum lysis test (Ham test). In both of these tests the hemolysis of PNH erythrocytes occurs by activation of the alternate complement pathway.

References

Henry JB, ed. *Clinical Diagnosis and Management by Laboratory Methods.* 18th ed. Philadelphia, Pa: WB Saunders Co; 1991.

Hillman RS, Finch CA. *Red Cell Manual.* 5th ed. Philadelphia, Pa: FA Davis Co; 1985.

Jandl JH. *Blood, Textbook of Hematology.* Boston, Mass: Little, Brown & Co; 1987.

Koepke JA, ed. *Laboratory Hematology.* New York, NY: Churchill Livingstone Inc; 1984.

Williams WJ, Bentley E, Erslev AJ, Lichtman MA, eds. *Hematology.* 4th ed. New York, NY: McGraw-Hill Inc; 1990.

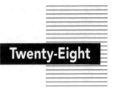

Twenty-Eight

Leukocyte Disorders

Key Points

1. The total leukocyte count and leukocyte differential aid in diagnosis of infectious and inflammatory diseases. Problems with the differential count include unequal distribution of leukocytes on a blood smear, morphological ambiguities, and statistical variation.
2. Neutrophilia is the most common cause of elevated leukocyte counts. Of the many physiological and pathological causes of neutrophilia, bacterial infections are the most common.
3. A blood leukemoid reaction is a marked leukocytosis with immature leukocytes. It is most commonly caused by severe infections and is associated with a marked acceleration of neutrophil production.
4. Neutropenia with counts below 1.0×10^9/L (1000/mm^3) places patients at increased risk of infection.
5. Some common associations include: eosinophilia—allergic diseases, parasitic infections, dermatitis; basophilia—myeloproliferative disorders; and monocytosis—chronic infections, recovery from acute infections, other unrelated disorders.
6. Lymphocytosis is associated with inflammatory reactions, particularly viral infections and chronic bacterial infections. Lymphopenia is associated with immune deficiency states and administration of glucocorticosteroids.
7. Immunophenotyping of blood lymphocytes aids the workup of immunodeficiency diseases and malignant lymphoid neoplasms.
8. Leukemias are diagnosed by morphological examination of bone marrow and blood. Immunophenotyping and cytogenetic studies provide valuable diagnostic and prognostic information.
9. Monoclonal gammopathies, diagnosed by serum and urine protein electrophoresis and immunoelectrophoresis, are associated with plasma cell myeloma and other neoplastic plasma cell and lymphocyte proliferations. Some normal individuals have monoclonal gammopathies of undetermined significance.

Table 28.1 WBC Terminology.

Leukocytosis: increased total blood leukocyte count

Leukopenia: decreased total blood leukocyte count

Granulocytosis: increased granulocytes
  Neutrophilia: neutrophilic leukocytosis
  Eosinophilia: eosinophilic leukocytosis
  Basophilia: basophilic leukocytosis

Granulocytopenia: decreased granulocytes
  Neutropenia: neutrophilic leukopenia
  Eosinopenia: eosinophilic leukopenia
  Basopenia: basophilic leukopenia

Lymphocytosis: increased lymphocytes

Lymphocytopenia: decreased lymphocytes

Monocytosis: increased monocytes

Monocytopenia: decreased monocytes

Pancytopenia: all leukocyte cell lines are decreased

Background

Quantitative studies of the blood's formed elements are commonly ordered laboratory tests. The red blood cell (RBC), white blood cell (WBC), and platelet counts may be performed manually, using a hemacytometer and microscope, but virtually all laboratories in this country employ automated blood cell counters. The total leukocyte count (WBC) quantitates the leukocytes in a blood sample. All five leukocyte types (neutrophil, eosinophil, basophil, lymphocyte, and monocyte) are grouped together. The reference range for the WBC varies with age. In adults, it is 5.0 to 10.0×10^9/L (5000-10,000/mm^3). WBC terminology appears in Table 28.1.

The differential leukocyte count provides additional information. It separates leukocytes into six types (segmented neutrophil, band neutrophil, eosinophil, basophil, lymphocyte, and monocyte) and gives the percent for each (Table 28.2). A medical technologist scans a blood smear and counts WBCs to get the percentages. Some laboratories have automated five-cell differential counters. The WBC, combined with the differential leukocyte count, provides the number and percent distribution of the blood leukocytes. The absolute differential count provides even more precise information about each morphological type. It is obtained by multiplying the percent of each cell type (provided by the differential count) by the total leukocyte count (provided by the WBC).

Some problems exist with the leukocyte differential count. Unequal distribution of leukocytes on a blood smear, ambiguities in recognition of cell types (ie, band vs segmented neutrophil and monocyte vs atypical lymphocyte), and statistical relevance of a differential count based on a 100-cell count are the major problems. These can lead to differential count inaccuracies and should be kept in mind when interpreting results. Therefore, the differential count should be used as a general guideline, always coupled with other clinical and laboratory information. The auto-

Table 28.2 Differential Leukocyte Count Reference Ranges.

	Differential	Absolute Value
Neutrophils, segmented	0.50-0.70 (50%-70%)	2.5-7.0 x 10⁹/L
Neutrophils, band forms	0.02-0.06 (2%-6%)	0.1-0.6 x 10⁹/L
Lymphocytes	0.20-0.40 (20%-40%)	1.0-4.0 x 10⁹/L
Monocytes	0.02-0.08 (2%-8%)	0.1-0.8 x 10⁹/L
Eosinophils	0.01-0.03 (1%-3%)	0.05-0.3 x 10⁹/L
Basophils	0.00-0.01 (0%-1%)	0.00-0.1 x 10⁹/L

mated differential cell counters overcome the statistical problems because they count 10,000 cells; however, they cannot distinguish mature (segmented) from immature (band) neutrophils and so they provide a five-cell differential.

Neutrophils

Neutrophil Kinetics

Neutrophils are present in three body compartments: (1) bone marrow, (2) peripheral blood, and (3) extravascular space of various body tissues.

In the bone marrow, neutrophils exist in two functional groups: the mitotic pool and the storage pool. In the mitotic pool, neutrophil precursors (myeloblast, promyelocyte, and myelocyte) are multiplying and maturing, while in the storage pool there is no mitotic division, only maturation and then storage of mature neutrophils (metamyelocyte, band, and segmented neutrophil). It is estimated that the granulocyte spends 2 to 3 days in the mitotic pool and 5 to 7 days in the storage pool. However, storage can be as short as 48 hours in the presence of infection.

The peripheral blood compartment is divided into the circulating granulocyte pool and the marginal granulocyte pool, where neutrophils are adherent to the wall of capillaries and postcapillary venules. Roughly half of the neutrophils within the blood vessels are in the marginal pool and half are circulating freely with the blood. This means that an absolute blood neutrophil count represents half of the peripheral blood neutrophil compartment. In most clinical situations, however, the measurement of the circulating granulocyte pool reflects the total blood neutrophil kinetics, because the circulating granulocyte pool and marginal granulocyte pool are in a state of dynamic equilibrium. The average neutrophil is present in the vascular compartment for approximately 10 hours before entering the tissues. Once in the tissues, neutrophil survival is approximately 24 hours.

Neutrophils move among the body compartments in one direction—from bone marrow to blood vessels to tissues. Neutrophils leave the blood in response to tissue demand. The migration of neutrophils from the blood is completely random; an "old" neutrophil is just as likely to enter the tissues as a "young" neutrophil.

There are normally far more mature neutrophils with segmented nuclei ("segs") in the blood than neutrophils with band-shaped nuclei ("bands"), because

Table 28.3 Causes of Neutrophilia.

Physiological neutrophilia
  Physical stimuli: temperature extremes, physical exercise, convulsions, cardiac arrhythmias, trauma, labor, vomiting, electric shock, pain
  Emotional stimuli: fear, psychological stress, depression with anxiety, catecholamine and glucocorticosteroid administration
Pathological neutrophilia
  Infections: acute and generalized bacterial, mycotic, parasitic, and viral infections
  Other inflammatory disorders: trauma, infarcts, surgery, necrosis, collagen vascular diseases, hypersensitivity states, and chronic inflammation
  Intoxications
    Metabolic: uremia, diabetic acidosis, thyroid storm, eclampsia, gout
    Chemical: certain drugs, chemicals, and venoms
  Malignant neoplasms: hematopoietic tumors; carcinoma of stomach, lung, uterus, liver, pancreas; brain tumors
  Miscellaneous: hemorrhage, hemolysis, transfusion reactions

segmented neutrophils are released from bone marrow in preference to band forms. When demand for neutrophils is accelerated, the bone marrow storage pool may become exhausted. When this occurs, the marrow increases production of neutrophils to compensate for storage pool loss. This results in the release of band neutrophils and occasionally even less mature forms. The presence of these immature neutrophils in the blood is often referred to as a left shift in the leukocyte differential count.

In addition to an increase in band neutrophils other changes are associated with early bone marrow release, particularly with infections. The neutrophils may contain more and larger granules than normal. This is referred to as toxic granulation. There may be small areas near the cytoplasmic border that are rich in endoplasmic reticulum and devoid of granules. These areas are called Döhle bodies and are recognizable by their light blue color in routinely stained blood smears.

Neutrophilia

A variety of physiological conditions may cause either transient or chronic neutrophilia (Table 28.3). A redistribution of neutrophils from the marginal pool to the circulating pool may be caused by exercise, hypoxia, stress, or the administration of catecholamines. Severe stress, glucocorticosteroid therapy, or injection of endotoxin may cause an influx of neutrophils from the bone marrow storage pool. Chronic glucocorticosteroid therapy can decrease the egress of neutrophils from the blood into the tissues. The overall consequence of these mechanisms is a physiological neutrophilia not involving a response to infection or tissue injury.

Change in the number and distribution of neutrophils as a result of infection and tissue damage constitutes pathological neutrophilia. There is chemotactic attraction of neutrophils to a site of tissue damage as part of the normal inflammatory response. The neutrophils egress from the marginal pool of the blood into the tissues. There is a concurrent shift of neutrophils from the circulating to the marginal pool. Depending on the severity of the inflammation, the bone marrow may release a variable number of neutrophils from the storage pool; neutrophilia may result.

Primarily acute systemic bacterial infection—but also fungal, parasitic, and some viral infections—may lead to neutrophilia. Individual host response and the particular microorganism determine the character and degree of cellular response. For instance, pyogenic bacteria are capable of inducing an intense neutrophilia. Infections due to fungi, rickettsia, or viruses are generally associated with less profound neutrophilia; a relative or absolute neutropenia may even be observed. Children usually respond to bacterial infections with a more profound neutrophilia than do adults. The capacity to mount a neutrophil response may be impaired by host factors that affect neutrophil production, such as folic acid or other deficiency states and underlying diseases that suppress marrow response or directly invade the bone marrow.

Noninfectious inflammatory processes may produce neutrophilia. Thermal burns and other trauma, surgical procedures, myocardial and pulmonary infarcts, extensive tissue necrosis from any cause, collagen vascular diseases, and chronic inflammatory disorders such as rheumatoid arthritis are included. Toxic and metabolic disorders, tissue injury, and neoplastic disease can induce neutrophilia. Neoplasms of the stomach, lung, pancreas, central nervous system, and lymphoid tissue have been known to induce elevated counts. The mechanism of the neutrophilia in neoplastic disease may be bone marrow injury or invasion, tumor necrosis, or host inflammatory response to the malignancy. Malignant diseases, when invasive into bone marrow, can cause uncontrolled overproduction of neutrophils and pronounced neutrophilia. Neutrophilic leukocytosis may be seen in a number of miscellaneous disorders, such as hemorrhage and hemolysis.

Leukemoid Reaction

Leukemoid reaction is a reactive leukocytosis characterized by a marked increase in leukocytes and/or circulating immature leukocytes, resembling the blood picture of leukemia. In some cases of severe infection or tissue damage, the blood neutrophil count may reach levels greater than 40.0×10^9/L (40,000/mm^3). There is increased neutrophil egress from bone marrow to blood to tissues maintained by accelerated bone marrow production of neutrophils. A leukemoid reaction must be distinguished from leukemia. Generally there are fewer immature cells present in a leukemoid reaction, and band forms, toxic granulation, and Döhle bodies are prominent. The patient's presenting signs and symptoms may point to a specific cause that has triggered the leukemoid reaction. In equivocal cases, a bone marrow examination may be necessary to distinguish the two processes.

Several features of leukocyte counts associated with infections are indicative of an unfavorable course of recovery. These are listed in Table 28.4.

Neutropenia

Neutropenia (Table 28.5) is a reduction below normal in the total number of neutrophils in the blood, usually less than 2.0×10^9/L (2000/mm^3). Marked neutropenia is termed agranulocytosis and there may be a depletion of eosinophils and basophils as well. Patients with neutrophil counts lower than 1.0×10^9/L (1000/mm^3) are vulnerable to infection; there is severe risk when the count is lower than 0.5×10^9/L (500/mm^3).

Physiological neutropenia may be caused by a shift of neutrophils from the circulating to the marginal pools, associated with endotoxemia, response to anes-

Table 28.4 Leukocyte Count and Infection.

Unfavorable signs
  Extreme leukocytosis with high percentage of neutrophils
  Failure to develop leukocytosis
  High proportion of immature cells
  Numerous toxic forms
  Marked absolute reduction of lymphocytes

Blood picture during recovery
  Decrease in total leukocyte count and neutrophils
  Decrease in immature forms
  Temporary increase in monocytes
  Increase in eosinophils
  Increase in lymphocytes
  Absence or decrease in toxic forms

thetic agents, and hemodialysis. Pathological neutropenia results from an increased rate of neutrophil destruction or inadequate production. Premature neutrophil destruction may be caused by an enlarged spleen and hyperactivity of the monocyte-macrophage system (hypersplenism) or by immune mechanisms due to antigen-antibody reactions. Drug-related mechanisms, excessive tissue demand for neutrophils (and inadequate marrow compensation) in cases of inflammation, and certain infections are regularly associated with neutropenia, often as a result of marrow suppression. Infections that lead to neutropenia include typhoid and paratyphoid fevers, brucellosis, tularemia, infectious mononucleosis, infectious hepatitis, malaria, yellow fever, measles and other viral infections, and rickettsial diseases. Neutropenia that occurs during the course of an active infection, such as gram-negative bacteremia, pneumococcal pneumonia, or miliary tuberculosis, is usually a poor prognostic sign.

Neutropenia is most often due to defective bone marrow production, either congenital or acquired. Constitutional abnormalities of granulocyte production occurring at or shortly after birth, such as Kostmann's syndrome and Shwachman's syndrome, are rare disorders. Cyclic familial or sporadic neutropenia is manifested by alternating periods of agranulocytosis and improved or normal neutrophil production. Acquired causes of inadequate neutrophil production include drugs, chemical and physical agents that damage the bone marrow, nutritional deficiencies that adversely affect bone marrow production, and diseases associated with a replacement of bone marrow tissue by either tumor cells or inflammatory foci.

Qualitative Genetic Abnormalities of Blood Neutrophils

These abnormalities are rare. They affect leukocyte motility, chemotaxis, phagocytosis, or capacity to kill ingested microorganisms. Chronic granulomatous disease (CGD), resulting in failure of neutrophils and monocytes to generate oxygen-derived radicals upon stimulation, is the most important. This defect can be readily detected by examining the capacity of the patient's stimulated neutrophils to (1) reduce the dye nitroblue tetrazolium or (2) undergo a chemiluminescence reaction that can be measured by a luminometer or ß-liquid scintillation counter. Children with CGD have repeated infections because their neutrophils have defi-

Table 28.5 Causes of Neutropenia.

Decreased bone marrow production
  Familial conditions
  Drug-induced
    Cytotoxic agents: alkylating drugs, DNA depolymerizers, mitotic inhibitors
    Antagonists of DNA synthesis: purine and pyrimidine analogs, phenothiazines, others
    Idiosyncratic: sulfonamides, phenylbutazone, benzene, chloramphenicol, others
  Hematopoietic disorders and myelophthisis
  Cachexia, extreme debilitation, irradiation

Decreased neutrophil survival
  Increased destruction within the circulation: hyperactive monocyte-macrophage system,
    microorganisms, drug-induced, immunologic destruction
  Increased utilization in the tissues: severe inflammations or infections

Production and survival problems
  Megaloblastic anemia, severe bacterial or mycobacterial infections
  Drug-induced: alcohol, aminopyrine, others
  Chronic intoxication: especially with heavy metals

---

cient H_2O_2 and therefore microbial killing is hindered. Catalase-positive microorganisms that break down what little H_2O_2 is present in the neutrophils or microorganisms that do not produce H_2O_2 most frequently cause infection. Staphylococcal, *Serratia*, mycobacteria, and *Candida* infections in the presence of CGD are particularly severe. Thus, one of these tests would be useful to screen infants and children having recurrent infections with these usually nonvirulent microorganisms.

Eosinophils

Eosinophil Kinetics
Eosinophil kinetics are like those of neutrophils, but eosinophil function is not as well understood. It is known that eosinophils play an important role in inflammation. They possess cytolytic properties, especially to helminth larvae, and modify and regulate the IgE-mediated inflammatory process. Eosinophils have an average half-life in the circulation of 3 to 8 hours, and in tissues they are at least 100 times as numerous as in the total circulating component.

Eosinophilia
Eosinophilia is defined as an absolute eosinophil count greater than 0.5×10^9/L (500/mm³). Persistent exposure to a large antigenic load or the presence of chronic inflammation triggers eosinophilia in allergic diseases, certain skin disorders, parasitic infections, neoplastic conditions, and collagen vascular diseases. Disease states associated with persistent eosinophilia, inflammation, and eosinophilic infiltration of various organs have been termed "hypereosinophilic syndromes." In a hospitalized adult patient population, a common cause of an eosinophilia is drug reaction (Table 28.6).

Table 28.6 Conditions Associated With Eosinophilia and Eosinopenia.

Eosinophilia
  Parasitic infestations
  Allergic disorders
  Dermatitis
  Malignant tumors
  Drug reactions
  Hereditary eosinophilia
  Hypereosinophilic syndrome
  Chronic myeloproliferative disorders
Eosinopenia
  Acute severe infections
  Endogenous or exogenous glucocorticoids
  Epinephrine administration
  Prostaglandins

Eosinopenia

Eosinopenia is a decreased absolute blood eosinophil count to less than 0.4×10^9/L (400/mm^3). It is generally associated with increased glucocorticoid and epinephrine secretion, seen acutely with stress or inflammation (Table 28.6).

Basophils

Basophils are the least numerous blood leukocytes. They are similar to tissue mast cells and release histamine in response to antigenic stimulation, particularly related to the reaction of surface-bound IgE with an antigen.

Basophilia

Basophilia is an increase in blood basophils to more than 0.2×10^9/L (200/mm^3). Mild basophilia may be seen in allergic disorders, hypothyroidism, chronic renal failure, chronic hemolytic anemia, and following irradiation or splenectomy. A persistent, substantial basophilia is generally associated with a myeloproliferative disorder such as chronic granulocytic leukemia, myelofibrosis, or polycythemia vera, and, more rarely, acute leukemia (Table 28.7). Basophilia may help differentiate myeloproliferative disorders from leukemoid reaction.

Basopenia

Basopenia is a decrease in basophils to less than 0.01×10^9/L (10/mm^3). The normally low number of blood basophils makes it extremely difficult to identify basopenia (Table 28.7). Basophils, like eosinophils, show diurnal variation, with lowest levels in the morning and highest levels at night.

Monocytes

Monocytes are cells of the mononuclear phagocytic system present in blood. When monocytes leave the blood for the tissues they mature into macrophages

Table 28.7 Conditions Associated With Basophilia and Basopenia.

Basophilia
  Myeloproliferative disorders, especially chronic myeloid leukemia
  Allergic disorders
  Hypothyroidism
  Chronic renal failure
  Following irradiation or splenectomy
Basopenia
  Sustained treatment with glucocorticoids
  Acute stress
  Acute infection
  Hyperthyroidism

or histiocytes, which are characteristically found at sites of inflammation, especially granulomatous inflammation, and within various body fluids. They ingest many different substances and microorganisms, ranging from bacteria and antibody-coated erythrocytes to inorganic compounds like silica.

Monocytosis
Monocytosis is an increase in the absolute blood monocyte count to more than 1.0×10^9/L (1000/mm^3). It is regularly present during the recovery phase of infections (Table 28.8). In tuberculosis, monocytosis is a poor prognostic sign.

Monocytopenia
Monocytopenia may be difficult to diagnose because of the normally low monocyte numbers in some individuals. Circulating monocytes less than 0.2×10^9/L (200/mm^3) is considered monocytopenia. There are rare conditions associated with monocytopenia (Table 28.9).

Lymphocytes

Blood lymphocytes are mononuclear cells derived from lymphoid stem cells. They are the cells driving humoral (B cell) and cell-mediated (T cell) immune

Table 28.8 Causes of Monocytosis.

Hematologic diseases: chronic neutropenia, hemolytic anemia, postsplenectomy state, hematologic malignancies

Collagen vascular diseases

Infections: tuberculosis, syphilis, subacute bacterial endocarditis, brucellosis, Rocky Mountain spotted fever, malaria, kala-azar

Recovery phase of common bacterial infections

Gastrointestinal disorders: inflammatory bowel disease, sprue

Miscellaneous: carbon tetrachloride poisoning, sarcoidosis, Gaucher's disease, cirrhosis

Table 28.9 Conditions Associated With Monocytopenia.

Aplastic anemia

Glucocorticoid therapy (transient)

Hairy cell leukemia

functions. Lymphocyte morphology spans a spectrum of size, nuclear, and cytoplasmic characteristics.

Lymphocytosis

The absolute lymphocyte count varies widely with age. Lymphocytosis exists when the absolute lymphocyte count is higher than 9.0×10^9/L (9000/mm^3) in a child and higher than 4.0×10^9/L (4000/mm^3) in an adult. A relative lymphocytosis accompanies most cases of neutropenia. Acute viral infections, chronic bacterial infections, the recovery phase of bacterial infections, and, rarely, hyperthyroidism are associated with increased numbers of lymphocytes (Table 28.10). Reactive or "atypical" lymphocytes in the peripheral blood are associated with infectious mononucleosis (Epstein-Barr virus) and other viral infections. Malignant lymphocytosis is associated with lymphocytic leukemia and malignant lymphoma.

Lymphocytopenia

Lymphocytopenia exists when the absolute lymphocyte count is lower than 1.5×10^9/L (1500/mm^3) in adults or lower than 3.0×10^9/L (3000/mm^3) in children. It is associated with rare congenital immunodeficiency disorders (Table 28.11). It may be generalized, with a reduction in all subsets of lymphocytes, or selective to certain types with a normal or only slightly reduced total lymphocyte count. Human immunodeficiency virus (HIV) infection with the resulting acquired immunodeficiency syndrome (AIDS) is a major clinical cause of lymphocytopenia. T helper lymphocytes are initially selectively reduced. A generalized lymphocytopenia may ensue later in the course of the illness.

Table 28.10 Causes of Lymphocytosis.

Physiological
  Recovery phase of acute infections

Infectious disease
  Acute bacterial: pertussis, brucellosis
  Viral exanthems: measles, varicella, mumps, rubella, roseola
  Other viral infections: infectious mononucleosis, cytomegalovirus infection, infectious hepatitis, herpetic infections
  Chronic infections: tuberculosis, syphilis, fungal infections, toxoplasmosis

Neoplastic disease: lymphocytic leukemia, lymphoma

Miscellaneous: stress, adrenocortical insufficiency, irradiation, drug reactions

Table 28.11 Causes of Lymphocytopenia.

Congenital immunodeficiency states

Acquired immunodeficiency syndrome (AIDS)

Administration of glucocorticoids and chemotherapeutic drugs

Irradiation

Advanced Hodgkin's disease and other malignancies

Lymphocyte Immunophenotyping

There are two major groups of lymphocytes, T cells and B cells, and several functional types of each. These can be categorized by their immune function and/or degree of maturation. Specific surface antigens or combinations thereof may be associated with or restricted to one lymphocyte type. Surface antigens can be identified by immunophenotyping methods: flow cytometry, immunofluorescence microscopy, and enzyme immunocytochemistry. Numerous monoclonal antibodies (MoAb) have been developed that react with specific lymphocyte surface antigens. By using a panel of MoAb with different antigen specificities, detailed characterization of lymphocyte populations can be accomplished. Table 28.12 shows general characteristics of the major types of T and B cells (further maturational and functional types of lymphocytes are not included in this table).

Immunophenotyping of lymphocytes is important in the characterization of congenital and acquired immunodeficiency diseases (including AIDS), immunoregulatory disorders, and reactive and malignant lymphoid diseases.

Table 28.12 Surface Marker Characteristics of T and B Lymphocytes.

	sIg	cIg	Pan B Cell Antigens	Pan T Cell Antigens	TdT Activity
T Lymphocytes					
Immature T cells	−	−	−	+	+
Blood helper T cells	−	−	−	+ (also have T helper antigens)	−
Blood suppressor/ cytotoxic T cells	−	−	−	+ (also have T suppressor antigens)	−
B Lymphocytes					
Immature B cells	−	± (μ chains only)	+	−	+
Mature blood B cells	+	−	+	−	−
Plasma cells	−	+	+	−	−

sIg = surface immunoglobulin; cIg = cytoplasmic immunoglobulin; TdT = terminal deoxynucleotidyl transferase

Table 28.13 Aids to Diagnosing/Classifying Leukemia.

Morphological examination of blood and bone marrow

Cytochemical studies on leukemic blasts

Immunophenotyping of the leukemic cells

Cytogenetic studies of the leukemic cells

In immunodeficiency diseases, one or more functional lymphocyte types may be altered or decreased. Identification of the specific deficiency may establish the diagnosis and guide management of the patient. Patients infected with HIV are often followed by periodic assessment of the absolute helper T lymphocyte count in the blood. As the level of helper T cells decreases, patients are at increasing risk for infectious complications and the onset of AIDS. The helper T cell count may also serve as an indicator to begin prophylactic therapies. The immunophenotyping of leukemias and lymphomas, particularly acute lymphoblastic leukemias, is important in establishing the diagnosis and assessing prognosis.

Leukemias

Leukemia is an acute or chronic neoplastic proliferation of hematopoietic cells involving the bone marrow and blood. The proliferative leukemic cells are of myeloid (granulocytic) or lymphocytic lineage. The four major leukemia categories are acute or chronic myeloid (granulocytic) and acute or chronic lymphocytic leukemia. There are variants or classes for each of these four categories, based on specific morphological, immunologic, or cytogenetic characteristics of the leukemic cells.

In acute leukemias, cell proliferation consists of early precursors of one or more types of leukocyte. Myeloblasts are generally the predominant cell in acute myeloid leukemias and lymphoblasts in acute lymphocytic leukemias. Acute leukemias are aggressive malignant neoplasms that progress rapidly, leading to death in a short time if untreated.

The cell proliferation in chronic leukemias consists of mature and maturing granulocytes or lymphocytes. Blast cells are absent or are a minority population. The onset of chronic leukemias is insidious and the clinical course often prolonged. In many cases, particularly with chronic lymphocytic leukemia, there is long survival even without treatment.

The diagnosis of leukemia is often made or suspected on the basis of a peripheral blood smear examination performed because of an abnormal complete blood count. The blood counts manifest a spectrum of abnormalities. The leukocyte count is usually elevated due to the circulating leukemic cells. The normal blood cell elements are usually decreased in acute leukemia because normal hematopoiesis is suppressed. In some cases of acute leukemia there are few or no leukemic blasts in the blood even though the bone marrow is heavily infiltrated. In chronic leukemia the leukocyte count is nearly always elevated, often markedly so, but the other blood counts may be normal.

Table 28.14 Distinction of Chronic Myeloid Leukemia and Leukemoid Reactions.

Chronic Myeloid Leukemia	Leukemoid Reaction
Higher leukocyte count (usually > 50 x 10⁹/L)	Lower leukocyte count (usually < 50 x 10⁹/L)
Morphology	Morphology
More immature forms (including myeloblasts)	Fewer immature forms (myeloblasts rare)
Lack toxic changes in neutrophils	Toxic changes (toxic granulation, Döhle's bodies) often present
Basophilia	Lack basophilia
Other Studies	Other Studies
Decreased neutrophil alkaline phosphatase	Normal or elevated neutrophil alkaline phosphatase
Bone marrow cytogenetic abnormality (eg, Philadelphia chromosome)	Normal bone marrow cytogenetics

Expertise in identifying morphological features of the various types of leukemia is essential for diagnosis (Table 28.13). Occasionally, a leukemoid reaction must be distinguished from leukemia (Table 28.14). This may be particularly problematic when chronic myeloid (granulocytic) leukemia is a considered diagnosis.

Laboratory Evaluation of Monoclonal Gammopathies

A gammopathy, or hypergammaglobulinemia, is the presence of an increased concentration of serum or urine gamma globulin, and it often requires further laboratory evaluation. Hypergammaglobulinemia may be polyclonal or monoclonal. A polyclonal gammopathy is a simultaneous increase of several immunoglobulin classes that differ from one another by immunoglobulin heavy and light chain type and antigen specificity. Polyclonal immunoglobulins are the products of many different clones of immunoglobulin-producing cells (plasma cells). The expansion of these clones and their immunoglobulin production is usually due to antigenic stimulation. This process is a feature of the inflammatory response, and may accompany a variety of infections and inflammatory disorders.

A monoclonal gammopathy is an increase of one specific class (or fragment) of the immunoglobulin molecule. The monoclonal immunoglobulin (or "M" component) is produced by a clone of plasma cells from a single precursor plasma cell. Monoclonal gammopathies are found in plasma cell neoplasms (eg, plasma cell myeloma), certain lymphoproliferative disorders, primary amyloidosis, occasionally in patients with carcinoma or other disorders, and as monoclonal gammopathies of undetermined significance. The distinction between polyclonal and monoclonal gammopathies is facilitated by serum protein electrophoresis (Figure 28.1).

Although serum protein electrophoresis is an important initial laboratory procedure for identification of a monoclonal gammopathy, further evaluation should be done with a serum protein immunoelectrophoresis and immunoglobulin quantitation. Immunoelectrophoresis provides immunologic identification of a monoclonal gammopathy by heavy and light chain types. However, the presence

Figure 28.1 Serum Protein Electrophoresis Patterns.

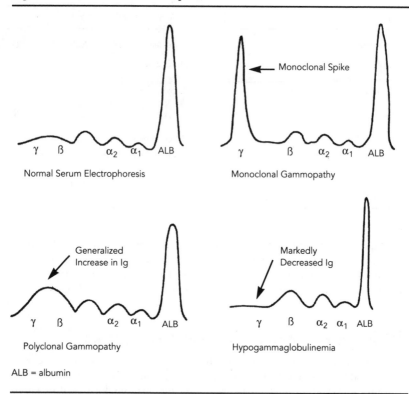

Monoclonal Spike

γ   ß   α₂   α₁   ALB
Normal Serum Electrophoresis

γ   ß   α₂   α₁   ALB
Monoclonal Gammopathy

Generalized
Increase in Ig

γ   ß   α₂   α₁   ALB
Polyclonal Gammopathy

Markedly
Decreased Ig

γ   ß   α₂   α₁   ALB
Hypogammaglobulinemia

ALB = albumin

of a heavy chain and a light chain does not insure that the immunoglobulin molecule is intact, and in some cases a monoclonal gammopathy may be present in amounts below the sensitivity of immunoelectrophoresis.

Monoclonal immunoglobulin light chains found in the urine in many cases of plasma cell myeloma are referred to as Bence Jones protein. The multiple reagent strips for urinalysis (dipsticks) are unsuited for detecting Bence Jones protein. Precipitation methods (eg, toluenesulfonic acid) are good screening tests but the best test for detecting Bence Jones proteinuria is urine protein electrophoresis. Bence Jones protein should be further characterized by urine protein immunoelectrophoresis. In some cases these urine light chains are the only identifiable monoclonal protein. This is true in approximately 15% of plasma cell myelomas. Immunoelectrophoresis of concentrated urine specimens and 24-hour quantitation of urinary light chains is often necessary in cases of suspected plasma cell myeloma.

References

Henry JB, ed. *Clinical Diagnosis and Management by Laboratory Methods*. 18th ed. Philadephia, Pa: WB Saunders Co; 1991.

Jandl JH. *Blood, Textbook of Hematology.* Boston, Mass: Little, Brown & Co; 1987.

Koepke JA, ed. *Laboratory Hematology.* New York, NY: Churchill Livingstone Inc; 1984.

Williams WJ, Bentley E, Erslev AJ, Lichtman MA, eds. *Hematology.* 4th ed. New York, NY: McGraw-Hill Inc; 1990.

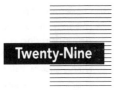

Twenty-Nine

Hemostasis

Key Points

1. A complete medical history and physical examination are the most important aspects of the assessment (evaluation) of a patient with a bleeding disorder.
2. The laboratory screening tests of the coagulation system include the prothrombin time (PT) and the partial thromboplastin time (PTT), which evaluate the integrity of the intrinsic (PT) and extrinsic (PTT) systems. Most congenital bleeding disorders (factor VIII and IX deficiency) prolong the PTT.
3. The most frequent inherited disorder of primary hemostasis is von Willebrand disease (vWD). Abnormalities of von Willebrand factor (vWF) cause impaired platelet adhesion, leading to petechiae and mucosal bleeding.
4. Acquired abnormalities of hemostasis that cause bleeding problems are more frequent than inherited disorders. Underlying diseases and drug therapy must be considered as causes when bleeding problems occur.
5. Inhibitors of individual coagulation factors are usually specific antibodies, which develop primarily in hemophiliacs requiring frequent replacement therapy. Approximately 10% of patients with hemophilia develop these inhibitors.
6. The lupus anticoagulant is an inhibitor that causes prolonged PTT in vitro. This is caused by phospholipid antibodies that neutralize the PTT reagent; however, there are no actual bleeding disorders associated with the lupus anticoagulant.
7. Several endogenous pathways function to limit the hemostatic response, and defects in any of those pathways can predispose individuals to thrombosis. These pathways include (a) ATIII and the enzyme inhibitors, (b) the protein C/protein S pathway, and (c) the fibrinolytic system.

8. Disseminated intravascular coagulation (DIC) is a syndrome caused by the inappropriate activation of the coagulation and fibrinolytic systems. An underlying disorder (eg, infection, malignancy) is always present.
9. Anticoagulant therapy is used for prophylaxis and treatment of vascular thromboembolic disorders. PTT assays are used to monitor heparin therapy; PT assay monitors oral anticoagulant therapy.
10. Fibrinolytic therapy is used to treat arterial and venous thrombosis. The exogenous plasminogen activators used for this purpose can induce a bleeding risk due to excess plasmin activity.

Background

Hemostasis results from the combined actions of vessel walls, coagulation proteins, and platelets to limit hemorrhage following vascular injury. When a blood vessel is injured, rapid vasoconstriction helps reduce blood flow and limit blood loss. Blood and plasma released locally into extravascular spaces increase tissue pressure and further contribute to vessel collapse. Rapid adherence of circulating platelets to exposed subendothelial connective tissue structures (eg, collagen) provides a scaffold for subsequent protein-mediated coagulant events and also stimulates platelet aggregation. Once the coagulation cascade has been localized by platelet phospholipid structures to the site of vascular injury, fibrin generation stabilizes the platelet plug and thus arrests hemorrhage. This platelet plug formation is known as primary hemostasis. Growth factors and other soluble mediators complete the repair process by stimulating cell growth in the vessel wall and endothelium at the injury site. The final step is platelet-fibrin thrombus dissolution and restoration of blood flow.

Many hemostatic disorders result in bleeding or thrombosis, requiring systematic evaluation to determine etiology. For example, spontaneous hemorrhage at an early age usually signifies a congenital problem, either a decrease or absence of a clotting factor or dysfunction due to clotting protein structural abnormalities. Bleeding disorders associated with platelet abnormalities may present as mucous membrane or postoperative hemorrhage. Bleeding due to intrinsic structural defects of blood vessels can present as purpura or as connective tissue disorders. Thrombotic episodes occur when pathways that down-regulate coagulation fail to limit the hemostatic mechanism.

The hemostatic disorders that result in bleeding or thrombosis are numerous and complex. Hemostasis regulation, including the coagulation cascade, will be discussed first, followed by clinical evaluation of the bleeding patient, inherited and acquired bleeding disorders, and the anticoagulation/fibrinolytic systems, including DIC and hypercoagulable states.

Coagulation and the Bleeding Patient

Secondary hemostasis initiates the physiological process of coagulation. This sequential and simultaneous cascade of events, preceded by platelet adhesion and aggregation, comprises a highly regulated set of interactions among the various plasma clotting factors (proteins), phospholipids (platelet factor 3) and calcium ions, ultimately resulting in conversion of the zymogen prothrombin to active protease thrombin. Thrombin catalyzes the conversion of fibrinogen, a soluble plasma protein, to fibrin, which undergoes spontaneous polymerization into the fibrin gel of a clot.

The coagulation proteins fall into three functional categories: enzymes-proenzymes (vitamin K–dependent serine proteases and a transpeptidase), cofactor proteins (Va, VIIIa, high-molecular-weight kininogen [HMWK], tissue factor), and fibrinogen, the structural protein necessary for clot formation. The individual clotting factors are represented by Roman numerals. The activated forms, which usually require limited, specific proteolysis, are represented with an additional lower case "a" following the individual factor numeral. Calcium ions are occasionally represented as factor IV. No factor has been designated as factor VI.

These coagulation factors require an appropriate stimulus to trigger activation. Two activating mechanisms are described, the intrinsic and extrinsic pathways. These are illustrated in Figure 29.1. The intrinsic pathway is assessed in the laboratory by the PTT and the extrinsic pathway by the PT.

The relative importance of each activation pathway in vivo is uncertain. Because patients with defects in the contact activation pathway of the intrinsic system rarely bleed, their deficiencies do not necessarily imply a bleeding tendency. More important in achieving hemostasis may be activation via the extrinsic system. The interaction of tissue factor and factor VII, resulting in factor VIIa activity, may be the important step in vivo. Also important is the in vivo activation of factor IX by VIIa–tissue factor. This interaction is the predominant mechanism of IX activation in vivo, while the in vitro activation of X by VIIa–tissue factor results from the high concentrations of tissue factor (thromboplastin) present in PT reagents. These findings would explain the absence of clinical bleeding with certain contact factor deficiencies but the presence of bleeding with factor VIII and IX deficiencies, since VIIa–tissue factor is a poor in vivo activator of factor X. Minor vascular injury with endothelial damage and collagen exposure may activate the intrinsic pathway, but in most cases primary hemostasis would probably be sufficient to prevent significant hemorrhage. Factor deficiencies of the intrinsic system or common pathway result in a prolonged PTT, where extrinsic pathway defects are identified by a prolonged PT. Patients with a prolonged PT and PTT should be evaluated for a defect in the common pathway or multiple defects.

Clinical Evaluation of the Bleeding Patient

Medical history and clinical features often identify the nature of a bleeding disorder and the laboratory findings may serve only to confirm the clinical impression. When the clinical findings are not specific the laboratory evaluation is more essential to the diagnosis. In all cases of bleeding disorders test ordering should be selective and based on the historical and clinical findings. This approach will allow a diagnosis to be made as quickly as possible at the lowest cost and expedite initiation of the appropriate therapy. The clinical assessment of a bleeding patient should identify the following:

Type of Bleeding. This is of critical importance. Small, pinpoint petechiae are characteristic of bleeding due to platelet defects, whereas ecchymoses and deep

Figure 29.1 Coagulation Cascade.

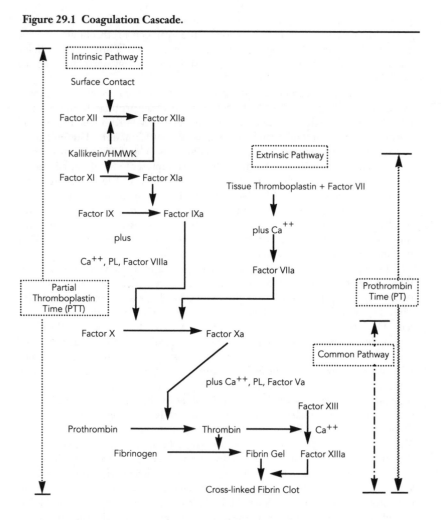

"a" denotes activated factor; HMWK = high-molecular-weight kininogen; PL = phospholipid, platelet factor 3

tissue hemorrhage are usually seen with plasma protein coagulation disorders. Diffuse oozing from multiple puncture sites can be seen with circulating inhibitors to clotting factors or in DIC.

Course of Bleeding. The date of bleeding onset, patient age, and outcome of previous episodes are important. Inquiries should be made about specific hemostatic challenges such as circumcision, dental extractions, menstrual history, trauma, and surgical procedures, as well as about previous transfusions and their indications. In the absence of previous hemostatic challenges the history may be indeterminate, but not necessarily negative.

Family History. With a positive family history for bleeding, emphasis should be placed on establishing an inheritance pattern by evaluating affected individuals in the family.

Previous or Current Therapy. Several prescribed and over-the-counter drugs can affect hemostasis. It is not unusual to perform an extensive hemostatic evaluation before learning that a patient is taking a drug with anticoagulant properties.

Associated Diseases. Many systemic diseases result in hemostatic defects by a variety of mechanisms, particularly uremia, hepatic disease, infections, and malignant neoplasms.

Other Physical Findings. Physical findings that might be important in diagnosis and etiology of a bleeding disorder include hepatomegaly and signs of hepatic failure, splenomegaly, lymphadenopathy, occult gastrointestinal blood loss, infection, and signs of uremia.

General Laboratory Evaluation of the Bleeding Patient

Laboratory tests should be selectively ordered in accordance with the type of bleeding and the patient's history. Initial evaluation should provide clues regarding the origin of the bleeding, eg, vascular, platelet, or coagulation. Because intrinsic vessel wall defects are not reflected in abnormalities of circulating blood, they cannot be directly diagnosed by laboratory evaluation. Specific diagnoses of platelet and coagulation disorders, however, can be assessed in the laboratory.

Platelets. Platelets are small fragments of membrane-enclosed cytoplasm derived from bone marrow megakaryocytes. Platelets are the major contributors to primary hemostasis. They may be quantitatively or qualitatively abnormal due to either congenital or acquired disorders. Bleeding due to platelet defects is manifested as epistaxis, gingival bleeding, and petechiae. Other types of bleeding, such as gastrointestinal, uterine, and intracranial, may occur but are not distinctive of platelet disorders. The two baseline tests used to assess primary hemostasis are the platelet count (for quantitative defects) and the bleeding time (for qualitative defects).

Platelet Counts. Platelet counts are determined on anticoagulated blood samples using a hemocytometer or an electronic particle counter. The platelet reference range is 150 to 450×10^9/L ($150\text{-}450\times10^3$/mm^3). Microscopic inspection of a peripheral smear is necessary to confirm platelet counts outside this range. Thrombocytopenia is the most common cause of serious bleeding. Platelet counts less than 50×10^9/L (50×10^3/mm^3) are considered severe thrombocytopenia. Patients with counts less than 20×10^9/L (20×10^3/mm^3) are at serious risk to develop spontaneous bleeding.

The coefficient of variation is approximately 30% for manual platelet counts and 10% with automated electronic particle counters. These variation values are important because day-to-day changes in a patient's platelet count outside these values are clinically significant, while changes within the coefficient of variation could represent inherent laboratory test performance variation.

Bleeding Time. The bleeding time is an in vivo assessment of platelet response to limited vascular injury and is reflective of the integrity of the primary hemostatic mechanism. Clinically significant platelet defects cause a prolonged bleeding time. The bleeding time is performed with a sphygmomanometer placed on the upper arm and inflated to 40 mm Hg pressure. A site for puncture on the volar surface of the forearm, free of superficial veins, scar tissue, and edema, is chosen then cleansed and dried. A uniform puncture wound is produced by using a disposable sterile blade. Time is recorded with a stopwatch beginning with the incision and ending with cessation of bleeding from the incision site. The reference range for bleeding time is 2 to 9 minutes. The test is prolonged with thrombocytopenia, qualitative platelet disorders, vWD, fibrinolytic states, afibrinogenemia, vasculitis, and aspirin therapy. No disorders resulting in shortened bleeding times have been identified. The bleeding time can be affected by individual technique and interpretation. There can be significant variation in bleeding time results when the test is performed on the same patient by different technicians.

Prothrombin Time and Partial Thromboplastin Time. These are important studies for evaluation of the coagulation aspect of hemostasis. The principles of these tests were discussed above.

Specialized laboratory evaluation for specific disorders of patients with abnormal screening tests should be performed by ordering specific tests based on the screening results and clinical findings. Suspected qualitative platelet abnormalities, when a patient has a prolonged bleeding time with a normal platelet count and morphology, should be evaluated by platelet aggregation studies, which detect various abnormalities based on the patterns of platelet aggregation responses to different agonists. Specific diagnoses such as vWD, Glanzmann's thrombasthenia, Bernard-Soulier syndrome, aspirin effect, granulocyte storage pool defects, and other rare disorders can be made.

Evaluation for blood coagulation disorders when an abnormality of the PT, PTT, or both is identified can be assessed by specific factor assays. Various mixing tests using patient plasma, normal plasma, and factor-deficient plasmas, can accurately assess the defect or defects as being factor deficiencies or factor inhibitors. Using various dilutions of the patient and reference plasmas, specific factor assays can be performed that measure the percentage of factor activity in a factor-deficient patient's plasma.

Bleeding Disorders: Clinical Features, Pathophysiology, and Diagnosis

Clotting factor deficiencies are inherited or acquired, the latter being more frequent. Hereditary deficiencies usually involve a single factor; acquired defects often involve more than one factor. The congenital deficiencies with autosomal inheritance patterns are rare, except for vWD. X-Linked disorders are characterized by synthesis of a defective protein or failure to synthesize the factor in detectable quantities. These types of disorders include afibrinogenemia, hypofibrinogenemia, and dysfibrinogenemia, as well as deficiencies of prothrombin, factor V (accelerator globulin), factor VII (proconvertin), factor X (Stuart-Prower deficiency), factor XI (hemophilia C), factor XII (Hageman trait), prekallikrein (Fletcher factor), high-molecular-weight kininogen (Williams-Fitzgerald-Flaujeac factor), and factor XIII (fibrin-stabilizing factor). The two most frequent causes of hereditary bleeding disorders, hemophilia A (factor VIII deficiency) and hemophilia B (factor IX deficiency), are both inherited as sex-linked recessive traits.

Factor VIII Deficiency

Factor VIII deficiency (hemophilia A) is the most common hereditary coagulopathy associated with serious bleeding, with approximately 1 in 10,000 individuals affected. With rare exception, hemophilia A is a disease of males and accounts for 80% to 85% of cases of hemophilia. Sons of affected males will be normal and their daughters will be obligate carriers of the trait. Because of the high mutation rate for this disease, one third of patients with hemophilia A have no family history of the disorder. Female carriers of the hemophilia A trait would be expected to have factor VIII levels of approximately 50%. However, the highly variable normal range of factor VIII levels in unaffected populations makes factor assay detection of carriers extremely inaccurate. Analysis of factor VIII defects is further complicated by the complexity of the molecule's circulating structure. The procoagulant activity of factor VIII, synthesized in the liver, circulates in plasma bound to vWF, which is synthesized and released from endothelial cells. The procoagulant, antihemophiliac component of factor VIII is decreased to absent in hemophilia A.

With appropriate assay techniques, the frequency and severity of bleeding problems in hemophilia A may be predicted from the plasma factor VIII level. Individuals with less than 1% activity (normal, 50%-200%) are classified as severe hemophiliacs and require intravenous factor VIII concentrate therapy two to four times a month. Factor VIII concentrates are prepared by affinity chromatography techniques from large volumes of pooled human plasma. The half-life of infused factor VIII, in the absence of inhibitors, is 8 to 12 hours. Individuals with greater than 5% activity, classified as mild hemophiliacs, usually hemorrhage in association with trauma or surgery. Individuals with factor VIII levels between 1% and 5% are considered moderately severe and have a variable clinical picture. The clinical hallmarks of classic hemophilia are (1) the lack of excessive hemorrhage from superficial cuts and abrasions, (2) spontaneous muscle and joint bleeding that may be difficult to control and is associated with severe morbidity, (3) easy bruising, and (4) severe postoperative bleeding. Hemarthroses most frequently involve the knees and elbows with lesser involvement of ankles, shoulders, hips, and wrists. Other sites of hemorrhage include the gastrointestinal tract, urinary tract (hematuria), soft tissue of the neck, and, rarely, epistaxis and gingival bleeding.

The diagnosis of hemophilia can be strongly suspected by the patient's history and physical findings. A prolonged PTT with a normal platelet count, bleeding time, and PT suggests a defect in the intrinsic system. Diagnosis is made by performing specific factor assays using mixing tests. Factor VIII levels are reliable predictors of bleeding problems in patients with hemophilia A. Complicating the laboratory evaluation is the fact that approximately 8% of patients with hemophilia A acquire specific antibodies that neutralize or inhibit factor VIII. This problem is more common in severe hemophilia.

Factor IX Deficiency

Factor IX deficiency (hemophilia B) is less common than classic hemophilia, with an incidence of 1 in 75,000 to 80,000 in the general population. Factor IX is a vitamin K–dependent zymogen that can be activated by factor XIa or the tissue-factor VIIa complex. It is required for in vivo hemostasis. Some patients have decreased levels of normal factor IX while others synthesize an abnormal, dysfunctional factor IX molecule. Approximately 10% of hemophilia B patients have material in their plasma that cross-reacts with factor IX antibodies while the other 90% have markedly reduced or undetectable levels. Spontaneous mutations causing hemophilia B may represent up to 30% of all cases. The disease presents with the same clinical features and inheritance pattern as hemophilia A. The severity of bleeding is related to the level of plasma factor IX procoagulant activity. Patients with hemophilia B usually have a prolonged PTT and normal PT.

Using mixing studies, the specific defect in hemophilia B can be determined and activity levels assayed. Identification of female carriers by activity assays is even less certain than in hemophilia A. Seven to ten percent of patients with hemophilia B who have received multiple transfusions develop antibody inhibitors to factor IX. Nearly all patients with severe (<1%) or moderate (1%-5%) hemophilia B need replacement therapy on a regular basis. The in vivo half-life of factor IX is 18 to 40 hours. Replacement therapy is provided by factor IX concentrates prepared by adsorption chromatography. Infectious complications associated with plasma factor VIII and IX concentrates include hepatitis, acquired immunodeficiency syndrome (AIDS), and other viral infections. Serious thrombotic complications can result from activated factors present in factor IX concentrates.

von Willebrand Disease

vWD results in bleeding problems due to abnormalities of vWF. Plasma vWF is a large multimeric glycoprotein synthesized and released into the circulation by endothelial cells. Megakaryocytes also synthesize vWF. vWF has no known enzymatic activity but is essential for normal platelet function. vWF performs its hemostatic function through several binding interactions with subendothelial structures and platelet surface glycoprotein receptors. Platelet glycoprotein Ib mediates adhesion of resting platelets to vWF bound to subendothelial connective tissue and the same receptor mediates the in vitro platelet aggregation response induced by ristocetin. After platelet activation a second platelet glycoprotein receptor, GPIIb/IIIa, is exposed on the surface and mediates aggregation through interaction with fibrinogen and possibly vWF. Collagen appears to best support vWF-mediated platelet adhesion, although other macromolecules may be important. During its synthesis, vWF is assembled into high-molecular-weight multimers, which are released constitutively or stored in the endothelium before being released into the circulation. In addition to its function in platelet aggregation/adhesion, vWF stabilizes plasma factor VIII.

The complexity of vWF is reflected in the clinical heterogeneity of vWD. Bleeding problems in vWD are associated with defects in platelet hemostatic function. With severe vWF defects, clinical problems of bleeding due to low factor VIII levels may also be present. In general, enough vWF is present to prevent the deep tissue bleeding and hemarthroses seen in hemophilia. In usual cases of vWD, bruising and bleeding in the skin, mucous membranes, and nasal passages are observed. Menorrhagia commonly occurs and postpartum hemorrhage may be severe. The number and severity of bleeding episodes generally decrease with age.

The laboratory evaluation of bleeding patients with vWD depends on the type of vWF defect. All types usually have a normal to decreased platelet count, normal platelet morphology, and a prolonged bleeding time. Laboratory findings for the variants of vWD are shown in Table 29.1. Type I vWD is characterized by a concordant reduction of factor VIII and ristoceten cofactor activities, reduced vWF antigen level, and a normal vWF multimer pattern. The inheritance pattern of this disorder is autosomal-dominant and the clinical symptoms are moderate to severe. The patient's platelet-rich plasma shows reduced ristocetin-induced platelet aggregation. The response to desmopressin (DDAVP) during bleeding episodes is usually good. Type II vWD is characterized by a more significant reduction of ristocetin cofactor activity compared with factor VIII activity and vWF antigen level. Several subgroups have been described based on multimer analysis. Most type II disorders show an autosomal-dominant inheritance pattern. In general, examination of plasma vWF multimers in patients with type II vWD shows a loss of the highest molecular-weight multimers. In addition, type II patients may show structural abnormalities of the monomers that form the multimeric polymers (type IIA). Type IIB patients also show a decrease of the highest molecular-weight multimers in their plasma, but most characteristically their platelet-rich plasma aggregates at much lower levels of ristocetin than normal. Patients with type IIB disease show inheritance as an autosomal-dominant trait and have moderate to severe bleeding problems, increased bleeding times, and occasionally manifest mild thrombocytopenia. The structural abnormality of vWF in these type IIB patients is thought to cause increased interactions with resting platelets and thereby result in their selective depletion in plasma. In response to DDAVP, these patients may develop a severe thrombocytopenia due to intravascular platelet aggregation.

Other type II disorders, all showing abnormalities in vWF multimer patterns, are rare and inherited in an autosomal-recessive pattern. Type III vWD patients have nearly undetectable amounts of vWF in their plasma, platelets, and endothelial cells. Low levels of factor VIII can be found. Consanguinity is frequent in patients with type III vWD. Patients with this disorder have a poor response to DDAVP and often develop anti-vWF antibodies after therapy with plasma or cryoprecipitate. The clinical symptoms are severe, the bleeding time is prolonged, and their plasma shows no platelet aggregation response to ristocetin.

Another disorder that can present as vWD clinically is called platelet-type vWD or pseudo-vWD. Patients with this disorder produce normal quantities of vWF, which bind to platelets at very low ristocetin concentrations to cause aggregation. In vivo, variable degrees of thrombocytopenia can be seen. Diagnostically, pseudo-vWD may resemble the type IIB disorder. The origin is

Table 29.1 Laboratory Findings in von Willebrand Disease (vWD).

Types of vWD	Clinical Symptoms	Platelet Count	Bleeding Time	Factor VIII Activity
I	Mild to moderate	Normal	Prolonged	Decreased or normal
IIA*	Moderate to severe	Normal	Prolonged	Normal
IIB*	Moderate to severe	Normal or decreased	Prolonged	Normal or slightly decreased
III†	Severe	Normal	Prolonged	Decreased

vWF = von Willebrand factor; DDAVP = desmopressin
* There are several other type II vWD variants that have been described in individual families, eg, II C, D, E, F, G, and H, and that vary in some minor repects from vWD II A and B.
† Type III vWD is considered type IS (severe) by some sources.

an abnormality of the platelet glycoprotein Ib receptor, which causes increased binding of vWF.

Acquired vWD can be seen in patients with immune-inflammatory disorders. These patients are usually older than 40 years and develop hemorrhage of their mucous membranes. Bleeding time is prolonged and multimer pattern abnormalities of vWF are nonspecific. Ristocetin cofactor activity may be reduced to 10% to 20% of normal. The mechanism of this disorder in some patients results from antibodies that neutralize ristocetin cofactor activity. Patients treated with steroids have shown improvement in some cases. Patients with acquired vWD associated with neoplasms (eg, lymphoma, Wilms' tumor) have shown improvement of their bleeding problems after therapy. Bleeding due to acquired vWD and/or qualitative platelet defects has also been described in patients with myeloproliferative disorders.

Acquired Bleeding Disorders

Acquired bleeding disorders are much more frequently encountered than congenital bleeding disorders. They include problems associated with acquired inhibitors to clotting factors, abnormalities of vitamin K activity, iatrogenic causes (particularly drugs), platelet disorders associated with various disease states, and consumptive processes involving platelets and coagulation factors.

Vitamin K is a fat-soluble compound that functions as a cofactor in a liver carboxylase system. It is necessary for the normal synthesis of several clotting factors as well as protein C and protein S. In the absence of vitamin K activity, bleeding problems can result. Numerous factors can induce vitamin K deficiency. In newborns, a transient clotting deficiency state can develop due to inadequate dietary intake of vitamin K (hemorrhagic disease of the newborn). Dietary deficiencies of vitamin K can develop in patients with malabsorption states and steatorrhea. Since several vitamin K compounds derived from intestinal organisms can be absorbed,

vWF Antigen	vWF Multimer Pattern	Ristocetin Cofactor Activity	Ristocetin-Induced Platelet Aggregation	Response to DDAVP
Decreased	Normal	Reduced	Reduced	Hemostasis restored
Decreased	Abnormal	Reduced	Reduced	Correction of hemostasis in approximately 50% of patients
Usually decreased	Usually normal	Normal	Increased	May develop thrombocytopenia
Markedly decreased	Absent	No response	Reduced	No response

treatment of nutritionally deprived patients with broad-spectrum antibiotics can result in vitamin K deficiency. Whether this antibiotic-associated hypocoagulable state is due to direct effects of antibiotics on the hepatic recycling of vitamin K or the loss of gut microorganisms and their vitamin K production is uncertain.

The most frequently encountered cases of vitamin K deficiency result from the use of the oral anticoagulants. These compounds (eg, coumarin), which act as competitive inhibitors, are structural analogs of vitamin K. They are used for prophylaxis and management of venous thrombosis and in the prevention of arterial embolization after cardiac valve replacement or mitral valve disease. Optimum anticoagulant therapy with these compounds requires proper monitoring of the patient's PT. In cases of extreme prolongation of the PT with coumarin, bleeding risks can be minimized with parenteral vitamin K administration.

Because most clotting factors are synthesized by liver hepatocytes, diseases of the liver may result in bleeding disorders. The disorders of hemostasis seen with liver disease can be multifactorial. Impaired synthesis, failure to clear activated factors, release of dysfunctional factors, and increased plasmin activity can contribute to bleeding.

Anticoagulants and the Fibrinolytic System

The control mechanisms that maintain blood in its normal fluid state are very important. Without their effects, repetitive episodes of minor vascular injury, which occur normally, would quickly cause massive and fatal thrombosis. The flow of blood itself is an important mechanism to prevent thrombosis. As blood flows rapidly by the site of thrombus formation, inactivated coagulation factors and unagglutinated platelets are removed from the thrombosis site, and activated coagulation factors become diluted in the vascular volume.

The liver and the phagocytic cells of the reticuloendothelial system also exert hemostatic controls by selectively removing activated coagulation factors and fibrin from the circulation. In addition, the liver synthesizes several plasma proteins that down-regulate the hemostatic system.

Anticoagulants and the fibrinolytic system control the coagulation system by regulating the three types of protein transformation that occur in the coagulation cascade: generation of serine proteases, production of activated cofactors, and polymerization of fibrin. These are illustrated in Figure 29.2. Inhibitors of serine proteases can bind to activated clotting factor enzymes to neutralize their proteolytic activity by forming complexes that are rapidly cleared from the circulation. These include antithrombin III, alpha$_2$-macroglobulin, alpha$_1$-antitrypsin, and other enzyme inhibitors. Deficiencies of these inhibitors can predispose to thrombosis.

The protein C–protein S system inhibits activated coagulation cofactors. Protein C is a vitamin K–dependent plasma zymogen that is slowly activated by thrombin to activated protein C. Activated protein C, with its cofactor protein S, exerts its anticoagulant effect by specifically degrading the activated cofactors of the clotting cascade, factors V and VIII. This results in the loss of factor X activation by factor IX (with factor VIIIa degradation) and prothrombin activation by factor Xa (with factor Va degradation). Removing these cofactors essentially inhibits further thrombin and fibrin formation. The specificity of activated protein C to the activated forms of factors V and VIII prevents bleeding risks since the unactivated clotting cofactors are not consumed.

The third natural pathway of down-regulation is the fibrinolytic system. This pathway is mediated by the proteolytic enzyme, plasmin. Plasmin breaks down fibrin to soluble degradation products, eventually leading to clot lysis. However, plasmin exhibits a rather wide specificity in vivo and can degrade fibrinogen and other clotting factors as well. Strict in vivo regulation of plasmin activity is required to prevent bleeding. Plasminogen is the precursor of plasmin and can be activated in vivo by various "activators." Exogenous plasminogen activators are now used therapeutically to limit ischemic damage due to venous or arterial thrombosis. Bleeding risks due to excess plasminogen activation are well documented and therapy with these drugs must be closely monitored.

Acquired inhibitors may evolve in patients with hemophilia and occasionally in other diseases. Approximately 10% of patients with hemophilia develop inhibitors. The antibodies bind to and neutralize the factor VIII protein. The most common of these are endogenous antibodies to factor VIII found in patients with hemophilia A. Characteristically, these patients are young with very low to absent endogenous factor VIII who require multiple transfusions of plasma or factor VIII concentrates. Inhibitors can also develop in patients with vWD who require replacement therapy. Nonhemophiliacs who develop factor VIII inhibitors tend to be older individuals or postpartum patients. Patients with factor IX deficiency (hemophilia B) can develop alloantibodies to factor IX, particularly if they require frequent transfusions. Rare instances of acquired inhibitors to clotting factors have been reported in patients with other systemic disorders, including collagen-vascular disease, severe infections, malignant neoplasms, and amyloidosis. Bleeding problems due to nonspecific inhibitors are seen in patients with plasma protein disorders such as macroglobulinemia, multiple myeloma, and cryoglobulinemia. The mechanism of bleeding in these disorders is usually due to

Figure 29.2 Regulation of Hemostasis.

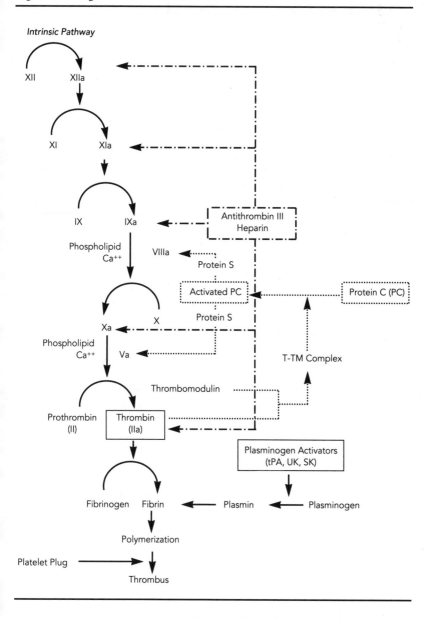

impaired primary hemostasis caused by protein deposition on platelet surfaces. The lupus anticoagulant is an inhibitor that prolongs the PTT in vitro. Phospholipid antibodies that neutralize the PTT reagent are the cause. Bleeding problems are not associated with the lupus anticoagulant. Fibrin split products, formed by plasmin digestion of fibrin and fibrinogen can interfere with fibrin polymerization and result in inhibition of coagulation.

Disseminated Intravascular Coagulation

DIC results from an uncontrolled formation of fibrin thrombi in the microcirculation, causing consumption of coagulation proteins and a secondary release of plasminogen activators. The high concentrations of plasmin cause fibrinolysis. Intravascular consumption of coagulation proteins and platelets together with secondary fibrinolysis and formation of fibrin split products leads to ineffective hemostasis. Clinical effects include a bleeding diathesis, ischemic tissue damage, often microangiopathic hemolytic anemia, and possibly shock. Characteristic laboratory features include hypofibrinogenemia, thrombocytopenia, abnormal blood coagulation studies, and increased circulating fibrin/fibrinogen degradation products.

Generalized endothelial damage appears to be the most common event triggering DIC. The endothelial damage exposes the subendothelium and releases tissue factor. These changes cause widespread activation of the coagulation system and platelet aggregation with resultant formation of microthrombi and consumption of platelets and proteins of coagulation. Another common initiating event is the release of tissue factor without endothelial damage. DIC complicating sepsis and shock is usually associated with endothelial damage, while DIC complicating massive trauma, extensive surgery, severe burns, and obstetric conditions is primarily mediated by the release of massive quantities of tissue factor. These different mechanisms often occur in concert. Activation of the fibrinolytic system is seldom the triggering mechanism of DIC though it may contribute to its hemorrhagic diatheses.

In acute DIC, patients are generally desperately ill, and the process lasts from a few hours to days. Bleeding and excessive bruising are common. Fibrin thrombi in renal capillaries may cause renal cortical necrosis, and fibrin thrombi in pulmonary vessels can cause respiratory failure. Destruction of erythrocytes by fibrin strands in capillaries can lead to microangiopathic hemolytic anemia. In chronic DIC, patients are chronically ill, and the process lasts from days to weeks. Bleeding is less severe than in acute DIC; most patients with chronic DIC have an underlying malignant neoplasm. The laboratory alterations are similar in both forms, but the alterations are less severe with chronic DIC. In both acute and chronic forms DIC is a secondary clinical event, and unless the initiating cause is controlled it will continue unabated.

Primary fibrinolysis, in contrast to DIC, is a rare disorder. It involves only activation of plasminogen without uncontrolled thrombosis.

Laboratory Evaluation of Disseminated Intravascular Coagulation and the Fibrinolytic System

Routine Coagulation Tests
Depletion of several hemostatic factors—mainly platelets, fibrinogen, coagulation enzymes, and factors V and VIII—contributes to the bleeding diathesis of

DIC. Typical laboratory findings are thrombocytopenia and prolongation of the PT and PTT.

Fibrinogen Levels

Fibrinogen, an acute phase reactant, may be increased or decreased in DIC. Conventional tests for plasma fibrinogen levels are useful to assess the degree of hypofibrinogenemia in DIC. Patients with congenital fibrinogen disorders may also manifest hypofibrinogenemia. Elevated fibrinogen levels occur with pregnancy, postoperative states, malignant neoplasms, and many inflammatory disorders.

Measurement of Fibrinogen/Fibrin Degradation Products

A variety of tests are available that measure the level of circulating degradation products. These tests are very useful screening procedures in the diagnosis of the DIC syndrome.

The diagnosis of DIC is often difficult. Subtle clinical and laboratory changes may be the only clues to the diagnosis. Development of more specific laboratory tests of fibrinolysis may become available in the near future and contribute to the assessment of perplexing clinical problems with underlying DIC.

Hypercoagulable States

Three congenital coagulation deficiencies and an acquired coagulation inhibitor are recognized to cause hypercoagulable states: protein C, protein S, and antithrombin III deficiency, and lupus anticoagulants. Most patients with one of the congenital deficiencies are young and have recurrent thromboembolic disease; a family history of thromboembolic disease is usually elicited. The majority of adult patients that have thrombophlebitis or other thrombotic disorders do not have a congenital hemostatic abnormality.

Lupus anticoagulants are antiphospholipid antibodies. They react with phospholipids involved in factor X and V interaction. They were first described in patients with systemic lupus erythematosus, but less than 10% of individuals with lupus anticoagulants have systemic lupus erythematosus. Most individuals with a lupus anticoagulant are asymptomatic without identifiable clinical abnormalities. Most commonly, the lupus anticoagulant is first recognized when a prolonged PTT is found in a presurgical laboratory screen. Instead of having a bleeding diathesis as expected with a coagulant inhibitor, patients with a lupus anticoagulant have increased risk of thrombosis. It is thought that the increase in thrombosis is related to inhibition of prostacyclin production or release by the lupus anticoagulant. Lupus anticoagulant in pregnant women has been associated with an increased incidence of intrauterine fetal death.

Anticoagulant Therapy

Heparins include a wide variety of negatively charged glycosaminoglycans, which function as anticoagulants. They act by accelerating the inhibition of thrombin and other clotting factors by antithrombin III and heparin cofactor II. Heparin is administered intravenously, intramuscularly, or subcutaneously for treatment or prevention of thromboembolic disease. Direct laboratory assays of plasma heparin levels are difficult to perform, making clinical monitoring of the drug problematic. Since several factors in the intrinsic system are inhibited by heparin, the PTT, which is prolonged by heparin therapy, is often used to monitor treatment. Overdosage of heparin can be neutralized by administration of protamine sulfate.

The coumarin drugs (warfarin and dicumarol) function as anticoagulants by inhibiting postribosomal carboxylation of vitamin K–dependent clotting factors (II, VII, IX, and X). Because addition of carboxyl groups is necessary for optimal functional activity of these factors, factor proteins released by the liver of patients taking coumarin drugs are ineffective in supporting the coagulation cascade. Monitoring coumarin anticoagulant therapy is usually performed by measuring the patient's degree of increase of the PT over baseline levels. Overdosage of coumarin compounds may result if careful monitoring is not performed, and hemorrhagic complications can occur. Therapy for overdose includes administration of vitamin K and plasma components.

Fibrinolytic Therapy

The fibrinolytic system is an important pathway of coagulation down-regulation that functions to digest insoluble fibrin. This system requires the conversion of plasminogen to plasmin by a plasminogen activator. The rate of plasminogen activation, or plasmin formation, is dependent on the level of various activators. The main endogenous activators are urokinase and tissue plasminogen activator. The site of synthesis of these activators is the vascular endothelial cells. These activators convert plasminogen to plasmin by hydrolysis of a single peptide bond in the plasminogen molecule.

Streptokinase is an important exogenous plasminogen activator used therapeutically as a fibrinolytic agent. It is a bacterial protein made by streptococcus (Lancefield group C, ß-hemolytic) that binds to plasminogen. The resulting streptokinase-plasminogen complex is a potent nonspecific plasminogen activator. Streptokinase can be an effective thrombolytic agent; however, occasionally resistance occurs due to preformed circulating antistreptococcal antibodies.

Laboratory monitoring of patients receiving fibrinolytic therapy is complicated by in vitro degradation of plasma proteins. This process can be minimized by adding plasmin and tissue plasminogen activator inhibitors to the specimen collection tube. Most hospital laboratories do not use specific specimen collection techniques for patients receiving thrombolytic therapy. However, if an anticoagulated specimen is immediately placed on ice after drawing and plasma is immediately separated by cold centrifugation, a reliable fibrinogen level can be obtained.

References

Bloom AL, Thomas DP. *Haemostasis and Thrombosis*. 2nd ed. New York, NY: Churchill Livingstone Inc; 1987.

Colman RW, Hirsh J, Marder VJ, Salzman EW. *Hemostasis and Thrombosis*. 2nd ed. Philadelphia, Pa: JB Lippincott Co; 1987.

George JN, Shattil SJ. The clinical importance of acquired abnormalities of platelet function. *N Engl J Med*. 1991;324:27-39.

Ratnoff OD, Forbes CD. *Disorders of Hemostasis*. 2nd ed. Philadelphia, Pa: WB Saunders Co; 1991.

Thirty

Blood Bank Tests and Blood Component Usage

Key Points

1. Most blood bank tests are performed to find compatible blood for transfusion, and involve testing for red blood cell (RBC) antigens and antibodies.
2. Proper labeling of the blood specimen for blood bank testing is of paramount importance in assuring a safe transfusion, as is proper identification of the recipient at the time of transfusion.
3. The presence of an antibody to an RBC antigen in a patient's serum complicates the procurement of compatible blood for transfusion. Additional time must be allowed prior to the anticipated transfusion.
4. The ABO blood group is the most important RBC antigen system clinically. Multiple tests in the pretransfusion workup are performed to ensure the ABO compatibility of blood components, because transfusion of ABO incompatible units may be life-threatening.
5. The D antigen in the Rh blood group is one of the most immunogenic RBC antigens known in humans. Therefore, units of blood compatible with the recipient's Rh (D) type are issued whenever possible.
6. The direct Coombs' test detects IgG antibody and/or C3 complement fragments on the surface of RBCs. The indirect Coombs' test detects RBC antibody free in the patient's serum.
7. During pregnancy, maternal IgG antibody to RBC antigens can cross the placenta into the fetal circulation and cause hemolysis of fetal RBCs bearing the antigen (hemolytic disease of the newborn). Prenatal screening is performed by the blood bank to identify fetuses at risk for this disease.

Background

Tests performed by the blood bank or transfusion service laboratory involve the detection of surface antigens on blood cells or antibodies to blood cells, most commonly RBCs. The antibodies detected may be either alloantibodies, directed against antigens absent from the patient's own cells (usually stimulated by previous exposure to these foreign antigens) or autoantibodies, directed against antigens present on the patient's own RBCs. These tests are usually part of the process of testing blood for compatible transfusion.

Surface antigens on RBCs are identified when agglutination occurs following mixture of patient RBCs with known reagent antisera containing antibodies. The presence of a RBC agglutinate or clump signifies the presence of the antigen for which testing is done. The lack of agglutination suggests the antigen is not present. Detection of RBC antibodies in the patient's serum is accomplished by adding patient serum to donor RBCs. The presence of RBC agglutination indicates that an antibody is present in the patient's serum.

ABO Grouping

The patient's RBCs are mixed with reagent antibodies anti-A and anti-B to determine ABO group. If the patient's RBCs have surface antigen A the anti-A will cross-link adjacent RBCs, causing agglutination. A patient with A antigen on his RBCs has group A blood. Agglutination with both anti-A and anti-B is seen with group AB blood. The absence of reaction with either anti-A or anti-B is seen with group O blood. This testing is called "forward ABO grouping" or "cell grouping."

Because of the importance of the ABO blood group for correct transfusion, the ABO group of each patient is double-checked using both serum and cells. The serum of all normal individuals should contain antibodies to those A or B antigens that they lack. In other words, a group O person (who lacks both A and B antigens) should have both anti-A and anti-B in his or her serum. A group A person should have anti-B in his or her serum, and so forth. Therefore, the blood bank tests the serum of every patient against RBCs of known ABO group. The serum of a group O person should agglutinate cells of group A, group B, and group AB. This testing is called "reverse ABO grouping" or "serum grouping."

The blood of infants cannot be ABO grouped accurately because the A and B antigens are not fully expressed on the RBCs of most newborns. These antigens do not fully develop until the age of 2 years. Therefore, infants may appear to have RBCs of group O if tested early in life, whereas over the next few months they may begin to express A or B antigen or both. Similarly, infants often do not have the appropriate antibodies to the A or B antigens they lack if tested early in life. Thus, reverse ABO grouping cannot generally be done on newborns.

Rh Typing

Rh typing is performed to establish the presence or absence of the D antigen, one of many Rh antigens. The D antigen is the most immunogenic RBC antigen present in humans. In other words, exposure to this antigen in persons who lack it is highly likely to result in formation of an alloantibody. Therefore, blood banks try to select blood for transfusion that is D antigen compatible.

Rh (D) typing is done by testing RBCs from the subject, using reagent antiserum containing strong anti-D antibodies. If agglutination takes place, the subject has the D antigen and is called "Rh positive." If agglutination does not take place with initial mixing of subject RBCs and reagent antiserum, some blood banks will perform a second test called the "D^u test." This test adds human antiglobulin serum, a further reagent, to promote agglutination in the presence of a weak D antigen. If the D^u test is positive for agglutination, the subject is also called "Rh positive." Only if both the initial D grouping and the D^u test are negative will the subject be called "Rh negative" in blood banks performing the D^u test.

"Reverse" grouping cannot routinely be done for the D antigen, because individuals do not automatically have an anti-D antibody when they lack the D antigen. Anti-D is formed only following exposure to RBCs expressing D during pregnancy or transfusion.

Antibody Screening

Antibody screening detects antibodies in the patient's serum directed against RBC antigens. The patient's serum is tested against reagent RBCs, which express all major, clinically significant RBC antigens on their surface. Generally, use of reagent cells from two or three carefully selected donors will allow detection of any clinically important RBC antibody. Further reagents are added to the RBC-serum mixture to enhance any agglutination of the cells. Incubation of the mixture at 37°C is performed to help detect antibodies reactive in vivo. If no agglutination or hemolysis is seen, the patient's serum is assumed to be free of any significant RBC antibodies.

Antibodies that are not clinically significant are sometimes detected during antibody screening. Often, these antibodies are active only at temperatures below normal body temperature. Many people have such cold-reacting RBC antibodies, but they are of no significance since they are inactive at 37°C. The blood bank usually disregards such antibodies when they are discovered.

Occasionally a patient has a negative RBC antibody screen yet actually has a clinically significant RBC antibody. This scenario may result for two reasons. First, the patient may have an antibody present at titers below the level of sensitivity of the antibody screen. Alternatively, the antibody may be directed against an uncommon RBC antigen that is lacking on the reagent RBCs used in the screening test. The RBCs used in the antibody screening express the most common clinically significant antigens, but cannot express every single RBC antigen in existence.

The antibody screening procedure is sometimes referred to as the "indirect Coombs' test" or "indirect antiglobulin test."

Antibody Identification

If the antibody screening test is positive, antibody identification must be done so that appropriate antigen-negative units of blood may be chosen at the time of transfusion. For antibody identification, a panel of reagent RBCs from at least 10 donors is tested with the patient's serum. Reagent RBCs from each donor have a variety of well-characterized antigens expressed on their surfaces. The antibody can generally be identified by comparing the pattern of agglutination with the antigens known to be expressed on each donor's cells. Mixtures of antibodies or unusual antibodies require more extensive testing and can necessitate hours of work. The patient's physician will be notified if such a situation exists, because transfusion should be delayed until the antibody identification is completed.

The most common clinically significant RBC antibodies react with antigens of the following blood groups: ABO, Rh (C, c, E, e, D), Kell, Duffy (Fy), Kidd (Jk), and MNSs. RBC antibodies less commonly of clinical importance include anti-I, anti-i, Lewis (Le) antibodies, Lutheran antibodies, and anti-P. However, because more than 300 RBC antigens have been described to date, additional antibodies of relevance are occasionally seen.

Some antibodies are "naturally occurring," that is, they seem to be present even if no previous exposure to foreign RBCs has occurred. The most common examples of such antibodies are anti-A and anti-B. Lewis antibodies, anti-P, and some examples of anti-M are also "naturally occurring." Most other antibodies occur only after stimulation of the patient's immune system following exposure to foreign RBC antigens via transfusion or pregnancy. Antibodies to Rh, Kell, Kidd, Duffy, and S/s antigens are generally the result of such previous exposure.

Group, Screen, and Hold

A group, screen, and hold (GSH) (also known as type and screen) is ordered when transfusion of a patient may be required at some time during the following 48 to 72 hours, but immediate transfusion is not anticipated, or when the probability of transfusion is remote. To perform a GSH, the blood bank laboratory needs a sample of blood, preferably a clotted specimen, although most laboratories can use an anticoagulated specimen as well. Serum separator tubes cannot be used, as the gel in them interferes with agglutination tests.

A GSH includes ABO and Rh(D) grouping of the patient's RBCs as well as an antibody screen. If the antibody screen is negative, the blood bank stores the specimen and awaits further word from the patient's physician about the need for transfusion. If the antibody screen is positive, most blood banks will notify the physician that further work needs to be done to identify the antibody. This work will be done if the possibility of transfusion remains. In this case, the GSH is converted to a type and crossmatch order. If transfusion is no longer a possibility, the workup may be stopped, or continued only at the convenience of the blood bank personnel.

Type and Crossmatch

A type and crossmatch is ordered when transfusion of a patient is certain or likely in the near future, or if any possibility of transfusion exists in a patient with an RBC antibody. The number of units of blood anticipated for transfusion is indicated, eg, "type and crossmatch 4 units of RBCs." The same type of patient specimen is required as for a GSH and the initial testing is the same. However, once the ABO and Rh grouping and antibody screening (and identification, if necessary) are complete, units of blood are located and tested for compatibility with the patient's serum through a process called "crossmatching."

Crossmatching involves mixing the patient's serum with a donor's RBCs and looking for agglutination. Other reagents may be added to promote RBC agglutination and enhance detection of weak antigens or antibodies of the IgG class. The presence of agglutination indicates that the unit of blood is not compatible with the patient's serum and so should not be transfused. If such a unit were transfused to a patient, the transfused RBCs might be destroyed following transfusion and possibly cause a hemolytic transfusion reaction. The purpose of the crossmatch is to double-check the ABO compatibility of the units to be transfused, and also to look for additional RBC antibodies that may not have been detected by the antibody screen.

The blood bank may provide blood specific for a patient's blood group or blood compatible with a patient's blood group. If the blood is group-specific, it is the same blood group as the patient's. If the blood is group-compatible, it is not the exact blood group, but the donor RBCs are compatible with the patient's serum and no adverse reaction due to the blood group will occur when transfused. For example, for ABO group: if a patient of group A gets group-specific RBCs, that patient receives group A RBCs. If a group A patient gets group-compatible RBCs, the blood may be of either group A or group O. Group O RBCs will not harm a group A recipient, whereas group AB RBCs (which are not compatible) would probably cause a hemolytic transfusion reaction due to the potent anti-B present in the group A recipient's serum.

RBC Phenotyping

For some patients, usually those in whom multiple RBC transfusions are anticipated, a complete RBC antigen phenotype may be useful. The patient's RBCs are tested against antisera for each of the most common, clinically important RBC antigens to identify which antigens (in addition to the ABO and D antigens) are present on his or her RBCs. The RBC phenotype, when performed early in the patient's course, can be extremely helpful in providing compatible blood when multiple RBC antibodies have developed later.

Direct Coombs' Test

The direct Coombs' test (direct antiglobulin test) will detect antibody (usually of IgG class) or complement (usually C3d) bound to the surface of the patient's circulating RBCs. The test, performed on an anticoagulated sample of blood, involves mixing anti–human globulin serum (rabbit anti–human IgG or monoclonal anti–human C3d) to the patient's RBCs. The antiglobulin serum will bind to immunoglobulin or complement bound to the RBCs and cross-link such RBCs, forming agglutinates.

The direct Coombs' test may be ordered by physicians suspecting RBC destruction due to an immune cause, or it may be instigated by the blood bank in the course of a transfusion workup. The test is useful to blood bank personnel when an antibody screening or antibody identification workup suggests that an antibody present in the patient's serum is agglutinating the patient's own cells. These agglutinated cells may be the patient's native RBCs in the presence of an autoantibody, or may be transfused RBCs in the presence of an alloantibody. In many cases, a direct Coombs' test positive for IgG will be followed by an RBC elution. A negative direct Coombs' test or a direct Coombs' test positive only for complement is usually not further investigated by an RBC elution.

The direct Coombs' test has limitations of sensitivity. Depending on the method used, 100 or more molecules of IgG or complement must be present on the surface of the RBC for the direct Coombs' test to be positive. The more molecules of immunoglobulin or complement that are present, the stronger the direct Coombs' agglutination result. The test reactions are graded from 1+ to 4+ in strength.

All normal persons are thought to have some small amount of immunoglobulin or complement molecules on their RBCs—few enough of these molecules that a direct Coombs' test would be negative. Positive direct Coombs' tests may result from antibodies specific for RBC antigens, either alloantibodies or autoantibodies. In addition, direct Coombs' tests may detect other immunoglobulin or immune complexes that have become nonspecifically adherent to the RBC surface. Many drugs can cause such a positive direct Coombs' test, as can autoantibodies to tissues in the body other than RBCs.

Most direct Coombs' tests will detect only IgG and certain portions of complement, such as C3d or both C3b and C3d. Detection of these molecules is usually adequate in the assessment of immune RBC destruction. Occasionally, a blood bank will use a reagent that detects other classes of immunoglobulin, such as IgM, or other components of complement, such as C4. Do not assume that the direct Coombs' test will detect IgM or IgA molecules.

RBC Elution Studies

This test is usually performed only after a positive direct Coombs' test with IgG detected on RBCs. The RBC elution will remove the antibody (detected in the direct Coombs' test) bound to the RBCs and collect it for further study. Antibody removed and collected in this manner can be tested against panels of reagent RBCs to determine the identity of the antibody. For example, depending on which reagent cells in the panel the antibody reacts with, the antibody may be identified as an anti-D or other alloantibody or as an autoantibody. The RBC elution also helps determine if the antibody present on the surface of the RBCs is not an antibody specific for RBCs. For example, administration of intravenous immunoglobulin in a patient may cause a positive direct Coombs' test due to the nonspecific adsorption of many Ig molecules on the RBC surface. However, this antibody will not react with any of the reagent RBCs following an elution procedure. Occasionally RBC elution may be informative following a negative direct Coombs' test. If antibody is present in amounts too small to be detected by the direct Coombs' test, elution may concentrate the antibody to detectable levels.

Prenatal Screening

Women routinely have testing performed by the blood bank early in a pregnancy. This testing, which includes ABO and Rh (D) grouping and an antibody screen, detects fetuses at risk for hemolytic disease of the newborn. In hemolytic disease of the newborn, an antibody present in the mother's blood (to an RBC antigen on the newborn's RBCs that the mother lacks) crosses the placenta and enters the blood of the fetus. It then binds to the antigen present on the RBCs of the fetus, causing premature RBC destruction. The severity of disease varies, depending on the reactivity of the antibody and which RBC antigen is involved. Only antibodies of the IgG class cross the placenta and enter fetal blood.

If a significant RBC antibody is identified in the mother's serum, serum dilutions are performed to determine the antibody titer. The titer is helpful to the obstetrician in determining how to monitor the pregnancy. For example, a pregnant patient with an anti-D of titer 2048 is more likely to have serial amniocentesis done than a patient with an anti-D of titer 2 who may just have serial antibody titers measured. A rising titer during pregnancy may indicate that the RBCs of the fetus do express that antigen and are stimulating the mother to make more antibody. Unfortunately, these titers do not correlate well with the risk of clinical disease. In other words, a Kell-positive infant born to one mother with an anti-Kell titer of 256 may have little or no anemia at birth, whereas a Kell-positive infant born to another woman with an anti-Kell titer of 32 may be moderately anemic and need transfusion.

Umbilical Cord Testing

At the time of birth, the blood bank may be asked to perform a direct Coombs' test (direct antiglobulin test) on cord blood. This screen may be helpful in infants at risk for neonatal jaundice. A positive direct Coombs' test at birth may identify infants suffering hemolytic disease of the newborn not previously identified. An RBC antibody that crosses the placenta and binds to the corresponding antigen on fetal RBCs should be detected as a positive direct Coombs' test in the cord blood. A weak (1+) positive result vs a stronger (3+ or 4+) result may indicate the severity of the RBC involvement, although the presence of antibody binding to the infant's RBCs does not always indicate that such RBCs are being destroyed prematurely.

If the cord blood RBCs test positive on the direct Coombs' test, further testing may be helpful. An ABO and Rh (D) grouping and elution studies of the infant's cord blood cells may determine if the positive direct Coombs' test is due to anti-A, anti-B, or anti-D. The blood bank may request an additional blood sample from the infant, such as a heel stick specimen, to confirm positive results.

Evaluation of Rh Immune Globulin Therapy

Screening for the presence of significant fetal-maternal hemorrhage will indicate whether a nonimmunized Rh (D)–negative pregnant patient who received Rh immune globulin at the time of delivery received an adequate dose of Rh immune globulin to prevent the mother from forming Rh antibodies. This may be done by various methods, all of which look for evidence of fetal cells in the maternal circulation. Some commonly used tests, such as the D^u test and the rosette test, look for the presence of D antigen on circulating RBCs. The detection of cells positive for the D antigen signifies that cells from an Rh positive fetus have leaked into the maternal blood. These two tests are qualitative only, and any positive results must be tested by a second method to determine the quantity of fetal RBCs present. If more cells are present than would be protected against by one vial of Rh immune globulin (the standard dose administered), additional vials of Rh immune globulin must be given to prevent alloimmunization to the D antigen.

The acid elution test (Kleihauer-Betke method) quantitatively evaluates the presence of fetal cells. This method looks for fetal hemoglobin, rather than D antigen, so certain conditions such as persistence of fetal hemoglobin in the mother can cause false-positive results.

Workup of Transfusion Reactions

With a suspected transfusion reaction, the transfusion should be stopped immediately, and all remaining blood in the bag and tubing set should be returned to the blood bank. In addition, a post-transfusion sample of blood and the first post-transfusion urine should be sent to the blood bank for evaluation. These specimens should be accompanied by a written report from the patient's physician, describing the nature of the transfusion reaction and the time course of any signs or symptoms. The blood bank has the pretransfusion blood sample for comparison.

The blood bank will try to determine the cause of the transfusion reaction. The first priority is to rule out an acute immune-mediated hemolytic reaction, which can be life-threatening. The blood bank checks its clerical records to assure that the correct unit of blood was issued to the correct patient. The post-transfusion serum and urine samples are examined for evidence of free hemoglobin. A direct Coombs' test is performed on the post-transfusion blood sample. If it is positive, the pretransfusion sample is also tested to see if a change has occurred.

Depending on the findings of these preliminary tests, further workup may be indicated. For example, repeated ABO grouping and crossmatching of the units may be worthwhile. In some situations, blood remaining in the bag may be cultured for microorganisms. Following interpretation of all findings, a report is issued from the blood bank physician summarizing the data with a conclusion about whether the reported reaction was indeed caused by the transfusion.

Evaluation of Warm Autoimmune Hemolytic Anemia

If a patient exhibits signs of RBC hemolysis without known cause, the blood bank may perform tests to determine if an autoantibody directed toward RBC antigens may be the underlying cause. Such autoantibodies are often optimally active at body temperature (37°C) as opposed to cooler, in vitro testing conditions, and thus are referred to as "warm" autoantibodies. Both a clotted and anticoagulated blood specimen should be submitted for testing along with pertinent patient history. The blood bank generally starts by performing a direct Coombs' test. An indirect Coombs' test (antibody screen) is also useful. These two tests will detect antibody to RBC antigens either bound to circulating RBCs or free in the serum. Many warm autoantibodies will demonstrate both free and bound immunoglobulin. An RBC elution study may be performed to demonstrate that the bound antibody is indeed an autoantibody to RBC antigens. Such an autoantibody usually reacts with every reagent and patient RBC sample tested.

Warm autoantibodies may react equally strongly with every RBC sample they are tested against, or they may show preferential reactivity with RBCs expressing certain RBC antigens. Autoantibodies with the latter behavior are said to mimic "specificity" for a particular blood group antigen. One of the more common examples is a warm autoantibody that reacts more strongly with RBCs expressing the Rh antigen e. Such an autoantibody is said to have anti-e specificity. This information may be helpful to the blood bank in finding RBCs that will survive in the patient's circulation longer should the patient require transfusion.

Evaluation for Cold Agglutinins

An autoantibody may demonstrate optimal activity at temperatures below normal body temperature. Such an antibody is referred to as "cold-reactive" or a cold autoantibody. Because these autoantibodies often cause RBC agglutination when active, they are also called cold agglutinins. Many normal persons have circulating cold autoantibodies that may be detected in routine blood bank testing. These autoantibodies are usually of no clinical relevance, however, because they are active only at very cold temperatures (eg, 4°C) and the subject's circulating blood never reaches such temperatures. However, some people may develop a cold autoantibody that reacts at higher temperatures, eg, 30°C or higher. The blood circulating in their extremities, especially in fingers, toes, ears, or nose, may drop to this temperature, leading to antibody activation and subsequent destruction of their RBCs.

To evaluate a patient for a cold autoantibody, the blood bank requires a clotted specimen kept at body temperature until reaching the laboratory. The blood must be kept warm to avoid activating the circulating autoantibody and causing it to bind to the RBCs in the sample before it reaches the laboratory. The blood bank needs to have the autoantibody in the serum to carry out the appropriate tests.

Cold Agglutinin Titer

A cold agglutinin titer may be performed, using serial dilutions of the patient's serum. This test indicates how much autoantibody is active in the serum at 4°C. The higher the titer, the more likely the autoantibody is of clinical significance. For example, a cold agglutinin titer of 2 is generally of no clinical relevance. However, a cold agglutinin titer of 2048 may very well be a clinical problem.

Thermal Amplitude Study

This test, like the cold agglutinin titer, uses serial dilutions of the patient's serum to detect the strength of antibody activity. However, this testing is done at higher temperatures. For example, the sample may be tested against reagent RBCs at room temperature and 30°C to see if reactivity persists at these temperatures. An autoantibody reactive at 4°C, 25°C, and 30°C is said to have a wide thermal amplitude. The stronger the reactivity at higher temperatures, the more likely the antibody is of clinical significance.

Donath-Landsteiner Test

This test is used to diagnose paroxysmal cold hemoglobinuria, a disorder caused by a specialized kind of cold-reactive autoantibody. To perform this test the blood bank needs a clotted specimen of blood maintained at body temperature until reaching the laboratory. The autoantibody causing paroxysmal cold hemoglobinuria is generally of IgG class and is "biphasic" in activity. In other words, at normal core body temperature the antibody does not bind to the patient's RBCs, but as the blood temperature drops (eg, in the extremities in cold weather) the antibody binds to the RBCs and fixes complement to the RBC surface. Then as the blood passes back into the warmer trunk of the body the antibody dissociates from the cells and the RBCs are hemolyzed. Therefore, testing for this antibody involves lowering the temperature of the blood and then rewarming it under controlled conditions to detect hemolysis.

Testing of Donor Blood

All donor blood must be typed for ABO and Rh (D) groups. Each unit of blood is labeled with its ABO and Rh group. In addition, at least in donors with a history of previous transfusion or pregnancy, an antibody screen must be performed. Many blood collection centers do such an antibody screen on all donors because it is easier logistically. The antibody screen is performed because the blood of any donor with a clinically relevant RBC antibody cannot be used to prepare any component containing a significant amount of plasma, such as fresh-frozen plasma or platelets.

As of March 1991, all whole blood collected in the United States must be screened by seven markers for infectious disease. The tests required are antibody to human immunodeficiency virus type 1, hepatitis B surface antigen, antibody to hepatitis B core antigen, antibody to hepatitis C virus, alanine aminotransferase, antibody to human T-lymphotropic virus types I/II, and a serologic test for syphilis (usually the rapid plasma reagin or Venereal Disease Research Laboratory test, followed by a treponemal test). Units that are repeatably reactive for any of these tests or have an elevated alanine aminotransferase level are not used for transfusion. Donors are generally notified of positive results.

Platelet Antigen Typing

Platelets may be tested to determine what platelet-specific antigens are present on their cell surfaces. This information is useful in patients with a known or suspected alloantibody directed against such antigens. Most platelet antigens have only recently been described and are not as well characterized as RBC antigens.

The most common antigens of clinical significance are Pl^A (Zw), Ko, Bak (Lek), Yuk (Pen), and Br. Platelet antigen typing theoretically may be useful in finding compatible platelets for transfusion into patients with a platelet alloantibody. This is rarely done in practice.

More frequently this test is useful in the diagnosis and management of neonatal alloimmune thrombocytopenia. This disorder is caused by a platelet alloantibody. If the platelets of a fetus express a platelet antigen toward which the mother has an antibody, the fetus is at risk for significant thrombocytopenia in utero and at birth due to fetal platelet destruction by the mother's antibody. In families with a history of neonatal thrombocytopenia, the mother's platelets and serum can be evaluated for the presence of the most common platelet antigens and antibodies. Because these antigens are genetically determined, typing the father's platelets may help provide information indicating whether a fetus is at risk.

Platelet Antibody Detection

Anti-platelet antibodies bound to circulating platelets or free in serum may be detected and quantitated through a direct platelet antibody test, while free antibody is detected by an indirect platelet antibody test. The antibody detected in these tests may be alloantibody to the platelet-specific antigens discussed above, or may be autoantibody such as those present in immune thrombocytopenic purpura. In addition, nonspecific adsorption of immunoglobulin to the platelet surface may be detected in platelet antibody testing.

Platelet Crossmatching

This technique may be used to provide a more compatible platelet transfusion in patients known to have anti-platelet antibodies and previous destruction of incompatible transfused platelets. The purpose is to select platelet donors whose platelets are compatible with the recipient's serum, hoping that these platelets will survive longer. Methods for this procedure vary greatly among laboratories. Platelet crossmatching is not done routinely in most blood banks, and many blood banks do not have the expertise to do it even when it may be useful. The effectiveness of platelet crossmatching is controversial and varies with the specific method used. If sent to a reference laboratory, results may not be available quickly.

Granulocyte Antigen/Antibody Tests

A few reference blood bank laboratories offer tests for detection of granulocyte antigens and antibodies. These tests may be useful in evaluation of patients with neutropenia due to leukoagglutinating alloantibodies and autoantibodies. Examples of such antibodies are seen in alloimmune neonatal neutropenia, autoimmune neutropenia, and multiply transfused patients who have developed anti-granulocyte antibodies.

Histocompatibility Typing

Many blood banks perform human leukocyte antigen (HLA) typing. The tests are generally performed on lymphocytes isolated from peripheral blood. Testing for class I and class II HLAs is useful in transplantation. Testing for class I antigens (A and B only) is used for procurement of HLA-matched platelets for transfusion to patients refractory to random platelet transfusion because of destruction of transfused platelets by HLA antibodies. HLA testing may also be utilized to resolve questions of paternity.

Paternity Testing

Many blood banks perform paternity testing. It is generally offered to resolve legal disputes over alleged paternity. Because the results of such testing have the potential to be presented in a court of law, the laboratory must be careful to document the source and continuous custody of all specimens. The purpose of paternity testing is to exclude the possibility of paternity of a falsely accused man. Paternity cannot be proven, although the probability of paternity can be calculated.

Paternity testing may include typing for RBC antigens. The most useful antigens are those with the greatest variability in the population, but must be inherited via mendelian genetics. Those RBC antigens most commonly used include ABO, Rh, Kell, Duffy, MNSs, and Kidd antigens. Use of these RBC antigen systems will exclude a wrongly accused man from paternity in approximately 70% of cases.

Because of the tremendous variability among the histocompatibility antigens in the population, HLA typing is useful in paternity testing. The use of HLA typing alone excludes paternity in over 90% of falsely accused men.

Other markers used to exclude paternity include isoforms of plasma proteins such as haptoglobin and transferrin, as well as isoforms of RBC enzymes such as glucose-6-phosphate dehydrogenase. As technology improves, more laboratories will be utilizing deoxyribonucleic (DNA) technology to assess paternity.

Blood Components for Transfusion

Because a person bleeds whole blood, transfusing whole blood seems logical, but it is usually not the best use of the few donated units physicians have to allocate. Using blood components allows a clinician to more closely monitor which deficient elements the patient receives, and to control intravascular volume more precisely. The following brief review of transfusion therapy can be supplemented by the in-depth references cited.

Whole Blood
Volume = 500 mL. Hematocrit = 0.40 (40%). Stored at 1°C to 6°C for up to 35 days.
Contains: RBCs, refrigerated plasma, anticoagulant, and preservative solution. Has little to no platelet activity, no viable granulocytes, and diminished factor VIII and factor V levels.

Use: Indicated for patients needing both RBC replacement and volume expansion with coagulation factors, eg, massive transfusion, heavy surgical bleeding, burn patients.

Possible hazards include: Viral transmission, RBC incompatibility with hemolysis, bacterial contamination, febrile reactions, volume overload, citrate toxicity, hyperkalemia, allergic response.

Dose: 1 unit for every 10 g/L (1 g/dL) rise in hemoglobin desired (for average-sized adult). More needed if patient actively bleeding. Donor must be ABO identical to recipient. Must be crossmatched.

RBCs in Citrate-Phosphate-Dextrose-Adenine-1 (CPDA-1) Preservative/Anticoagulant

This is the classic "packed" RBC unit. Volume = 250 mL. Hematocrit = 0.75 to 0.80 (75%-80%). Stored at 1°C to 6°C for up to 35 days.

Contains: RBCs, minimal amount of refrigerated plasma, anticoagulant, and preservative solution. Has little to no platelet activity, granulocyte activity, or clotting factors.

Use: RBC replacement for increased oxygen-carrying capacity. Generally used for symptomatic anemia or preoperatively. Beware of transfusing RBCs based only on hemoglobin or hematocrit levels.

Possible hazards include: Viral transmission, RBC incompatibility with hemolysis, bacterial contamination, febrile reactions, hemosiderosis, allergic response, graft-versus-host disease.

Dose: Same as whole blood. Donor RBCs must be ABO compatible with recipient plasma. Must be crossmatched.

RBCs in Additive Solution (AS-1, AS-3, AS-5)

Volume = 350 mL. Hematocrit = 0.65 (65%). Stored at 1°C to 6°C for up to 42 days.

Contains: RBCs and preservative solution with anticoagulant. No platelet or granulocyte activity present; basically no plasma present.

Use: Indicated for replacement of RBCs in patients who can also tolerate or benefit from extra volume. Lower viscosity than traditional "packed" RBCs, so better flow for emergency department or surgical use. May want to avoid in neonates because of possible adverse effects of the additive solution.

Possible hazards include: Viral transmission, RBC incompatibility with hemolysis, bacterial contamination, febrile reactions, volume overload, allergic response.

Dose: Same as whole blood. Donor RBCs must be ABO compatible with recipient plasma. Must be crossmatched.

Platelets Pooled From Individual Donors of Whole Blood

These are separated by centrifugation in the laboratory. Volume = 50 mL per individual unit. Stored at 20°C to 24°C for up to 5 days with agitation.

Contains: Platelets, white blood cells, fairly fresh plasma (with coagulation factors), anticoagulant/preservative solution.

Use: Patients with thrombocytopenia or platelet dysfunction. Only rarely needed if platelet count is greater than 20×10^9/L (20,000/mm^3), unless an invasive procedure is planned or dysfunctional platelets are documented. Also replaces clotting factor deficiency.

Possible hazards include: Viral transmission, bacterial contamination, febrile reactions, volume overload, allergic response, graft-versus-host disease.

Dose: One unit per 10 kg of body weight, pooled. The plasma of the donor should be ABO compatible with the recipient's RBCs. Not usually crossmatched.

Apheresis ("Single Donor") Platelets

Only platelets and some plasma are harvested from the donor in a 1½ to 2 hour procedure. The RBCs are returned to the donor after separation centrifugally. Volume = 250 mL. Stored at 20°C to 24°C for up to 5 days with agitation.

Contains: Platelets, white blood cells, and fairly fresh plasma in acid citrate dextrose anticoagulant/preservative.

Use: Same as pooled platelets.

Possible hazards include: The same as for pooled platelets, except that the risk of viral disease transmission is significantly less because the recipient is exposed to only one donor rather than seven or eight.

Dose: One apheresis unit = 1 dose. Contains an equivalent number of platelets as six to eight individual units of platelets from whole blood. Plasma of donor should be ABO compatible with the recipient's RBCs. Not usually crossmatched.

Fresh-Frozen Plasma

Volume = 250 mL. Stored at -18°C or colder for up to 1 year. Must be thawed prior to transfusion. After thawing, may store at 1°C to 6°C for up to 24 hours.

Contains: Fresh plasma, including all coagulation factors, and anticoagulant-preservative solution. Contaminating RBCs and most leukocytes do not survive the freezing and thawing process.

Use: Replacement of coagulation factors in patients with multiple factor deficiencies, undefined factor deficiencies, or factor deficiencies for which no concentrated replacement is available. Also used for thrombotic thrombocytopenic purpura. Never used solely for volume expansion or nutritional repletion.

Possible hazards include: Viral transmission, allergic reactions, volume overload, hemolysis.

Dose: One unit contains approximately 250 units of activity of all clotting factors and 400 mg of fibrinogen. Calculate dose accordingly. Plasma of donor must be ABO compatible with RBCs of recipient. Not crossmatched.

Cryoprecipitate

Volume = 15 mL per unit. Stored at -18°C or colder for up to 1 year. Must be thawed and pooled prior to transfusion. After thawing and pooling, may store at 1°C to 6°C or at room temperature for up to 4 hours. The preferred temperature of storage after thawing is under investigation.

Contains: Factor VIII, factor XIII, fibrinogen, fibronectin, and von Willebrand factor.

Use: In a pool, indicated for replacement of any of the specific coagulation factors listed above. Most commonly used for fibrinogen deficiency or von Willebrand disease. A single unit is sometimes used topically with thrombin in surgery for local hemostasis ("fibrin glue").

Possible hazards include: Viral transmission, allergic reactions.
Dose: One unit contains at least 80 units of factor VIII activity and 200 units of fibrinogen activity. Calculate dose accordingly. Generally issued as a pool of units. ABO type not important. Not crossmatched.

Granulocytes

Special apheresis collection must be arranged. Volume = 250 mL. Stored at 20°C to 24°C for up to 24 hours. Transfuse immediately.
Contains: Fresh, viable granulocytes and other leukocytes, plasma, and anticoagulant/preservative. May contain significant numbers of platelets. Some RBC contamination usually present.
Use: Patients with severe neutropenia with active infection and no response to antibiotics. In adults, use is controversial and utilized most commonly in neutropenic, infected patients receiving chemotherapy or infected patients with congenital granulocyte dysfunction. Has been used for both bacterial and fungal infection. A pediatric dose is used for septic, neutropenic neonates with good results.
Possible hazards include: Febrile, nonhemolytic reactions, viral transmission, pulmonary reactions, hemolysis.
Dose: One apheresis collection = one adult dose. Generally should give several doses over consecutive days. A neonatal dose may be prepared from a single unit of whole blood. RBCs of donor must be ABO compatible with plasma of recipient. Must be crossmatched.

Albumin/Plasma Protein Fraction

Volume is variable. Albumin may come as 5% solution in 250- or 500-mL bottles or as 25% solution in 50- or 100-mL bottles. Plasma protein fraction comes as a 5% solution in 250- or 500-mL bottles. Stored at room temperature for months to years.
Contains: Plasma proteins obtained through Cohn fractionation and pasteurized. Plasma protein fraction is approximately 88% albumin and 12% alpha and beta globulins. Albumin solution is more purified. Neither preparation contains significant amounts of gamma globulins.
Use: Indicated for volume expansion in patients needing colloid.
Possible hazards include: Allergic reactions. No risk of viral transmission known.
Dose: In grams based on patient weight and colloid needs.

Coagulation Factor VIII Concentrate

Prepared in lyophilized form, reconstituted with sterile saline; each vial marked with measured number of activity units present. Stored at 1°C to 6°C for months prior to reconstitution. Must be stored at room temperature and used within 3 hours after reconstitution.
Contains: Factor VIII. Made from pools of plasma from large numbers of donors.
Use: For patients with hemophilia A.
Possible hazards include: Hemolysis, immunosuppression, factor VIII inhibitor formation. Current concentrates appear to be safe from viral transmission.

Dose: Calculate using desired rise in factor VIII levels and plasma volume of patient.

Prothrombin Complex Concentrate
Also known as coagulation factor IX complex concentrate. Volume and storage are the same as factor VIII concentrate.
Contains: Factors II, VII, IX and X.
Use: Patients with factor IX deficiency and reversal of the anticoagulant effect of coumarin.
Possible hazards include: Viral transmission, thrombosis.
Dose: Calculate using desired rise in factor IX levels and plasma volume of patient.

Activated Prothrombin Complex Concentrate
Volume and storage are the same as factor VIII concentrate.
Contains: Activated factors II, VII, IX and X.
Use: Patients with hemophilia A and antibodies to factor VIII.
Possible hazards include: Serious risk of thrombosis; viral transmission.
Dose: See package insert.

Porcine Coagulation Factor VIII Concentrate
Volume is the same as factor VIII. Stored at -18°C for months prior to reconstitution.
Contains: Factor VIII harvested from pigs.
Use: Patients with hemophilia A and antibodies to factor VIII.
Possible hazards include: Thrombocytopenia, allergic reactions.
Dose: Calculate based on level of antibody to porcine factor VIII and patient weight.

Rh Immune Globulin
Volume is approximately 2 mL for one standard 300-μg dose. Stored at 1°C to 6°C for months.
Contains: Anti-D harvested from alloimmunized donors.
Use: To prevent anti-D formation in Rh (D)-negative persons who do not have an anti-D antibody but are at risk for exposure to Rh (D)-positive RBCs. Generally, these patients are pregnant or postpartum women or persons receiving Rh (D)-positive platelet concentrates.
Possible hazards include: Allergic reactions, discomfort at injection site. No risk of viral transmission.
Dose: One intramuscular 300-μg dose should protect against exposure to 15 mL of Rh (D)-positive RBCs.

Intravenous Immunoglobulin Concentrate
Volume: comes lyophilized, must be reconstituted with sterile saline before use. Stored at room temperature for up to several months prior to reconstitution.
Contains: Immunoglobulin, mostly IgG, derived from pools of human plasma.
Use: Patients with immunoglobulin deficiency; patients with immune thrombocytopenic purpura.

Possible hazards include: Allergic reactions, headache.

Dose: Calculate dosage based on disease process being treated and weight of patient.

Special Kinds of Blood Components

Leukocyte-Poor Blood. Most transfusion centers now prepare leukocyte-poor blood by using a leukocyte-depletion filter rather than by washing the unit. Filtration is generally easier and faster, and removes significantly more white blood cells. Leukocyte-depletion filters are available for both platelets and RBC components. Leukocyte depletion is not necessary for fresh-frozen plasma or cryoprecipitate. No method available can remove all of the leukocytes in a unit of blood.

Uses: (1) Prevention of nonhemolytic, febrile reactions in a recipient who has had previous febrile reactions (usually two or more), especially if such reactions occur despite premedication with antipyretics. (2) Prevention of formation of HLA antibodies in patients who will be multiply transfused and will need future platelet transfusions. (3) Reduce the risk of cytomegalovirus (CMV) and other leukocyte-associated viral infections.

Gamma Irradiation of Blood. Irradiation of any blood component containing viable leukocytes may be done to prevent transfusion-transmitted graft-versus-host disease.

Uses: Patients with immunodeficiencies, especially those with congenital T cell immunodeficiencies, bone marrow transplant recipients, and fetuses and premature infants. Also recommended by some authorities for transfusions from related donors to prevent graft-versus-host disease due to HLA haplotype similarity between first-degree relatives.

Cytomegalovirus Antibody–Negative Blood. Donors who test negative for antibodies to CMV comprise 20% to 60% of the donor population, depending on the geographical region.

Uses: Blood from these donors should be used to prevent CMV infection in CMV seronegative immunocompromised patients. Examples of such patients include fetuses, newborns, and transplant recipients receiving organs from CMV antibody–negative donors.

Autologous Blood. If blood transfusion is anticipated, the use of the patient's own blood for transfusion should always be considered. Use of the patient's own blood alleviates many, but not all, of the risks related to blood transfusion. Because the risks of volume overload, bacterial contamination, and mislabeling of the unit may also occur with the patient's own blood, transfusion even of autologous units should never be undertaken except when absolutely necessary.

Uses: Three forms of autologous blood use are available. The first, preoperative, deposit is the most widely used. Units of whole blood are donated by the patient prior to an elective surgical procedure which will likely require transfusion. Patients with systemic bacterial infections, significant anemia, and severe medical conditions precluding sudden loss of one unit of blood are excluded from preoperative deposit. The second method of autologous blood use is intraoperative salvage. Blood from the surgical field is collected, washed, and returned to the patient. The surgical field must be clean of tumor cells, bacteria, and other contaminants to utilize this procedure. Finally, hemodilution involves removal of one or more units of whole blood immediately prior to surgery with crystalloid replacement. The blood may then be reinfused after the procedure is over.

References

Judd WJ, Luban NLC, Ness PM. Prenatal and perinatal immunohematology: recommendations for serologic management of the fetus, newborn infant, and obstetric patient. *Transfusion.* 1990;30:175-183.

McCullough J. *Granulocyte Serology: A Clinical and Laboratory Guide.* Chicago, Ill: ASCP Press; 1988.

Mueller-Eckhardt C, Kiefel V, Santoso S. Review and update of platelet alloantigen systems. *Transfusion Med Rev.* 1990;4:98-109.

Petz LD, Swisher SN, eds. *Clinical Practice of Transfusion Medicine.* 2nd ed. New York, NY: Churchill Livingstone Inc; 1989.

Rossi EC, Simon TL, Moss GS, eds. *Principles of Transfusion Medicine.* Baltimore, Md: Williams & Wilkins; 1991.

Silver H. Paternity testing. *Crit Rev Clin Lab Sci.* 1989;27:391-408.

Walker RH. *Technical Manual.* 10th ed. Arlington, Va: American Association of Blood Banks; 1990.

Index

B

Bacteremia, 19
Bacteriuria, 155, 159
  colony counts, 21
Basopenia, 220, **221**
Basophilia, 220, **221**
Basophils, 220
Bence Jones proteins, 67, 151-152, 226
Benign prostatic hyperplasia (BPH),
  66
Bentiromide test, 112-113
Beta-thalassemia minor, 199
Bile salt absorption, 111
Bile secretion, 119-122
Bilirubin, 154, **155**
  secretion, 119-121
Biomarkers, tumor, 65-68, **66**
Bleeding
  disorders, 234-239
  general lab evaluation of, 233-234
  time, 234
  type of, 231-232
Blood
  in cerebrospinal fluid, 90
  components, 256-262
  donor testing, 254
  irradiation, 261
  tests for malabsorption, 113
  urea nitrogen (BUN), 164
  whole, 256-257
Blood bank tests, 245-256
Bone marrow
  analysis, chromosomal, 12, **12-13**,
    14-15
  failure, 202-203, **202-203**
Bordetella pertussis, 34
Breath tests, 110-111, 113
Brucellosis, 33-34

C

^{14}C-D-xylose breath test, 111
Calcitonin, 67, 172
Calcium, 167-168
  in cerebrospinal fluid, 94
  homeostasis, **168**, 169-171
  metabolism, 167-173
Carcinoembryonic antigen (CEA),
  66-67

Carcinoma
  adrenocortical, 185
  pancreas, 130
  prostate, 66
Cardiolipin antibodies, 104
Casts
  epithelial cell, 158
  erythrocyte, 158
  fatty, 159
  granular, 158
  hyaline, 158
  leukocyte, 157-158
  waxy, 159
CD4 cell counts, 41
CD4 to CD8 ratio, 41
Cerebrospinal fluid (CSF), 87-95
  cell counts in, 91-92
  chloride in, 94
  computed tomography (CT), 88-89
  C-reactive protein in, 94
  electrolytes in, 94
  findings, **88-89**
  glutamine in, 94
  infectious disease, 19-20, 34-35
  magnetic resonance imaging (MRI),
    88-89
  pCO_2 in, 94
  pH of, 94
  pO_2 in, 94
  protein in, 92-93
  syphilis, **46-47**, 47
  turbidity of, **88**, 90-91
  visual interpretation of, 89-90
Ceruloplasmin, 126
Chancroid, 24
Cholesterol, 78, **79**, 80-86, **84**
Cholyl-^{14}C-glycine breath test,
  110-111
Chorionic villus sample, 10, 15
Chromatography, 62
  in toxicology, 55-56
Chromosome
  abnormalities, 8-13, **10**, **12-13**
    acquired, 11-12, **12-13**
    constitutional, 8-11, **10**
  -breakage syndrome, 11
  myelodysplastic state, **13**
  postnatal analysis, 11

Fluorescent antinuclear antibody (ANA) test, 102
Fluorescent treponemal antibody absorption test (FTA-Abs), 45
Folate deficiency, 199-202, **201**
Fragile X syndrome, **10**, 11
Free erythrocyte protoporphyrin (FEP), 198
Froin's syndrome, 93
Fungal infections, 34-35

G

Galactosemia, 153
γ-Glutamyltransferase (GGT), 124
Gas chromatography, 56
Gastric acid output, 115-117
Gastric secretion tests, 115-118
Gastrin levels, 117-118
Giemsa stain, 24, 27
Glomerular filtration rate, 161-164
Glomerulonephritis, 32-33
Glucose
  in cerebrospinal fluid, 93-94
  concentration, 136-137
  tolerance, oral, 134, **134-135**, 137
Glucosuria, 146, 152-153
Glutamine, 94
Glycosylated hemoglobins, 137-138
Gonococcal pharyngitis, 21
Gram's stain, 20, 22-24, 27, 34, 94
Granulocyte concentrate, 259
Grave's disease, 176-177, **177**
Growth hormone, 188-190
Guillain-Barré syndrome, 93

H

HCO₃⁻, 140
Heinz bodies, 208
Hematology ranges, adult, **195**
Hematuria, 153-154
Hemoglobinopathies, 207-208
Hemoglobinuria, 153
Hemolytic anemia, 203-204, **204**
  acquired, 209-211
  autoimmune, 252-253
  due to drugs and chemical agents, 210
  hereditary, 206-208

microangiopathic, 209, **210**
Hemophilia, 235-236, 240
  component therapy, 259-260
Hemostasis, 229-244
Henle's loop, 166
Heparin, 14, 98, 243-244
Hepatitis
  B e antigen (HBeAg), 124
  B surface antigen (HBsAg), 124
  C antigen (HCAg), 124
High-density lipoproteins (HDLs), 78, 83-85, **84**
High-pressure liquid chromatography, 56
Histocompatibility typing, 256
Homovanillic acid (HVA), 67
Human chorionic gonadotropin (HCG), 59-61
Human immunodeficiency virus (HIV), 222
  antibody
    HIV-1, 37-39
    HIV-2, 38-40
  antigen, HIV-1, 40
  infections, 37-41
  in infants, 40
Hydrogen breath test, 110
5-Hydroxyindoleacetic acid (5-HIAA), 67
Hyperbilirubinemia, 204-205, **205**
Hypercalcemia, 170
Hypercholesterolemia, 80, 81
Hypercoagulable states, 243-244
Hyperlipidemia, 80, 81
Hyperlipoproteinemias, **79**, 80-82
Hyperphosphatemia, 171
Hyperthyroidism, 176-178, **177**
Hypertriglyceridemia, 80, 81
Hypocalcemia, 170
Hypoglycemia, 136
Hypoparathyroidism, 170
Hypothyroidism, 81, 178

I

IgG, 93, 104
Immunoglobulin concentrate, 260-261
Infectious disease
  darkfield microscopy, 26

Myocardial injury, laboratory tests for, 69-76
Myoglobinuria, 154

N

Nasopharynx specimen, 21
Neurosyphilis, 47
Neutropenia, 217-218, **219**
Neutrophilia, **216**, 216-217
Neutrophils, 215-219
  abnormalities, 218-219
Nitrite test, 155
Nontreponemal antibody tests, 44-45
Normal values, 2-4
Nuclear antigens, 103, **103**

O

Oliguria, 145, 150
Osmolality, 149-150, 191
Ouchterlony double-immunodiffusion techniques, 103
Oxytocin, 190

$PaCO_2$, 140
Pancreas tests, 112-113, 127-131
Parasites, 35, 159
Parathyroid hormone (PTH), **168**, 169-172
Paroxysmal cold hemoglobinuria, 254
Paroxysmal nocturnal hemoglobinuria (PNH), 211
Partial thromboplastin time (PTT), 234
Paternity testing, 256
Pertussis, 21
pH, 140-141
Philadelphia chromosome, 12
Phosphate, 168-169
Phosphorus metabolism, 167-173
Pituitary
  adenomas, 188
  function tests, 187-191
Plasma
  fresh-frozen, 258
  protein fraction, 259
Platelet, 233
  antibody detection, 255
  antigen typing, 254-255

apheresis, 258
counts, 233-234
crossmatching, 255
pooled from whole blood, 257-258
Pleocytosis, **89**, 91-92
Polymerase chain reaction, 41
Polyuria, 145
Posterior pituitary disorders, 190-191
Postnatal constitutional chromosome analysis, 11
Predictive value, 4-5, **5**
Pregnancy-related tests, 59-62
Prenatal
  antibody screen, 251
  constitutional chromosome analysis, 10-11
Prolactin, 189
Prostate-specific antigen (PSA), 66
Prostatic-fraction acid phosphatase (PAP), 66
Protein C, 240
Protein electrophoresis patterns, 225-226, **226**
Proteinuria, 150-152
Prothrombin time (PT), 122, 234
Pyuria, 155-156

Q

Q fever, 35-36
Quantitative stool fat determination, 109-110

R

Radioimmunoassay
  of serum insulin levels, 138
  in toxicology, 56
Radioimmunoprecipitation assay, 38
Rapid plasma reagin (RPR) test, 44, **46**
Red blood cell (RBC)
  in additive solution (AS-1, AS-3, AS-5), 257
  catabolism, 196, **197**
  in citrate-phosphate-dextrose-adenine-1, 257
  elution studies, 250
  enzymopathies, 208
  impaired production, 198-203, **199**
  indices, 194-211

membrane abnormalities, 206-207
production, 195-196
phenotyping, 249
Renal
concentrating capacity, 165-166
diluting capacity, 166
function tests, 161-166
Respiratory
acidosis, 140-141, **141**
alkalosis, 141, **141**
tract specimens, 21-23
Reticulocyte counts, 195-196,
196, 198
Rh
immune globulin, 260
therapy, 251-252
typing, 254
Rheumatic fever, 32-33
Rheumatoid arthritis, 104
Rheumatoid factors, 104
Rickettsial infections, 35-36
Rocky Mountain spotted fever, 35

S
Schilling test, 111-112, 201
Secretin
levels, 118
test, 112, 129
Sensitivity, 4-5, **5**
Sexually transmitted disease (STD), 24
Sickle cell anemia, 207
Specificity, 4-5, **5**
Specimen
chromosomal, 10-11, 13-15
drug screen, 55
ear, 21
infectious disease, 17-26
for myocardial injury, 70-75, **71-72**
throat, 21-22
transportation of, 18
Spherocytosis, 206-207
Steatorrhea, 109-110
Streptococcus pyogenes, 32-33
Streptokinase, 244
Streptozyme, 33
Subarachnoid hemorrhage, 90, **90**
Substance abuse testing, 53-57
Sudan III stain, 109

Surfactant, 62
Susceptibility, antimicrobial testing,
28-29
Synovial fluid, 97-99, **98-99**
Syphilis, 23-24
cerebrospinal fluid test for, 95
congenital, 46-47
darkfield microscopy, **46**
diagnostic test recommendations, **46**
nontreponemal antibody tests, 44-45
serologic tests, 43-47
Systemic lupus erythematosus (SLE),
102-104, **103**

T
Tamm-Horsfall protein, 158
Terminal ileal function, 111-112
Thalassemia syndromes, 208
Therapeutic drug monitoring (TDM),
49-52
Thermal amplitude study, 253-254
Thin-layer chromatography, 55
Thrush, 23
Thyroid
function tests, 175-178
-stimulating hormone (TSH),
175-178
Thyroliberin (TRH), 175, 177-178
Thyroxine, 175-178
-binding globulin (TBG), 176, **176**
Total iron-binding capacity (TIBC),
198-199, **200**
Total serum iron (TSI), 198-199, **200**
Toxicology, 53-57
Toxoplasma gondii, 35
Transferrin saturation, 198-199
Transfusion
components, 256-262
reaction workup, 252
Transtracheal aspiration, 22
Treponemal antibody tests, 45-46
Triglycerides, 78, **78**, 80-83, 85
Trisomy, 9-11, **10**
Troponin-T, 76
True-negative results, 4, **5**
True-positive results, 4, **5**
Trypsin, 129

Tuberculosis, 25-26
  meningitis, 90-91, 95
Tubular function tests, 164
Tularemia, 33-34
Tumor biomarkers, 65-68, **66**
Turner syndrome, **10**, 11
Tympanocentesis, 21
Type and crossmatch, 248-249
Typhus, 35

U
Umbilical cord testing, 251
Unstable hemoglobins, 208
Urethra, 23
Urinalysis, 145-160
Urine
  bilirubin, 121
  casts in, 157-159
  cells in, 156-157
  clarity of, 147
  color of, 147
  contaminants in, 160
  crystals in, 159, **160**
  epithelial cells in, 157
  erythrocytes in, 156-157
  fungal infection in, 159
  glucose, 137
  infectious disease, 20-21
  microorganisms in, 159-160
  odor, 147
  pH of, 147-148, **149**
  protein, 150-152
  sample, drug screen, 55
  sediment constituents of, 156-160,
    160
  specific gravity, 148-149

tumor cells in, 160
viral inclusions, 160
Urobilinogen, 121-122, 154, **155**

V
Vanillylmandelic acid (VMA), 67
Venereal Disease Research Laboratory
  (VDRL) test, 44-47, **46**
Very-low-density lipoproteins
  (VLDLs), 78, **78-79**, 80-83
Viral disease tests, 36-41
Vitamin
  B_{12}, 200-202, **201**
  D, 172-173
  K, 238-240
von Willebrand disease, 236-238,
  238-239

W
Warfarin, 244
Warm autoantibodies, 252-253
Western immunoblot, 38-40
Wet mounts, 26-27
Whipple's triad for hypoglycemia, 136
White blood cell (WBC), 214-215
  count, 47
  differential counts, **215**
  terminology, **214**
Whooping cough, 34
Wright's stain, 24, 27

X
Xanthochromia, 90

Z
Zollinger-Ellison syndrome, 117